Patient Care in Imaging Technology

Seventh Edition

Patient Care in Imaging Technology

SEVENTH EDITION

LILLIAN S. TORRES, RN, M.S., CNS, NP
Professor Emeritus, Chaffey College
School of Health Science
Rancho Cucamonga, California

ANDREA GUILLEN DUTTON, M. Ed., ARRT (R, M), CRT (R, F, M)
Program Director, Radiologic Technology Program
Professor, Chaffey College
School of Health Science
Rancho Cucamonga, California

TERRIANN LINN-WATSON, M.Ed., ARRT (R, M) CRT (R, M, F)
Clinical Coordinator, Radiologic Technology Program
Professor, Chaffey College
School of Health Science
Rancho Cucamonga, California

Wolters Kluwer | Lippincott Williams & Wilkins
Health
Philadelphia • Baltimore • New York • London
Buenos Aires • Hong Kong • Sydney • Tokyo

Acquisitions Editor: Pete Sabatini
Editorial Manager: Eric Branger
Managing Editor: Amy Millholen, Kevin Dietz
Associate Marketing Manager: Allison Noplock
Compositor: Aptara, Inc.
Printer: C & C Offset Printing Co.

Library of Congress Cataloging-in-Publication Data

Torres, Lillian S.
   Patient care in imaging technology / Lillian S. Torres, Andrea Guillen Dutton, TerriAnn Linn-Watson. — 7th ed.
      p.   ;   cm.
   Rev. ed. of: Basic medical techniques and patient care in imaging technology / Lillian S. Torres, TerriAnn Linn-Watson Norcutt, Andrea Guillen Dutton. 6th ed., c2003.
   Includes bibliographical references and index.
   ISBN-13: 978-0-7817-7183-2 (alk. paper)
   ISBN-10: 0-7817-7183-8 (alk. paper)
   1. Radiology, Medical. 2. Radiologic technologists. 3. Nursing. I. Dutton, Andrea Guillen.
II. Linn-Watson, TerriAnn. III. Torres, Lillian S. Basic medical techniques and patient care in imaging technology. IV. Title.
   [DNLM: 1. Technology, Radiologic—methods. 2. Patient Care—methods. WN 160
T693p 2009]
   RC78.T67 2009
   616.07'57—dc22
                                                                                    2008030349

CCS1208

• **To Joseph** •

It has been 30 years since the first edition of this text was published. It was first named *Basic Medical Techniques and Patient Care for Radiologic Technologists*. The author and her consultants had no idea of the degree or magnitude of changes that would take place in the profession of radiologic technology. Each edition of this textbook has made significant contributions to this profession to meet the changing needs of students and educators in this field and to the improvement in patient care.

The seventh edition of this text, now called *Patient Care in Imaging Technology*, has been dramatically altered to serve the needs of the beginning student in this profession as well as those who desire advanced courses in imaging technology. It includes the latest techniques used in imaging and meets the current requirements of the ASRT and the ARRT. The patient's safety is emphasized in each chapter.

HIGHLIGHTS OF THE SEVENTH EDITION

- All tables and displays have been updated; most photos are in color with extensive radiographic images included to enhance information presented.
- Procedures are placed in a step-by-step format for quick and easy reference for students and instructor use.
- CALL OUTS and WARNINGS provide students with notice of vital concepts.
- Infection control in imaging is stressed and includes the current threats to the health care of patients and all health care workers. Methods of protecting all involved in patient care from nosocomial infections are emphasized.
- Radiation safety is intensified to include the pregnant health care worker as well as the patient.
- The responsibilities of the radiographer during cardiac monitoring are included.
- The pharmacology and drug administration chapter has been completely revised to reduce the amount of material not relevant to the radiographer, and administration of contrast agents is emphasized.
- A course in venipuncture is included. Procedural charts and photos are also included.
- PowerPoint presentations and electronic learning resources are available for each chapter to reinforce concepts for improved student education.

It is the hope of the authors that the changes in the seventh edition will assist radiologic technology students to be safe and sensitive practitioners in every aspect of patient care.

Please feel free to contact us regarding the use of this textbook. We will appreciate your feedback.

Lillian S. Torres, RN, M.S., CNS, NP

Andrea Guillen Dutton, M. Ed., ARRT (R, M), CRT (R, F, M)

TerriAnn Linn-Watson, M.Ed., ARRT (R, M) CRT (R, M, F)

User's Guide

This User's Guide shows you how to put the features of
Patient Care in Imaging Technology, 7th Edition *to work for you.*

CHAPTER OPENING ELEMENTS

Each chapter begins with the following elements, which will help orient you to the material.

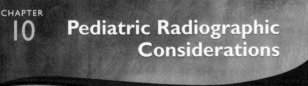

CHAPTER
10 **Pediatric Radiographic Considerations**

STUDENT LEARNING OUTCOMES

After studying this chapter, the student will be able to:

1. Define the pediatric patient.
2. Discuss professional, appropriate, age-specific, and effective communication strategies for pediatric patients, parents, and guardians during radiographic procedures.
3. Discuss transporting infants and children.
4. Demonstrate safe methods of immobilizing a pediatric patient with commercial available devices and other positioning aids.
5. Describe proper radiation protection and safety measures, techniques, and practices used in pediatric radiography (ALARA principle).
6. Discuss your role as the radiographer in a suspected child abuse procedure.
7. Discuss administering medication to the pediatric patient in radiographic imaging procedures.

KEY TERMS

Adolescent: The period of life beginning at puberty and ending with physical maturity

Child abuse: The psychological, emotional and sexual abuse of a child

Disinfectant: A solution capable of destroying pathogenic micro-organisms or inhibiting their growth

Enhance: Increase

Hand hygiene: Handwashing with soap and water or the use of alcohol-based products that do not require water

Hypothermia: Significant loss of body heat below 98.6 °F

Immobilization: The act or process of fixing or rendering immobile

Infant: Newborn baby or a child under the age of 1 year

Isolette: A type of bed used in the newborn intensive care unit to keep babies warm and protected from the environment

Neonate: Newborn infant up to 1 month of age

NICU: Neonatal intensive care unit

Pigg-O-Stat: Commercial mechanical immobilizer device

Preschooler: A child who is not old enough to attend kindergarten

School age: Age at which the child is considered old enough to attend school

Toddler: Young child learning to walk

185

Student Learning Outcomes provide a quick overview of the content to be covered.

Key Terms are listed and defined at the beginning of each chapter.

SPECIAL FEATURES

Unique chapter features will aid readers' comprehension and retention
of information—and spark interest in students and faculty.

Procedures Boxes with Accompanying Videos
help you master the steps needed to ensure the safety
of both you and your patient.

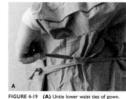

PROCEDURE

Removing Contaminated Garments

1. Untie waist ties of gown (Fig. 4-19A).

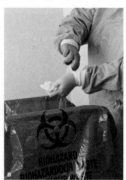

FIGURE 4-19   **(A)** Untie lower waist ties of gown.

2. Remove gloves according to the procedure for removing contaminated gloves, and place them in the waste receptacle (Fig. 4-19B).

FIGURE 4-19   **(B)** Remove gloves as described earlier in this chapter.

3. Untie top gown ties (Fig. 4-19C).

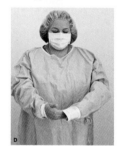

FIGURE 4-19   **(C)** Untie top gown ties.

4. Remove the first sleeve of the gown by placing fingers under the cuff of the sleeve and pulling it over the hand (Fig. 4-19D).

FIGURE 4-19   **(D)** Remove the first sleeve.

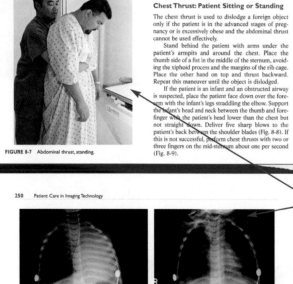

FIGURE 8-7   Abdominal thrust, standing.

certain to direct the thrust directly up and not deviate to the left or right. This maneuver acts in the same way for the patient who is sitting or standing.

Chest Thrust: Patient Sitting or Standing

The chest thrust is used to dislodge a foreign object only if the patient is in the advanced stages of pregnancy or is excessively obese and the abdominal thrust cannot be used effectively.

Stand behind the patient with arms under the patient's armpits and around the chest. Place the thumb side of a fist in the middle of the sternum, avoiding the xiphoid process and the margins of the rib cage. Place the other hand on top and thrust backward. Repeat this maneuver until the object is dislodged.

If the patient is an infant and an obstructed airway is suspected, place the patient face down over the forearm with the infant's legs straddling the elbow. Support the infant's head and neck between the thumb and forefinger with the patient's head lower than the chest but not straight down. Deliver five sharp blows to the patient's back between the shoulder blades (Fig. 8-8). If this is not successful, perform chest thrusts with two or three fingers on the mid-sternum about one per second (Fig. 8-9).

FIGURE 14-11   **(A)** Radiographic image demonstrating a collapsed left lung due to incorrect endotracheal tube placement. **(B)** This image shows that the left lung has now reinflated when the ET tube was withdrawn and the tip of the tube is above the carina.

Full-Color Photos and Radiographic Images
enable you to visualize key techniques and procedures.

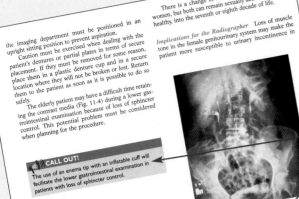

the imaging department must be positioned in an upright sitting position to prevent aspiration.

Caution must be exercised when dealing with the patient's dentures or partial plates in terms of secure placement. If they must be removed for some reason, place them in a plastic denture cup and in a secure location where they will not be broken or lost. Return them to the patient as soon as it is possible to do so safely.

The elderly patient may have a difficult time retaining the contrast media (Fig. 11-4) during a lower gastrointestinal examination because of loss of sphincter control. This potential problem must be considered when planning for the procedure.

There is a change in sexual response in men and women, but both can remain sexually active, if they are healthy, into the seventh or eighth decade of life.

Implications for the Radiographer Loss of muscle tone in the female genitourinary system may make the patient more susceptible to urinary incontinence in

CALL OUT!

The use of an enema tip with an inflatable cuff will facilitate the lower gastrointestinal examination in patients with loss of sphincter control.

The Hepatic System

Normal Changes of Aging
- Liver size decreases.
- Enzyme activity decrease.
- Bile storage is r

---

134   Patient Care in Imaging Technology

100%. Values of less than 85% indicate that the tissues are not receiving adequate oxygen. The pulse oximeter is used in all areas of acute health care as well as in the special procedures areas of radiographic imaging.

Hazards of Oxygen Administration

Oxygen is considered to be a medication and, like all other forms of medical therapy, must be prescribed by a physician. Excessive amounts of oxygen may produce toxic effects on the lungs and central nervous system or may depress ventilation.

Varying degrees of oxygen toxicity may result from inhalation of high concentrations of oxygen for more than a brief period of time. Mild oxygen toxicity may produce reversible tracheobronchitis. Severe oxygen toxicity may cause irreversible parenchymal lung injury. Because of the potential for adverse effects from excessive amounts of oxygen, oxygen should be administered as prescribed and in the lowest possible amount to achieve adequate oxygenation.

Special care is necessary when oxygen is administered to patients who have **chronic obstructive pulmonary disease (COPD)**. Excessive oxygen in the blood of the patient who has COPD may depress the respiratory drive, and the patient may stop breathing.

WARNING!

Oxygen is combustible, so great care must be taken to prevent sparks from occurring while radiographing a patient with the mobile unit.

Oxygen Delivery Systems

Oxygen is administered by artificial means when the patient is unable to obtain adequate amounts from the atmosphere to supply the needs of the body. If the patient requires supplementary oxygen, it is delivered to the respiratory tract under pressure. When the flow rate is high, the oxygen is humidified to prevent excessive drying of the mucous membranes. Passing the oxygen through distilled water can do this, because oxygen is only slightly soluble in water. The procedure for moisturizing oxygen varies somewhat from one institution to another, but often, the receptacle for distilled water is attached at the wall outlet, and the oxygen passes through the water and then into the delivery system.

In most hospitals, oxygen is piped into patient rooms, post-anesthesia areas, emergency suites, and the diagnostic imaging department. Wall outlets make

Call Out and Warning Boxes alert you to important facts and steer you away from common pitfalls.

CHAPTER 10: Pediatric Radiographic Considerations   187

DISPLAY 10-2

Caring for Children during Radiographic Procedures

Infants (Birth–12 Months)
Identify the patient. Educate by explaining the procedure to the parents or guardians. Maintain trust, assess need, maintain safe surroundings, and never leave unattended.

Toddlers (1–3 years)
Identify the patient. Educate by explaining the procedure to the parents and patient, assess needs and level of independence, have concern for privacy, maintain safe surroundings, and never leave unattended.

Preschooler (3–5 years)
Identify the patient. Educate parents and patient, assess needs, support independence, have concern for privacy, maintain safe surroundings, and never leave unattended.

School Age (6–12 years)
Identify the patient. Educate parents and patients, assess needs, and have concern for privacy.

carry a toy or security item to the radiographic room, he or she should be allowed to do so if at all possible. If it is not practical, explain to the child that the toy will be placed so the child can see it during the procedure. Return the toy to the child immediately after the procedure.

When explaining a procedure to a child, tell him what part of the body will be examined, why, and who will be performing the procedure. Also explain how the examination will proceed, what part of the child's body must be touched to accomplish the procedure, and why he must hold still during the process.

Some children are very modest. If a child's body must be exposed for an examination, only the necessary part should be exposed. The radiographer must guard against allowing the child to become chilled while in his care. This is particularly important for infants, because they lose body heat rapidly and **hypothermia** may occur.

Parents or guardians who accompany the child will feel less anxious if they are given an explanation of the procedure. Enlist their cooperation by encouraging them to explain the child's special needs and sensitivities. If the adult can be allowed to remain with the child during the procedure without jeopardizing the child's safety or the successful completion of the procedure, provide the appropriate protective apparel and other radiation protective measures. Also, give parents or guardians specific instructions about what is expected of them during the procedure. It is important to follow the department policies and procedures addressing the parents' or guardians' role during the radiographic examinations.

Explicit instructions must be provided for the adults involved in the exam in all aspects. The adult holding the child must assure the child will not fall from the x-ray table. If the parents are holding the child during the imaging procedure, they must wear the proper protective apparel, which includes a lead apron and possibly lead gloves. In addition to explaining the importance of wearing the protective apparel, the radiographer should explain how to secure the apron and assist them with the garments. Make sure that the child is not left unattended while this is being done. The radiographer must never assume that the parent is watching the child on an x-ray table and must instruct parents in the exact measures they need to take. For instance:

RADIOGRAPHER: *I would like you to stand on this side of the table with your hands on your child [use child's name] at all times. It will be necessary for you to wear this lead apron while I am x-raying your child as a radiation protective measure. I will hold the child while you put on the apron. The apron fastens with Velcro attachments on the sides. Now, if you will please keep your hands on the child at all times.*

If the child refuses to follow directions and is emotionally distraught, it may be necessary for the accompanying adult to leave the room. In this case, the child must be made to understand that the doctor and his or her parents want the examination to be done and that it will be done. Then, repeat the directions and proceed. Do not belittle or criticize the child's behavior; remain nonjudgmental and matter-of-fact and accomplish the

Display Boxes highlight important accreditation, competency, or skills information.

CHAPTER CLOSING ELEMENTS

Each chapter closes with the following elements, which will help aid in further study.

A Summary highlights the important topics that were discussed in the chapter.

SUMMARY

There are two types of contrast agents: positive and negative. The most commonly used contrasts are the positive type. Studies using barium and barium in combination with air are frequently conducted in the radiographic imaging department to diagnose pathological conditions of the upper and lower gastrointestinal tracts. Correct preparation for these examinations is essential for a successful outcome. The radiographer's professional responsibility is to teach the patient the correct methods of preparing for barium studies and the care and precautions that he or she must take after these or any diagnostic imaging procedures. The radiographer has a professional obligation to instruct other members of the health care team regarding the correct preparation of patients for diagnostic imaging examinations.

Scheduling for a series of diagnostic imaging examinations requires careful planning so that the studies can be completed in as brief a time as possible. Imaging examinations must also be scheduled so that they will not conflict with other therapeutic procedures that may be prescribed. Knowledge concerning which diagnostic imaging examinations will interfere with other tests will expedite the process for the patient by allowing the schedule to move forward smoothly. The very young, the elderly, and the patient with diabetes mellitus must be

scheduled to accommodate their dietary restrictions and frailties.

Preparation for examinations of the lower GI tract using barium as a contrast agent usually requires that the bowel be cleansed with enemas. The types of cleansing enemas are saline, hypertonic, oil-retention, tap water, and SS enemas. The tap water and SS enemas are the most often prescribed to precede lower GI examinations. The radiographer may be required to perform the cleansing enema if the patient is not properly prepared after arriving in the imaging department. Proper care must be taken to prevent injury to the patient during the administration of a cleansing enema.

The patient with an ostomy may also require a barium enema. The procedure and the tip used vary for these patients. The radiographer must be sensitive in his or her care of ostomy patients because they are often in the process of grieving over the recent alteration in body image. Recent ostomy patients must be related to in a therapeutic manner.

Barium studies of the upper GI tract are frequently done to diagnose pathological conditions of the pharynx, esophagus, stomach, duodenum, and jejunum. The preparation before and after these studies varies somewhat from that of the lower GI series.

CHAPTER 13 TEST

1. Before removing the retention-style enema tip, what is the most important thing to remember?
2. Barium is a relatively nontoxic contrast agent.
   a. True
   b. False
3. Mr. and Mrs. Ob Noxious bring their 3-year-son into the department for an upper GI examination. They have been concerned because he has been spitting out all of his food saying that he is not hungry. They suspect that he has a tumor in his stomach. The child immediately begins screaming that he will not drink any of "that stuff." What is your best response in this situation?
   a. Ask the parents to wait outside while you do the examination
   b. Try to calm the child down
   c. Tell the family to leave and return when the child is under control
   d. Ask for sedation for the child
4. What would be the worst response in the above scenario?

5. A double-contrast study of the gastrointestinal tract includes all of the following. Circle all that apply.
   a. Use of room air
   b. Use of barium
   c. Use of nitrogen
   d. Use of carbon dioxide
   e. Use of a water-soluble contrast agent
6. If the patient has the large bowel removed at the sigmoid area and the opening is made on the anterior surface of the abdomen, the patient is said to have a:
   a. Colostomy
   b. Ileostomy
   c. Sigmoidostomy
   d. Colonostomy
7. After a barium study, the patient must receive the following after-care instructions. Circle all that apply.
   a. Increase fluid intake for the next 24-48 hours
   b. Call the physician if no bowel movement has occurred within the next hour

A Chapter Test at the end of each chapter lets you assess your knowledge and put your new skills into practice.

ADDITIONAL LEARNING RESOURCES

This powerful tool also includes a host of resources for instructors and students on the Point. companion website at http://thepoint.lww.com/torres7e. See the inside front cover for details on how to access these resources.

Student Resources include videos, a question bank, pronunciation glossary, skills checklists, lab activities, and more!

Instructor Resources include PowerPoint slides, lesson plans, an image bank, a test generator, and answers to the chapter tests and situational judgement questions.

Acknowledgements

Completing the seventh edition of this textbook is a deeply satisfying accomplishment for us, the authors. We needed the assistance of many students and professionals to assure its accuracy and completeness.

Special thanks to the following:

Charles Salemi, MD, and Trina L. Rich, MSN, ARNP, Director of Infection Control at Riverside County Regional Medical Center, Riverside, California. They are at the forefront of hospital epidemiology and were of valuable assistance to us in updating infection control and its ever-increasing medical problems.

Our photographer, Keith Skelton, who worked tirelessly to create the best photos possible.

The radiologic technology classes of 2008 and 2009 at Chaffey College who gave us of their time and constructive suggestions in methods of meeting student needs.

We also wish to thank Dr. Dan Vasili at San Antonio Hospital Urgent Care Center, Edith Bromley, ARRT(R), Brian Bethel, ARRT, Susan Diaz, ARRT, Sue Herman, RN, MSN, and Sylvia Pompura, RN, MS, who were valuable professional consultants.

To Peter Sabatini, Andrea Klinger, and the Lippincott Williams & Wilkins staff who were so gracious during our visit to Baltimore and for their continuing support. Thanks to Kevin Dietz, who was so helpful and patient during this arduous process.

We are grateful to our managing editor, Amy Millholen, for her exceptional work in putting this all together. She will be long remembered by the three of us for a difficult job well done.

Brief Contents

Expanded Table of Contents

Professional Issues in Imaging

STUDENT LEARNING OUTCOMES

After completing the chapter, the student will be able to:

1. Explain the criteria of a profession, and explain how the profession of imaging technology has evolved to meet these criteria.

2. List the members of the health care team with whom the radiographer may frequently interact and briefly describe the role of each.

3. Discuss the purpose of professional organizations, and explain why the radiographer should join the professional organizations in his field.

4. Explain Practice of Standards and professional growth in radiologic technology.

5. Define ethics and discuss ethics as it applies to radiologic technology.

6. Explain the legal obligations that the radiographer has toward his patients, peers, and other members of the health care team.

7. Define the *Patient Care Partnership* and *A Patient's Bill of Rights*.

8. Explain the patient's expectations, rights, and responsibilities when he seeks medical care and the role the radiographer has in protecting these expectations, rights, and responsibilities.

9. Describe the legal responsibilities of the radiographer when using immobilizing techniques, informed consent, incident reports, and Good Samaritan laws.

10. Explain the need for professional malpractice insurance.

KEY TERMS

Adhere: To stay fixed or firm

Automatic external defibrillator: An electrical or battery-operated device applied to the chest of a victim who is suffering a particular heart dysrhythmia to counter-shock them; available to the general public who has been trained to its use

Bias: An inclination or temperament based upon personal judgment; prejudice

Bioethics: Moral issues dealing with human life and death

Common law: Decisions and opinions of courts that are based on local customs and habits of an area within a particular country or state

Continuing education: Professional education received following completion of a training to maintain skills

Defaming: To attack or injure a person's reputation

Diagnostic imaging: Modern term for radiography, encompassing all specialties devoted to producing an image of a body part

Ethical: Conforming to the standards of conduct of a given profession or group

Holistic: The view that an organic or integrated whole has a reality independent of and greater than the sum of its parts

Immobilization device: A piece of equipment that assures restricting patient movement

In-service: Training given to employees in connection with their work or profession to update or maintain knowledge

Liability: Something that a person is obligated to do or an obligation required to be fulfilled by law; usually an obligation of financial nature

Malpractice: Professional negligence that is the cause of injury or harm to a patient

Mentor: A teacher, coach, or advisor of conduct

Practitioner: Any individual practicing in a specific area or discipline

11. Describe the patient's need for confidentiality and the legal implications for the radiographer.
12. Explain the need for accurate documentation in health care and the radiographer's obligations in this aspect of health care.
13. List and define the current methods of health care delivery in the United States.

Preceptor: A teacher; directs action or conduct of another individual

Profession: A calling that requires specialized knowledge and intensive academic preparation

Radiographer: A radiologic technologist who uses critical thinking, problem solving, and judgment to perform diagnostic images

Regulatory compliance: Control of a situation or group of laws that supervise a profession

Statutory law: Established law that is enacted by a legislative body and punishable by the court system

Therapeutic: Healing or palliative

Unethical: Not conforming to the standards of conduct of a particular profession or group

Radiologic technology has evolved to meet the criteria of a **profession**. As in all professions, radiographers are expected to **adhere** in conduct and behavior to the particular **ethical** and legal standards of the field. Any person who does not adhere to this code may lose his or her license as well as the privileges of the profession.

As a **radiographer**, one will not work alone in caring for the patient. One will work and interact with members of a health care team whose goal is to improve or restore the patient to good health. The health care team consists of physicians, nurses, therapists, social workers, and other health care professionals, all of whom work within their scope of practice and are accountable for performing their professional responsibilities.

The student, who has made the decision to enter the profession of radiologic technology, must realize that he/she is committed to accepting the code of ethics of this profession and must work within the scope of practice. He must also understand that he is accountable for what he does as a radiographer and may be held legally liable for any errors made while caring for patients.

Radiologic technology is a profession oriented toward the diagnosis and treatment of trauma and disease. This means the radiologic technologist, or radiographer, will work in intimate contact with people on a daily basis. He must be prepared to work collaboratively with people of all cultures, religions, and socioeconomic backgrounds and to relate to them in an unbiased, nonjudgmental manner.

Anyone contemplating a career in radiologic technology needs to examine the reasons why he has chosen this profession. It would be helpful to ask oneself the following questions before proceeding:

- Am I prepared to accept and practice the profession of radiologic technology and support the American Registry of Radiologic Technologists (ARRT) and American Society of Radiologic Technologist Standards of Ethics?
- Am I prepared to avoid violations of the law in practicing this profession?
- Will I be willing and able to learn to relate to my patients in a professional and nonjudgmental manner at all times?

If these questions cannot be answered positively, this career choice must be reconsidered.

THE CRITERIA FOR A PROFESSION

Radiologic technology has evolved from an undereducated workforce of x-ray technicians in the early 1900s to the continued advances as a profession in the 21st century (Display 1-1). This progression took place over a number of years with the efforts and dedication of the persons who worked in this field. The term profession implies a body of work that requires extensive training

Chronology of Events in the History of the Radiologic Technology Profession

1895	Wilhelm Conrad Roentgen discovered x-rays in Wurzburg, Germany.
1920	The American Association of Radiological Technicians, the first society for the profession, was created by a group of technologists in Chicago, Illinois. The society was dedicated to the advancement of radiologic technology.
1921	The society's first annual meeting was held. Membership totaled 47.
1922	The American Registry of Radiological Technicians originated.
1930s–1940s	Radiographer education was primarily by apprenticeship.
1932	The name of the American Association of Radiological Technicians was formally changed to the American Society of X-ray Technicians (ASXT).
1936	The ASXT was authorized to make appointment to the Registry Board of Trustees.
1952	The ASXT provided a basic minimum curriculum for training schools.
1955	The ASXT created a new membership category—Fellow of AXST—which recognized individual members who have made significant contributions to the profession.
1959	The ASXT membership reached 8,600 members.
1960	Registry applicants were required to have at least 2 years of training or experience.
1963	The American Registry of Radiological Technicians changed its name to the American Registry of Radiologic Technologists (ARRT).
1964	The ASXT changed its name to the American Society of Radiologic Technologists.
1966	Registry applicants were required to be graduates of training programs approved by the American Medical Association's Council on Medical Education.
1967	The Association of University Radiologic Technologists was established to stimulate an interest in radiologic technology through the academic environment.
1968	The Society membership reached 14,000. 1970 Registry Certificate No. 1 was awarded by the Registry to Sister Mary Beatrice.
1984	The Association of University Radiologic Technologists changed its name to The Association of Educators in Radiological Sciences (AERS). Current membership is around 1,000 educators from the United States and other countries.
1988	The Summit on Radiologic Sciences and Sonography met in Chicago to develop strategies to alleviate the personnel shortage in the profession.
1995	The American Registry of Radiologic Technologists announced that, beginning in 1995, x-ray technologists would henceforth be obligated to obtain 12 continuing education units per year to maintain their licenses.
1996	The Society membership reached 47,000 members.
1997	ARRT marked its 75th anniversary.
1998	ASRT launched an aggressive campaign to protect patients from overexposure to radiation during radiologic procedures and help reduce the costs of health care.
2001	ASRT introduced a bill, known as the Consumer Assurance of Radiologic Excellence (CARE) bill, during the 2001 congressional session. It ensures that the people performing radiologic examinations are qualified.
2002	ASRT membership reached 100,000 members.
2003	CARE bill reintroduced.
2005	CARE/RadCARE bill is enacted.
2006	RadCARE (S.B. 2322) bill is introduced and passes unanimously.

and the mastery of study by its members who have specialized skills, has a professional organization and ethical code of conduct, and serves a specific social need. The criteria for a group of **practitioners** to identify themselves as a profession was summarized by Chitty (2004) as the following:

1. A vital human service is provided to the society by the profession.
2. Professions possess a special body of knowledge that is continuously enlarged through research.
3. Practitioners are expected to be accountable and responsible.
4. The education of professionals takes place in institutions for higher education.
5. Practitioners have an independent function and control their own practice.
6. Professionals are committed to their work and are motivated by doing well.
7. A code of ethics guides professional decisions and conduct.
8. A professional organization oversees and supports standards of practice.

All professions have a code of ethics and professional organizations that control the educational and practice requirements of its members. The two organizations that assume these roles for radiographers are the American Society of Radiologic Technologists (ASRT) and the American Registry of Radiologic Technologists (ARRT). If applicable, the professional radiographer is registered by ARRT and by state licensure or certification.

Radiologic technology fulfills the basic requirements of a profession and is becoming increasingly autonomous in professional practice. The status of a profession demands certain responsibilities and educational requirements that former "x-ray technicians" did not possess. An individual contemplating radiologic technology as a profession must examine the criteria of a profession listed above to make certain that he is willing to uphold the high standards of a professional. These standards include responsibility, accountability, competence, judgment, ethics, professionalism, and lifelong learning. The professional radiographer is expected to demonstrate all of these qualities.

PRACTICE STANDARDS AND PROFESSIONAL GROWTH IN RADIOGRAPHY

ASRT states, "Professional practice standards define the role of the practitioner and establish the criteria used to judge performance." *Practice Standards for Medical Imaging and Radiation Therapy* is a guide for the

appropriate practice of medical imaging. The practice standards define the practice and establish general criteria to determine compliance (Display 1-2). Practice standards are authoritative statements enunciated and promulgated by the profession for judging the quality of practice, service, and education. They include desired and achievable levels of performance against which actual performance can be measured (ASRT, 2006). Radiographers are the primary liaison between patients, licensed independent practitioners, and other members of the health care team. Radiographers must remain sensitive to the physical and emotional needs of the patient through good communication, patient assessment, patient monitoring, and patient care skills. Radiographers use independent, professional, ethical judgment and critical thinking. Quality improvement and customer service allow the radiographer to be a responsible member of the health care team by continually assessing professional performance. Radiographers engage in continuing education to enhance patient care, public education, knowledge, and technical competence while embracing lifelong learning. In addition, the radiographer must include professional values in effective oral and written communication skills; critical thinking and problem-solving skills; and a broad knowledge base in developing technology.

The preparatory education for the radiographer has evolved from a hospital-based, **preceptor** training to formal educational programs. Hospital-based programs, as well as college- or university-based programs of study, are now available. To become a registered radiographer, one must successfully complete an accredited educational program.

Programmatic accreditation by the Joint Review Committee on Education in Radiologic Technology (JRCERT) assures that the program will provide the knowledge and skills for quality patient care in compliance for the JRCERT accreditation standards. Currently, approved and accredited programs operate under nine standards effective January 1, 2002. Included in the nine standards are sixty-one objectives that educational programs must clearly present documentation assuring compliance. The initial accreditation process for a program takes about 18–21 months from the receipt of the application/self-study reports. The accreditation process has several steps, which include a site visit, report of team findings, response to report of findings, and program notification of accreditation. Eight years is the maximum number of years awarded to programs; thereafter, accredited programs provide periodic self-studies and interim reports. Depending on the accreditation status, JRCERT conducts periodic site visits.

The formal educational programs include the didactic and clinical competency requirements. Two-year certificate, associate degree, and 4-year baccalaureate

American Society of Radiologic Technologist— Practice Standards–2006

Introduction to Radiography

Radiographers must demonstrate an understanding of human anatomy, physiology, pathology, and medical terminology.

Radiographers must maintain a high degree of accuracy in radiographic positioning and exposure technique. He or she must maintain knowledge about radiation protection and safety. Radiographers prepare for and assist the radiologist in the completion of intricate radiographic examinations. They prepare and administer contrast media and medications in accordance with state and federal regulations.

Radiographers are the primary liaison between patients and radiologists and other members of the support team. They must remain sensitive to the physical and emotional needs of the patient through good communication, patient assessment, patient monitoring, and patient care skills.

Radiographers use professional, ethical judgment and critical thinking when performing their duties. Quality improvement and customer service allow the radiographer to be a responsible member of the health care team by continually assessing professional performance. Radiographers embrace continuing education for optimal patient care, public education, and enhanced knowledge and technical competence.

Professional Performance Standards define the activities of the practitioner in the areas of education, interpersonal relationships, personal and professional self-assessment, and ethical behavior.

Standard One—Quality: The practitioner strives to provide optimal care to all patients.

Standard Two—Self-Assessment: The practitioner evaluates personal performance, knowledge, and skills.

Standard Three—Education: The practitioner acquires and maintains current knowledge in clinical practice.

Standard Four—Collaboration and Collegiality: The practitioner promotes a positive, collaborative practice atmosphere with other members of the health care team.

Standard Five—Ethics: The practitioner adheres to the profession's accepted Code of Ethics.

Standard Six—Exploration and Investigation: The practitioner participates in the acquisition, dissemination, and advancement of the professional knowledge base.

Radiography Clinical Performance Standards

Standard One—Assessment: The practitioner collects pertinent data about the patient and about the procedure.

Standard Two—Analysis/Determination: The practitioner analyzes the information obtained during the assessment phase and develops an action plan for completing the procedure.

Standard Three—Patient Education: The practitioner provides information about the procedure to the patient, significant others, and health care providers.

Standard Four—Implementation: The practitioner implements the action plan.

Standard Five—Evaluation: The practitioner determines whether the goals of the action plan have been achieved.

Standard Six—Implementation: The practitioner implements the revised action plan.

Standard Seven—Outcomes Measurement: The practitioner reviews and evaluates the outcome of the procedure.

Standard Eight—Documentation: The practitioner documents information about patient care, the procedure, and the final outcome.

Quality Performance Standards define the activities of the practitioner in the care of patients and delivery of diagnostic or therapeutic procedures and treatments. The section incorporates patient assessment and management with procedural analysis, performance, and evaluation.

Standard One—Assessment: The practitioner collects pertinent information regarding equipment, the procedures, and the work environment.

Standard Two—Analysis/Determination: The practitioner analyzes information collected during the assessment phase and determines whether changes need to be made to equipment, procedures, or the work environment.

Standard Three—Education: The practitioner informs patients, the public, and other health care providers about procedures, equipment, and facilities.

Standard Four—Implementation: The practitioner performs quality assurance activities or acquires information on equipment and materials.

Standard Five—Evaluation: The practitioner qualifies assurance results and establishes an appropriate action plan.

Standard Six—Implementation: The practitioner implements the quality assurance plan.

Standard Seven—Outcomes Measurement: The practitioner assesses the outcome of the quality assurance action plan in accordance with established guidelines.

Standard Eight—Documentation: The practitioner documents quality assurance activities and results.

degree programs are available in the United States. Within 5 years of successful completion of an accredited formal educational program in radiologic technology, candidates are eligible to participate in the American Registry of Radiologic Technologist national certification examinations.

Radiography program curriculum includes an extensive set of courses for the production of diagnostic images for interpretation by a radiologist. The course work includes: anatomy, patient positioning, examination techniques, equipment protocols, radiation safety, radiation protection, and basic patient care. Entry-level radiographers need the skills and abilities to perform the following functions:

1. Apply modern principles of radiation exposure, radiation physics, radiation protection, and radiobiology to produce diagnostic images.
2. Use knowledge of medical terminology, pathology, cross-sectional anatomy, topographic anatomy, anatomy and physiology, and positioning procedures to produce diagnostic images.
3. Provide direct patient care such as ECG, contrast media, and other drug administration.
4. Evaluate recognized equipment malfunctions.
5. Evaluate radiographic images.
6. Achieve a level of computer literacy.
7. Teach educational courses at the technical level.
8. Communicate with other members of the health care team.
9. Provide patient and family education.
10. Participate in community affairs.

In addition, the entry-level radiographer must possess the following qualities: an ability to think in a critical manner; a willingness to participate in lifelong learning, including becoming an active member of professional organizations; ethical behavior, from a holistic caregiver perspective; a broad computer knowledge base; problem-solving skills; and the ability to communicate effectively orally and in writing.

As one becomes more experienced, he will possess all of the qualities and abilities listed above as well as the following:

1. The ability to supervise, evaluate, and counsel staff
2. The ability to plan, organize, and administer professional development activities
3. Superior decision-making and problem-solving skills to assess situations and identify solutions for standard outcomes
4. The ability to promote a positive, collaborative atmosphere in all aspects of radiography
5. Skills as a **mentor**

6. Knowledge in areas of supervision, **in-service** and/or **continuing education**, and **regulatory compliance**

As a health care professional, one must acquire and maintain current knowledge to preserve a high level of expertise. Continuing education will provide educational activities to enhance knowledge, skills, performance, and awareness of changes and advances in the field of radiologic technology. Continuing education supports professionalism, which fosters quality patient care.

Previously voluntary for radiographers, continuing education became a mandate in 1995 for all who are licensed by ARRT. The radiologic technologist is now required to earn 24 continuing education credits. These credits must be accepted by ARRT and are to be earned every 2 years. The licensing body must verify these credits before license renewal. Continuing education credits, such as seminars, conferences, lectures, departmental in-service education, directed readings, home study, and college courses, may be achieved by participating in educational activities that meet the criteria set forth by ARRT. Twenty-four credits may be earned by taking an entry-level examination in another eligible discipline that was not previously passed. The entry-level examinations are in radiography, nuclear medicine, or radiation therapy. Another way to earn 24 credits is by passing an advanced-level examination in the field after proving eligibility. The advanced-level examinations are in mammography, cardiovascular-interventional technology, magnetic resonance, computed tomography, quality management, and sonography. By participating in continuing education activities, professional knowledge and professional performance are enhanced and provide a higher standard of patient care.

PROFESSIONAL ORGANIZATIONS IN RADIOLOGIC TECHNOLOGY

Participation in professional organizations is the responsibility of all practicing professionals, regardless of their field. Membership in professional organizations provides a pathway to continued successful professional development. It also provides comprehensive opportunities to remain current in a constantly changing technological career. Professional organizations provide pathways for technical growth and the development of leadership skills as well as an arena for professional interaction and problem solving, especially in career issues. The mission statement for ASRT "is to lead and serve its members' profession, other health care providers and the public on all issues that affect the radiologic sciences." ASRT offers many program and member services, including continuing education, a job bank and career information, events, conferences and seminars, government relations and collective legislative power, group professional liability insurance, and other member benefits and services. In addition, ASRT works with professional certification bodies and accreditation agencies for radiographers. Ultimately, membership in professional organizations enables the radiographer to continue providing quality patient health care in accordance with the standards of the profession.

There are various levels of professional organizations in radiologic technology. Internationally, there is the International Society of Radiographs and Radiologic Technologists. In the United States, ASRT is the national organization for radiologic technology. ASRT has affiliated societies at state levels, and the state societies have district affiliates. A chronology of the events that stimulated the radiologic technology profession is interesting to review.

■ THE HEALTH CARE TEAM

The radiographer will interact on a daily basis with his peers in diagnostic imaging and with other members of the health care team (Display 1-3).

■ PROFESSIONAL ETHICS

Ethics may be defined as a set of moral principles that govern one's course of action. *Moral principles* are a set of standards that establish what is right or good. All individuals have a personal code of ethics that evolves based on their cultural and environmental background. This same background has taught us to place *values* on behaviors, as well as on objects in our environment; that is, to assign a judgment of either good or bad to an action.

Ethics is a combination of the attributes of honesty, integrity, fairness, caring, respect, fidelity, citizenship, competence, and accountability. As one can quickly see, the terms "ethics," "principles," and "values" are closely linked and may be used interchangeably from time to time.

Bioethics is a relatively new branch of ethics that was established because of the advanced technical methods of prolonging life. It pertains solely to ethics in the field of health care and "narrows ethical inquiry to the moral 'oughts' of those who work in professional clinical practice, basic research, or the education of health care professionals. Bioethics affects all health professionals and those who seek their knowledge and skills" (O'Neil, 1995).

The student entering the profession of radiologic technology brings with him a personal code of ethics, moral principles, and personal values. All professionals have a set of professional values, and all professionals have a set of ethical principles or a code of ethics that governs professional behavior. This is true of radiologic technology.

The Standard of Ethics is made up of two parts: the Code of Ethics and the Rules of Ethics. The Code of Ethics was developed, revised, and adopted by ASRT

DISPLAY 1-3

The Health Care Team

Members of other health care professions with whom the radiographer will interact are:

Physicians: A doctor of medicine or doctor of osteopathy. They often specialize in a specific area of practice and, following licensing, are able to prescribe and supervise the medical care of the patient.

Registered nurses: Provide patient care, which is often required 24 hours a day. They also provide home health care and case management; educate; act as a patient advocate; administer medications and treatments as ordered by physicians; monitor the patient's health status; and coordinate and facilitate all patient care when the patient is hospitalized. Advance practice nurses work as clinical nurse specialists and nurse practitioners.

Vocational nurses: Work with patients under the supervision of a registered nurse.

Occupational and physical therapists: Members of a profession that work in the rehabilitative area of health care.

Pharmacist: Prepares and dispenses medications and oversees the patient's drug therapy.

Respiratory therapist: Maintains or improves the patient's respiratory status.

Laboratory technologist: Analyzes laboratory specimens for pathological conditions.

Social workers: Counsel patients and refer them for assistance to appropriate agencies.

There are also many unlicensed assistive personnel including nursing assistants, ward clerks, pharmacy technicians, electrocardiogram technicians, and many more.

and ARRT in July 1998. It serves as a guide in maintaining ethical conduct in all aspects of the radiologic sciences. The rules of ethics were added in 2001. Considered to be mandatory and enforced by ARRT, the 22 Rules of Ethics are designed to promote protection, safety, and comfort of the patient (Display 1-4).

Together, these documents represent the application of moral principles and moral values to the practice of the profession and are considered to be the minimum acceptable standards of conduct. They are concerned with the duties and responsibilities that the radiographer must have toward him, his patients, and professional peers and associates. These responsibilities deal with rights and correlated responsibilities and are discussed in the following section.

Unfortunately, as the world of health care becomes increasingly complex and the ability to prolong life expands, there are more difficult choices to be made. This leads to a growing number of ethical conflicts and dilemmas. The radiographer will not be immune to these as he performs his professional duties. Professional standards of ethics must be adhered to at all times, even though doing so will, at times, present difficult problems to be resolved.

A set of ethical principles has been derived from the basic ethical philosophies. These are *utilitarianism, deontology,* and *virtue.* Utilitarianism is often called *consequentialism* and advocates that actions are morally correct or right when the largest number of persons is benefited by the decision made. An example of this is as follows:

A large accident occurs and a number of persons are critically injured. The triage team assigns a higher priority to the less injured patients and, since the chance of survival is less for the most severely injured, attends last to those who are critically injured.

This is an acceptable philosophy if one benefits from the decision. In this example, the important element is the result of the action. This is based on the principal known as *teleological theory* (meaning end or completion). In other words, it is based on consequences with the highest good with the greatest happiness for the largest number of people.

Deontology upholds the philosophy that the rules are to be followed at all times by all individuals. Deontology comes from a Greek word meaning "duty"; therefore, one judges an action by deciding if it is an obligation. When making decisions using this school of thought, one generally does not take consequences into consideration even if it proves to be beneficial to the patient. Following the rules at all times may be too restrictive, especially when specific circumstances surrounding a situation do not fit a set of rules.

An example of deontology is illustrated by the accident portrayed above. Since the health care provider has the duty to "do no harm," then assigning a low priority number to the most critical patients would be wrong. Since deontology and utilitarianism are more or less opposite, the more critically injured patients would get the highest priority, and the most likely to survive would be attended to last because they would survive longest without care.

Virtue is a new philosophical belief that focuses on using wisdom rather than emotional and intellectual problem solving. With **holistic** medicine gaining popularity in recent years, virtue ethics incorporates certain principles of both utilitarianism and deontology to provide a broader view of issues. Analysis, review of consequences, and societal rules are essential to forming decisions using virtue. Again, using the accident example to illustrate, with virtue ethics, the triage of the patients would take into account the significance of each individual. How the family and friends of the victims would be affected by the triage decisions would be the deciding factor in who gets first treatment.

Ethical Principles

To resolve ethical dilemmas, one may apply this established set of principles to decision making:

Autonomy: Refers to the right of all persons to make rational decisions free from external pressures. Patients have the right to make decisions concerning their lives, and all health care workers must respect those decisions. In practice, the radiographer will act as the liaison between the radiologist and the patient. In these circumstances, the radiographer must act on behalf of the patient.

Beneficence: Refers to the fact that all acts must be meant to attain a good result or to be beneficial. As a radiographer, you must always plan patient care to ensure safe outcomes and avoid harmful consequences. Beneficence requires action that either prevents harm or does the greatest good for the patient. This may require you to side with the patient and against his co-workers.

Confidentiality: Refers to the concept of privacy. All patients have the right to have information concerning their state of health or other personal information kept in confidence unless it will benefit him or her, or unless there is a direct threat to society if not disclosed. The radiographer must not disclose facts concerning the patient's health or other personal information to anyone uninvolved with the patient's care.

American Registry of Radiologic Technologist—Standards of Ethics

From the July 1, 2005 revision. Please note, the Standards of Ethics were revised again on August 1, 2008. Please refer to the ARRT website (www.arrt.org) for the most recent version.

Preamble

The *Standards of Ethics* of The American Registry of Radiologic Technologists shall apply solely to persons holding certificates from ARRT who either hold current registrations by ARRT or formerly held registrations by ARRT (collectively, "Registered Technologists"), and to persons applying for examination and certification by ARRT in order to become Registered Technologists ("Candidates"). The *Standards of Ethics* are intended to be consistent with the Mission Statement of ARRT and to promote the goals set forth in the Mission Statement.

A. Code of Ethics

The Code of Ethics forms the first part of the *Standards of Ethics*. The Code of Ethics shall serve as a guide by which Registered Technologists and Candidates may evaluate their professional conduct as it relates to patients, health care consumers, employers, colleagues, and other members of the health care team. The Code of Ethics is intended to assist Registered Technologists and Candidates in maintaining a high level of ethical conduct and in providing for the protection, safety, and comfort of patients. The Code of Ethics is aspirational.

1. The radiologic technologist conducts herself or himself in a professional manner, responds to patient needs, and supports colleagues and associates in providing quality patient care.
2. The radiologic technologist acts to advance the principle objective of the profession to provide services to humanity with full respect for the dignity of mankind.
3. The radiologic technologist delivers patient care and service unrestricted by the concerns of personal attributes or the nature of the disease or illness, and without discrimination on the basis of sex, race, creed, religion, or socioeconomic status.
4. The radiologic technologist practices technology founded upon theoretical knowledge and concepts, uses equipment and accessories consistent with the purposes for which they were designed, and employs procedures and techniques appropriately.
5. The radiologic technologist assesses situations; exercises care, discretion, and judgment; assumes responsibility for professional decisions; and acts in the best interest of the patient.

6. The radiologic technologist acts as an agent through observation and communication to obtain pertinent information for the physician, to aid in the diagnosis and treatment of the patient, and recognizes that interpretation and diagnosis are outside the scope of practice for the profession.
7. The radiologic technologist uses equipment and accessories, employs techniques and procedures, performs services in accordance with an accepted standard of practice, and demonstrates expertise in minimizing radiation exposure to the patient, self, and other members of the health care team.
8. The radiologic technologist practices ethical conduct appropriate to the profession and protects the patient's right to quality radiologic technology care.
9. The radiologic technologist respects confidences entrusted in the course of professional practice and respects the patient's right to privacy and reveals confidential information only as required by law or to protect the welfare of the individual or the community.
10. The radiologic technologist continually strives to improve knowledge and skills by participating in continuing education and professional activities, sharing knowledge with colleagues, and investigating new aspects of professional practice.

B. Rules of Ethics

The Rules of Ethics form the second part of the *Standards of Ethics*. They are mandatory standards of Ethics of minimally acceptable professional conduct for all present Registered Technologists and Candidates. Certification is a method of assuring the medical community and the public that an individual is qualified to practice within the profession. Because the public relies on certificates and registrations issued by ARRT, it is essential that Registered Technologists and Candidates act consistently with these Rules of Ethics. These Rules of Ethics are intended to promote the protection, safety and comfort of patients. The Rules of Ethics are enforceable. Registered Technologists and Candidates engaging in any of the following conduct or activities, or who permit the occurrence of the following conduct or activities with respect to them, have violated the Rules of Ethics and are subject to sanctions as described hereunder:

1. Employing fraud or deceit in procuring or attempting to procure, maintain, renew or obtain reinstatement of certification or registration as issued by ARRT; employment in radiologic technology; or, state permit license or registration certificate to practice radiologic

(continued)

technology. This includes altering in any respect any document issued by ARRT or any state or federal agency, or by indicating in writing certification or registration with ARRT when it is not the case.

2. Subverting or attempting to subvert ARRT's examination process. Conduct that subverts or attempts to subvert ARRT's examination process includes, but is not limited to:
   (i) conduct that violates the security of ARRT examination materials, such as removing or attempting to remove examination materials from an examination room, or having unauthorized possession of any portion of or information concerning a future, current or previously administered examination of ARRT; disclosing information concerning any portion of a future, current, or previously administered examination of ARRT; or, disclosing what purports to be, or under all circumstances is likely to be understood by the recipient as, any portion of or "inside" information concerning any portion of a future, current, or previously administered examination of ARRT;
   (ii) conduct that in any way compromises ordinary standards of test administration, such as communicating with another Candidate during administration of the examination, copying another Candidate's answers, permitting another Candidate to copy one's answers, or possessing unauthorized materials;
   (iii) impersonating a Candidate or permitting an impersonator to take the examination on one's own behalf.

3. Convictions, criminal proceedings or military court-martials as described below:
   (i) Conviction of a crime, including a felony, a gross misdemeanor or a misdemeanor with the sole exception of speeding and parking violations. All alcohol and/or drug related violations must be reported.
   (ii) Criminal proceeding where a finding or verdict of guilt is made or returned, but the adjudication of guilt is either withheld or not entered, or a criminal proceeding where the individual enters a plea of guilty or nolo contendere.
   (iii) Military court-martials that involve substance abuse, any sex-related infractions, or patient-related infractions.

4. Failure to report to ARRT that:
   (i) charges regarding the person's permit, license or registration certificate to practice radiologic technology or any other medical or allied health profession are pending or have been resolved adversely to the individual in any state, territory or country (including but not limited to,

imposed conditions, probation, suspension, or revocation); or
   (ii) the individual has been refused a permit, license, or registration certificate to practice radiologic technology or any other medical or allied health profession by another state, territory, or country.

5. Failure or inability to perform radiologic technology with reasonable skill and safety.

6. Engaging in unprofessional conduct, including, but not limited to:
   (i) departure from or failure to conform to applicable federal, state, or local governmental rules regarding radiologic technology practice; or, if no such rule exists, to the minimal standards of acceptable and prevailing radiologic technology practice;
   (ii) any radiologic technology practice that may create unnecessary danger to a patient's life, health, or safety; or
   (iii) any practice that is contrary to the ethical conduct appropriate to the profession that results in the termination from employment.

Actual injury to a patient or the public need not be established under this clause.

7. Delegating or accepting the delegation of a radiologic technology function or any other prescribed health care function when the delegation or acceptance could reasonably be expected to create an unnecessary danger to a patient's life, health, or safety. Actual injury to a patient need not be established under this clause.

8. Actual or potential inability to practice radiologic technology with reasonable skill and safety to patients by reason of illness; use of alcohol, drugs, chemicals, or any other material; or as a result of any mental or physical condition.

9. Adjudication by a court of competent jurisdiction as mentally incompetent, mentally ill, chemically dependent, or a person dangerous to the public.

10. Engaging in any **unethical** conduct, including, but not limited to, conduct likely to deceive, defraud, or harm the public; or demonstrating a willful or careless disregard for the health, welfare, or safety of a patient. Actual injury need not be established under this clause.

11. Engaging in conduct with a patient that is sexual or may reasonably be interpreted by the patient as sexual, or in any verbal behavior that is seductive or sexually demeaning to a patient; or engaging in sexual exploitation of a patient or former patient. This also applies to any unwanted sexual behavior, verbal or otherwise, that results in the termination of employment. This rule does not apply to pre-existing consensual relationships.

12. Revealing privileged communication or relating to a former or current patient, except when otherwise required or permitted by law.

13. Knowingly engaging or assisting any person to engage in, or otherwise participate in, abusive or fraudulent billing practices, including violations of federal Medicare and Medicaid laws or state medical assistance laws.

14. Improper management of patient records, including failure to maintain adequate patient records or to furnish a patient record or report required by law; or making, causing, or permitting anyone to make false, deceptive, or misleading entry in any patient record.

15. Knowingly aiding, assisting, advising, or allowing a person without a current and appropriate state permit, license or registration certificate, or a current certificate of registration with ARRT to engage in the practice of radiologic technology in a jurisdiction which requires a person to have such a current and appropriate state permit, license, or registration certificate, or a current and appropriate certification of registration with ARRT.

16. Violating a rule adopted by any state board with competent jurisdiction, an order of such board, or state or federal law relating to the practice of radiologic technology, or any other medical or allied health professions, or a state or federal narcotics or controlled substance law.

17. Knowingly providing false or misleading information that is directly related to the care of a former or current patient.

18. Practicing outside the scope of practice authorized by the individual's current state permit, license, or registration certificate, or the individual's current certificate of registration with ARRT.

19. Making a false statement or knowingly providing false information to ARRT or failing to cooperate with any investigation of ARRT of the Ethics Committee.

20. Engaging in false, fraudulent, deceptive, or misleading communications to any person regarding the individual's education, training, credentials, experience, or qualifications, or the status or the individual's state permit, license, or registration certificate in radiologic technology or certificate of registration with ARRT.

21. Knowing of a violation or a probable violation of any Rule of Ethics by any Registered Technologist or by a Candidate and failing to promptly report in writing this to ARRT.

22. Failing to immediately report to his or her supervisor information concerning an error made in connection with imaging, treating, or caring for a patient. For purposes of this rule, errors include any departure from the standard of care that reasonably may be considered to be potentially harmful, unethical, or improper (commission). Errors also include behavior that is negligent or should have occurred in connection with patient's care, but did not (omission). The duty to report under this rule exists whether or not the patient suffered any injury.

Double Effect: Refers to the fact that some actions may produce both a good and a bad effect. Four criteria must be fulfilled before this type of action is ethically permissible:
  a. The act is good or morally neutral.
  b. The intent is good, not evil, although a bad result may be foreseen.
  c. The good effect is not achieved by means of evil effects.
  d. The good effect must be more important than the evil effect, or at least there is favorable balance between good over bad.

Radiation exposure may be harmful; however, the diagnosis obtained by the exposure will aid in restoring the patient to health.

Fidelity: Refers to the duty to fulfill one's commitments and applies to keeping promises both stated and implied. The radiographer must not promise patients results that cannot be achieved.

Justice: Refers to all persons being treated equally or receiving equal benefits according to need. One patient must not be favored over another or treated differently from another, regardless of personal feelings.

Nonmaleficence: Refers to the duty to abstain from inflicting harm and also the duty to prevent harm. The radiographer is obligated to practice in a safe manner at all times.

Paternalism: Refers to the attitude that sometimes prompts health care workers to make decisions regarding a person's care without consulting the person affected. If one is tempted to make such a unilateral decision, he must consider whether the action is justifiable based on potential outcomes. The radiographer is justified in taking action in instances in which not acting would do more harm than the lack of patient input into the decision.

Sanctity of life: Refers to the belief that life is the highest good and nobody has the right to judge that another person's quality of life is so poor that his or her life is not of value and should be terminated. One cannot make life-and-death decisions for patients based on personal values.

Veracity: Refers to honesty in all aspects of one's professional life. One must be honest with patients, co-workers, and oneself.

Respect for property: Refers to keeping the patients' belongings safe and taking care not to intentionally damage or waste equipment or supplies with which one works.

Ethical Issues in Radiography

A radiographer is expected to conduct oneself in a professional manner. He must be reliable; he is expected to report for work on time and complete his assigned share of the workload in a timely, competent, and efficient manner. He is also to work as a cooperative member of the health care team. He must be articulate in his speech and free of vulgar expressions or inappropriate slang. He must treat all patients as persons of dignity and worth and not demonstrate preference for one patient over another.

The student radiographer may observe behavior and patient care problems that may seem ethically questionable in clinical laboratory practice in health care institutions. Some of the problems that might be encountered are protecting professional colleagues who are violating codes of professional ethics, unequal medical resource allocation based on a patient's age or socioeconomic status, lack of respect for a patient, breaches of privacy and confidentiality, and over-treatment or under-treatment of patients. In other words, what is observed is not what is taught in the classroom.

In such cases, the student radiographer should observe the issues that are believed to be violations of the ethical code and discuss them with colleagues and instructors in private conference. These issues can become learning situations to contemplate as a group and decide how they should be resolved.

As the scope of practice and the professional responsibilities of radiologic technology grow, so do the ethical responsibilities of radiographers. Often, an ethical decision involves a choice between two unsatisfactory solutions to a problem. This is often the case with health care. If one conscientiously follows his professional code of ethics and ethical principles previously listed to make difficult decisions as they arise, he will be able to resolve ethical dilemmas in a manner that allows for peace of mind. Combine this approach with critical thinking and the problem-solving process that will be discussed in Chapter 2 of this text.

For ethical dilemmas of some magnitude, most health care institutions have ethics committees that meet on a regular basis to solve problems and formulate policies that provide guidelines to facilitate decision making. If an ethical dilemma is encountered in the workplace that cannot be readily resolved by following one's professional code of ethics, a person is obliged to present the problem to such a body.

LEGAL ISSUES IN IMAGING TECHNOLOGY

While ethics refers to a set of moral principles, law refers to rules of conduct as prescribed by an authority or group of legislators. The *New World Webster's Dictionary* defines *law* as all rules of conduct established and enforced by the authority, legislation, or custom of a given community or group (Agnes and Guralnik, 2001). The group, in the case of the radiographer, includes ARRT and ASRT. The rules of conduct refer to the Practice Standards in Display 1-2. These standards define the practice and establish general criteria to determine compliance with the law as it applies to imaging technology.

The standards are general in nature by design to keep pace with the rapidly changing environment in which we live and work. They have been divided into three sections:

1. The *Professional Performance Standards* define the activities of the practitioner in the areas of education, interpersonal relationships, personal and professional self-assessment, and ethical behavior.
2. The *Clinical Performance Standards* define the activities of the practitioner in the care of patients and the delivery of diagnostic or **therapeutic** procedures and treatment. The section incorporates patient assessment and management with procedural analysis, performance, and evaluation.
3. The *Quality Performance Standards* define the activities of the practitioner in the technical areas of performance including equipment and material assessment, safety standards, and total quality management.

Patient Rights

The radiographer has a legal responsibility to relate to his colleagues, other members of the health care team, and the patient in a manner that is respectful of each person with whom he interacts and to adhere to the *Patient's Bill of Rights* and *The Patient Care Partnership* (Displays 1-5 and 1-6). These bills delineate the rights of the patient as a consumer of health care. Because all health care workers are required to adhere to the provisions of these bills, they must be familiar with them. The radiographer must also be aware of the areas of practice in which health care workers may infringe upon the patient's rights and be held legally liable. Some of these are as follows:

- Acting in the role of a diagnostician and providing a patient with results, impressions, or diagnoses of **diagnostic imaging** examinations
- Failing to obtain appropriate consent from women of childbearing age before performing a diagnostic imaging procedure
- Failing to obtain a complete history from a patient before administering an iodinated contrast agent

DISPLAY 1-5

A Patient's Bill of Rights

Introduction

Effective health care requires collaboration between patients and physicians and other health care professionals. Open and honest communication, respect for personal and professional values, and sensitivity to differences are integral to optimal patient care. As the setting for the provision of health services, hospitals must provide a foundation for understanding and respecting the rights and responsibilities of patients, their families, physicians, and other caregivers. Hospitals must ensure a health care ethic that respects the role of patients in decision making about treatment choices and other aspects of their care. Hospitals must be sensitive to cultural, racial, linguistic, religious, age, gender, and other differences as well as the needs of persons with disabilities.

The American Hospital Association presents A Patient's Bill of Rights with the expectation that it will contribute to more effective patient care and be supported by the hospital on behalf of the institution, its medical staff, employees, and patients. The American Hospital Association encourages health care institutions to tailor this bill of rights to their patient community by translating and/or simplifying the language of this bill of rights as may be necessary to ensure that patients and their families understand their rights and responsibilities.

Bill of Rights

These rights can be exercised on the patient's behalf by a designated surrogate or proxy decision maker if the patient lacks decision-making capacity, is legally incompetent, or is a minor.

1. The patient has the right to considerate and respectful care.
2. The patient has the right to and is encouraged to obtain from physicians and other direct caregivers relevant, current, and understandable information concerning diagnosis, treatment, and prognosis. Except in emergencies when the patient lacks decision-making capacity and the need for treatment is urgent, the patient is entitled to the opportunity to discuss and request information related to the specific procedures and/or treatments, the risks involved, the possible length of recuperation, and the medically reasonable alternatives and their accompanying risks and benefits.

   Patients have the right to know the identity of physicians, nurses, and others involved in their care, as well as when those involved are students, residents, or other trainees. The patient also has the right to know

the immediate and long-term financial implications of treatment choices, insofar as they are known.
3. The patient has the right to make decisions about the plan of care prior to and during the course of treatment and to refuse a recommended treatment or plan of care to the extent permitted by law and hospital policy and to be informed of the medical consequences of this action. In case of such refusal, the patient is entitled to other appropriate care and services that the hospital provides or can transfer to another hospital. The hospital should notify patients of any policy that might affect patient choice within the institution.
4. The patient has the right to have an advance directive (such as a living will, health care proxy, or durable power of attorney for health care) concerning treatment or designating a surrogate decision maker with the expectation that the hospital will honor the intent of that directive to the extent permitted by law and hospital policy.

   Health care institutions must advise patients of their rights under state law and hospital policy to make informed medical choices, ask if the patient has an advance directive, and include that information in patient records. The patient has the right to timely information about hospital policy that may limit its ability to fully implement a legally valid advance directive.
5. The patient has the right to every consideration of privacy. Case discussion, consultation, examination, and treatment should be conducted in a manner that protects a patient's privacy.
6. The patient has the right to expect that all communications and records pertaining to his/her care will be treated as confidential by the hospital, except in cases such as suspected abuse and public health hazards when reporting is permitted or required by law. The patient has the right to expect that the hospital will emphasize the confidentiality of this information when it releases it to any other parties entitled to review information in these records.
7. The patient has the right to review the records pertaining to his/her medical care and to have the information explained or interpreted as necessary, except when restricted by law.
8. The patient has the right to expect that, within its capacity and policies, a hospital will make reasonable response to the request of a patient for appropriate and medically indicated care and services. The hospital must provide evaluation, service, and/or referral as

(continued)

14 Patient Care in Imaging Technology

indicated by the urgency of the case. When medically appropriate and legally permissible, or when a patient has so requested, a patient may be transferred to another facility. The institution to which the patient is to be transferred must first have accepted the patient for transfer. The patient must also have the benefit of complete information and explanation concerning the need for, risks, benefits, and alternatives to such a transfer.

9. The patient has the right to ask and be informed of the existence of business relationships among the hospital, educational institutions, other health care providers, or payers that may influence the patient's treatment and care.

10. The patient has the right to consent to or decline to participate in proposed research studies or human experimentation affecting care and treatment or requiring direct patient involvement, and to have those studies fully explained prior to consent. A patient who declines to participate in research or experimentation is entitled to the most effective care that the hospital can otherwise provide.

11. The patient has the right to expect reasonable continuity of care when appropriate and to be informed by physicians and other caregivers of available and realistic patient care options when hospital care is no longer appropriate.

12. The patient has the right to be informed of hospital policies and practices that relate to patient care, treatment, and responsibilities. The patient has the right to be informed of available resources for resolving disputes, grievances, and conflicts, such as ethics committees, patient representatives, or other mechanisms available in the institution. The patient has the right to be informed of the hospital's charges for services and available payment methods.

The collaborative nature of health care requires that patients, or their families/surrogates, participate in their care. The effectiveness of care and patient satisfaction with the course of treatment depends, in part, on the patient fulfilling certain responsibilities. Patients are responsible for providing information about past illnesses, hospitalizations, medications, and other matters related to health status. To participate effectively in decision making, patients must be encouraged to take responsibility for requesting additional information or clarification about their health status or treatment when they do not fully understand information and instructions. Patients are also responsible for ensuring that the health care institution has a copy of their written advance directive if they have one. Patients are responsible for informing their physicians and other caregivers if they anticipate problems in following prescribed treatment.

Patients should also be aware of the hospital's obligation to be reasonably efficient and equitable in providing care to other patients and the community. The hospital's rules and regulations are designed to help the hospital meet this obligation. Patients and their families are responsible for making reasonable accommodations to the needs of the hospital, other patients, medical staff, and hospital employees. Patients are responsible for providing necessary information for insurance claims and for working with the hospital to make payment arrangements, when necessary. A person's health depends on much more than health care service. Patients are responsible for recognizing the impact of their lifestyle on their personal health.

Conclusion

Hospitals have many functions to perform, including the enhancement of health status, health promotion, and the prevention and treatment of injury and disease; the immediate and ongoing care and rehabilitation of patients; the education of health professionals, patients, and the community; and research. All these activities must be conducted with an overriding concern for the values and dignity of patients.

DISPLAY 1-6

The Patient Care Partnership: Understanding Expectations, Rights, and Responsibilities

When you need hospital care, your doctor and the nurses and other professionals at our hospital are committed to working with you and your family to meet your health care needs. Our dedicated doctors and staff serve the community in all its ethnic, religious, and economic diversity. Our goal is for you and your family to have the same care and attention we would want for our families and ourselves.

The sections below explain some of the basics about how you can expect to be treated during your hospital stay. They also cover what we will need from you to care for you better. If you have questions at any time, please ask them. Unasked or unanswered questions can add to the stress of being in the hospital. Your comfort and confidence in your care are very important to us.

What to Expect During Your Hospital Stay

- **High-quality hospital care.** Our first priority is to provide you the care you need, when you need it, with skill, compassion, and respect. Tell your caregivers if you have concerns about your care or if you have pain. You have the right to know the identity of doctors, nurses, and others involved in your care, as well as when they are students, residents, or other trainees.

- **A clean and safe environment.** Our hospital works hard to keep you safe. We use special policies and procedures to avoid mistakes in your care and keep you free from abuse or neglect. If anything unexpected and significant happens during your hospital stay, you will be told what happened and any resulting changes in your care will be discussed with you.

- **Involvement in your care.** You and your doctor often make decisions about your care before you go to the hospital. Other times, especially in emergencies, those decisions are made during your hospital stay. When they take place, making decisions should include:

  - *Discussing your medical condition and information about medically appropriate treatment choices.* To make informed decisions with your doctor, you need to understand several things:
    - The benefits and risks of each treatment
    - Whether it is experimental or part of a research study
    - What you can reasonably expect from your treatment and any long-term effects it might have on your quality of life
    - What you and your family will need to do after you leave the hospital
    - The financial consequences of using uncovered services or out-of-network providers

      Please tell your caregivers if you need more information about treatment choices.

  - *Discussing your treatment plan.* When you enter the hospital, you sign a general consent to treatment. In some cases, such as surgery or experimental treatment, you may be asked to confirm in writing that you understand what is planned and agree to it. This process protects your right to consent to or refuse a treatment. Your doctor will explain the medical consequences of refusing recommended treatment. It also protects your right to decide if you want to participate in a research study.

  - *Getting information from you.* Your caregivers need complete and correct information about your health and coverage so that they can make good decisions about your care. That includes:
    - Past illnesses, surgeries, or hospital stays
    - Past allergic reactions
    - Any medicines or diet supplements (such as vitamins and herbs) that you are taking
    - Any network or admission requirements under your health plan

  - *Understanding your health care goals and values.* You may have health care goals and values or spiritual beliefs that are important to your well-being. They will be taken into account as much as possible throughout your hospital stay. Make sure your doctor, your family, and your care team know your wishes.

  - *Understanding who should make decisions when you cannot.* If you have signed a health care power of attorney stating who should speak for you if you become unable to make health care decisions for yourself, or a "living will" or "advance directive" that states your wishes about end-of-life care, give copies to your doctor, your family, and your care team. If you or your family need help making difficult decisions, counselors, chaplains, and others are available to help.

- **Protection of your privacy.** We respect the confidentiality of your relationship with your doctor and other caregivers, and the sensitive information about your health and health care that are part of that relationship. State and federal laws and hospital operative policies protect the privacy of your medical information. You will receive a Notice of Privacy Practices that describes the ways that we use, disclose, and safeguard patient information and that explains how you can obtain a copy of information for our records about your care.

- **Help preparing you and your family for when you leave the hospital.** Your doctor works with hospital staff and professionals in your community. You and your family also play an important role. The success of your treatment often depends on your efforts to follow medication, diet, and therapy plans. Your family may need to help care for you at home.

  You can expect us to help you identify sources of follow-up care and to let you know if our hospital has a financial interest in any referrals. As long as you agree we can share information about your care with them, we will coordinate our activities with your caregivers outside the hospital. You can also expect to receive information and, where possible, training about the self-care you will need when you go home.

- **Help with your bill and filing insurance claims.** Our staff will file claims for you with health care insurers or other programs such as Medicare and Medicaid. They will also help your doctor with needed documentation. Hospital bills and insurance coverage are often confusing. If you have questions about your bill, contact our business office. If you need help understanding your insurance coverage or health plan, start with your insurance company or health benefits manager. If you do not have health coverage, we will try to help you and your family find financial help or make other arrangements. We need your help with collecting needed information and other requirements to obtain coverage or assistance.

  While you are here, you will receive more detailed notices about some of the rights you have as a hospital patient and how to exercise them. We are always interested in improving. If you have questions, comments, or concerns, please contact _____.

- Failing to correctly identify a patient before performing an examination
- Failing to explain a diagnostic imaging procedure to a patient before the examination
- Failing to document technical factors used to facilitate dose calculations for a procedure
- Failing to maintain a patient's physical privacy during an examination
- Failing to maintain the highest quality of images with the lowest possible radiation dose for the patient

The radiographer must never assume the role of other medical personnel in the department. It is not within his scope of practice to read radiographs or other diagnostic tests or to impart the results of these to the patient or the patient's family. This constitutes medical diagnosis and is the physician's responsibility. If a patient is injured in the diagnostic imaging department in any manner, the radiographer must not dismiss the patient from the department until the patient has been examined by a physician and deemed safe for discharge.

Patient Responsibilities

Just as the radiographer has to abide by the *Patient Bill of Rights* and *The Patient Care Partnership,* the patient has responsibilities when he or she presents for health care. These responsibilities are as follows (Grieco, 1996):

1. The patient has the responsibility to provide, to the best of his or her knowledge, an accurate and complete health history.
2. The patient is responsible for keeping appointments and for notifying the responsible practitioner or the hospital when unable to do so for any reason.
3. The patient is responsible for his or her actions when refusing treatment or not following the practitioner's instructions.
4. The patient is responsible for fulfilling the financial obligations of his or her health care as promptly as possible.
5. The patient is responsible for following hospital rules and regulations affecting patient care and conduct.
6. The patient is responsible for being considerate of the rights and property of others.

Legal Concerns

Many types of laws affect people in daily life; however, statutory law and common law are the most significant for the radiographer in professional practice. **Statutory** **laws** are derived from legislative enactments. **Common law** usually results from judicial decisions.

Two major classifications of the law are criminal law and civil law. An offense is regarded as criminal behavior and in the realm of criminal law if it is an offense against society or a member of society. If the accused party is found guilty, he or she is punished.

Criminal law protects the entire community against certain acts. An example of this would be a terrorist bombing that results in the destruction of public property and the death of one or more persons. The crime is a crime against society and is a felony. A felony is a crime of a serious nature punishable by a fine higher than $1,000.00 and a prison sentence of more than 1 year or, in extreme cases, by death.

A misdemeanor is a crime of a less serious nature punishable by a fine or imprisonment for less than 1 year. In some instances, driving under the influence of drugs or alcohol may be a misdemeanor provided that no accident or injury has resulted.

Civil law has been broken if another person's private legal rights have been violated. The person who is found guilty of this type of offense is usually expected to pay a sum of money to repair the damage done. An example of a violation of civil law might be a suit by an individual against a physician for a misdiagnosis that results in injury. This injury is to one person and not to the entire society.

Tort law exists to protect the violator of a law from being sued for an act of vengeance, to determine fault, and to compensate the injured party. A tort involves personal injury or damage resulting in civil action or litigation to obtain reparation for damages incurred. A tort may be committed intentionally or unintentionally. An intentional tort is a purposeful deed committed with the intention of producing the consequences of the deed. **Defaming** a colleague's character or committing assault or battery are examples of intentional torts. It is possible for a radiographer to be found guilty of a criminal act in professional practice. Generally, in this situation, the radiographer is likely to be legally liable for malpractice in the commitment of a tort. Battery may be charged by a patient to whom the radiographer has administered treatment against the patient's will. Assault and battery are often linked together, meaning that a threat of harm existed before the actual contact; however, assault may be charged without any physical contact if the patient fears that this will occur. Other examples of intentional tort include:

- Immobilizing a patient against his or her will (false imprisonment)
- Falsely stating that a patient has AIDS (defamation of character)
- Causing extreme emotional distress resulting in illness through outrageous or shocking conduct

An unintentional tort may be committed when a radiographer is negligent in the performance of patient care and the patient is injured as a result. The following are examples of unintentional torts:

- Improperly marking radiographic images, such as incorrectly labeling intravenous pyelography images for right and left, which could result in the surgeon removing the healthy kidney, leaving only the diseased kidney
- Omitting to apply gonadal shielding on a female patient with a femur fracture who is subsequently discovered to be pregnant
- Improperly positioning a trauma patient for tibia and fibula projections so that the projections do not adequately demonstrate the entire lower leg, resulting in a fracture being "missed" by the orthopedic physician and the radiologists
- Handing the radiologist the incorrect syringe during a procedure, which results in the injection of Xylocaine (lidocaine) instead of the contrast media
- Leaving an unconscious patient on a gurney while the radiographer leaves the room, thus allowing the patient to jar the siderails and fall off the gurney because the safety belt was not secure
- Improperly positioning a footboard on an x-ray table, which results in the patient sliding off the table when the table is placed in the upright position during an examination
- Not providing parents of pediatric patients with the proper protective attire when they are aiding in immobilizing their child, especially during fluoroscopic procedures

Radiographers most often have suits brought against them in cases of patient falls. Although the institution where the accident occurs (the employer) may be found liable for the actions of the radiographer (employee) under the principle of *respondent superior* ("let the master answer"), the technologist is responsible for his or her actions if named in a lawsuit.

Ethical and legal issues are frequently combined in the practice of imaging. The radiographer must be aware of this and take precautions to prevent situations that may lead to problems of this nature. Discrimination and **bias** shown toward a particular person constitute an example of this. It is unlawful to discriminate against any patient or co-worker on the basis of race, color, creed, national origin, ancestry, sex, marital status, disability, religious affiliation, political affiliation, age, or sexual orientation. Health care must be practiced in a totally nonjudgmental manner. No decisions must be made or any action taken based on these issues.

Use of Immobilization Techniques

Patients may not be immobilized for radiographic imaging procedures simply as a matter of convenience for the radiographer. An order must be obtained from the physician in charge of the patient for immobilization. A defined period of time must be specified to protect the patient's safety. The method of immobilization must be one that is the least restrictive to the patient's movement and freedom. There must be a need to immobilize the patient to achieve the most satisfactory outcome. The term "restraint" is often substituted for immobilization techniques; the two are used interchangeably in this text.

Only when the radiographer has exhausted all other safe methods of obtaining a radiograph should immobilizing the patient be considered. If a combative patient threatens the radiographer, security personnel may be called to assist in the immobilization of the patient. All patients who have been immobilized must be carefully monitored.

Immobilizers must be appropriate to the individual needs of the patient. When **immobilization devices** are necessary, documentation of the reasons for use and a description of specific patient actions, alternatives considered/attempted, the type used, and the length of time applied must be made. In addition, the immobilization used should be explained to the patient or family attending the patient. Immobilizers must be released for specified periods of time when they are in use. Documentation of the time and conditions of immobilizer release are required.

The use of medication as a restraining technique (chemical restraint) occurs only in extreme circumstances and only as prescribed by the patient's physician. Using immobilization techniques improperly or without a physician's orders can be considered false imprisonment and therefore cause for legal action. An institutional policy for the use of immobilization must be present in all departments, and user instructions must be clearly visible on all immobilizing devices. The technical aspects of application of immobilizers for adults and children are discussed later in this text.

CALL OUT!

Unauthorized use of immobilization techniques can be construed as false imprisonment—a tort.

Incident Reports

An injury to a patient or any error made by personnel in the diagnostic imaging department must be documented in an *incident report* as soon as it is safe to do so. The document may also be called an *unusual occurrence report* or an *accident notification report* (Display 1-7).

Incident or Unusual Occurrence Reports—Sample form:

This is a confidential report

Section 1

Name of the individual reporting the incident: _____

Institution where the incident occurred: _____

Date of incident: _____ Time of incident: _____ A.M. _____ P.M. _____

Exact location of incident: _____

Section 2

Incident occurred to: _____

☐ Staff   ☐ Student   ☐ Patient - ID# _____ ☐ Equipment

Other Explain: _____

_____

If staff, student, or patient is checked, see sections 3 & 5.
If equipment is checked, see sections 4 & 5.

Section 3

Occurrence: _____ Type of incident: _____

☐ Back injury from lifting patients   ☐ Reaction to foreign substances
☐ Miscellaneous back injury   ☐ Contagious disease
☐ Injury from a patient   ☐ Laceration
☐ Needle stick   ☐ Contusion
☐ Unsafe/defective equipment   ☐ Burn
☐ Improper use of equipment   ☐ Fracture
☐ Patient contact   ☐ Sprain/strain
☐ Fall (attended)   ☐ Puncture
☐ Fall (unattended)   ☐ Other
☐ Fire
☐ Other

Did the injury require treatment by a physician?
Was the incident reported to the appropriate personnel?

Section 4

Type of equipment damaged: _____

How was equipment damaged: _____

Result of damage (e.g., equipment down time for repair): _____

Section 5

Briefly describe the incident factually (what happened): _____

_____

_____

Name(s) of person(s) notified: _____

Name(s) of witness(es): _____

I certify that the above information is correct: _____ /title: _____

Home address: _____ Date of birth: _____ Telephone: _____

Signature of person filling out the form: _____ Date: _____

Witness Signature: _____ Date: _____

An injury may seem slight and not worthy of such a report, but all injuries—whether to patients, visitors, students, or staff or accidents involving equipment regardless of severity—must be reported according to the department procedure. An error in medication administration, imaging the wrong patient, performing the wrong procedure, a patient falling, or any error in treatment or significant change in patient status must be documented in an incident report.

When filing an incident report, write in simple terms what occurred, at what time, on what date, in which room or department, to whom, who was present, and what was done to alleviate the situation at the time. If a patient or person is injured, report the condition of the individual involved in the situation. Any injured patient must be examined by a physician before they are allowed to leave the department. Injured health care workers or visitors must be examined according to the agency's policy.

The incident report should be factual regarding the nature of the injury or situation and signed by all who participated or witnessed the event. All incidents resulting in patient or personnel injury must be reported according to the policy and procedures developed by the institution's risk management department. Filing an incident report is not an admission of negligence, but simply a record of an event that was not routine in nature.

Patient Safety Reporting

The Patient Safety and Quality Improvement Act of 2005 was signed by President Bush and enacted to amend title IX of the Public Health Service Act to provide for the improvement of patient safety and to reduce the incidence of events that adversely affect patient safety. The act created a voluntary system for health care providers to report medical errors and other patient safety information to improve patient safety. The reported information is confidential and privileged under the Patient Safety and Quality Improvement Act. Therefore, adverse actions may not take place against individual(s) for good faith reporting to recognized patient safety organizations.

Good Samaritan Laws

All states in the United States now have Good Samaritan laws. These laws were enacted to protect persons who give medical aid to persons in emergency situations from civil or criminal **liability** for their actions or omissions under these circumstances. State laws vary, but generally if one stops to render aid at the scene of an accident, he is not held liable for any adverse results of his actions, provided that he acts within accepted standards and without gross negligence.

Automatic external defibrillators (AEDs) have been added to emergency medical procedures, and the equipment for this procedure is now available in many areas of public use such as in airplanes and city buildings. "To permit and encourage the use of AEDs by the lay public, nearly all states have enacted facilitating legislation. In addition, the Cardiac Arrest Survival Act provides immunity for lay rescuers who use AEDs and for businesses or other entities or individuals who purchase AEDs for public access defibrillation" (American Heart Association, 2005). The radiographer will be instructed to use the AED as part of his or her Basic Life Support for Healthcare Providers education.

Informed Consent

Many procedures performed in diagnostic imaging departments require special consent forms to be signed by the patient or, in the case of minor children or other special cases, by parents or legal representatives. The radiographer must be familiar with the procedures that require special consent forms and not confuse these with the blanket consent forms, which are often signed when the patient enters the hospital, as these are not valid if an informed consent is required.

A consent is a contract wherein the patient voluntarily gives permission to someone (in this case, the imaging staff) to perform a procedure or service. The legal aspect of obtaining consent deals with the imaging staff's "duty to warn" and the ethic "do no harm." The medical aspect of consent hopes to establish rapport with the patient through communication to secure a successful outcome. Informed consent is required for the following procedures:

- Invasive procedures such as a surgical incision, a biopsy, a cystoscopy, or paracentesis
- Procedures requiring sedation and/or anesthesia
- A nonsurgical procedure such as an arteriography that may carry risk to the patient
- Procedures that involve radiation

Consent is not legal if the patient is not informed of all aspects of the procedure to be performed. These include the potential risks, benefits, and suggested alternatives. The patient must also be informed of the consequences if the suggested procedure is not completed. Because a patient usually consents or refuses a procedure based on the information that the health care professional provides, the duty of obtaining the informed consent involves the patient's physician or radiologist and the radiographer.

Although special consent forms may be signed before the patient comes to the diagnostic imaging department, it is the duty of the radiographer to recheck the patient's chart to be certain that this has been accomplished. The radiographer must also make sure that the patient understands what is going to be done and the essential nature of the choices available to him. If the patient, parent, or legal representative denies knowledge of the procedure or withdraws consent, notify the radiologist and/or the patient's physician. The procedure should be postponed until the matter is satisfactorily resolved. It is not the radiographer's responsibility to determine whether a procedure should be terminated. It is his responsibility to bring the problem to the physician or supervisor in charge for resolution.

There are several levels of informed consent:

1. *Simple consent* is a matter of obtaining a patient's permission to perform a procedure without knowledge of that procedure. Simple consent is divided into express and implied consent.

    a. *Express consent* occurs when the patient does not stop the procedure from taking place. By allowing the procedure to occur, the patient has given his or her express consent to the radiographer; however, legally, silence is not an agreement.

    b. *Implied consent* occurs in emergency situations when it is not possible to obtain consent from the patient, his or her parents, or a legal representative. The health care provider operates under the belief that the patient would give permission if able; it is "implied" that permission would be given.

2. *Inadequate consent* is also known as *ignorant consent*. This occurs when the patient has not been informed adequately to make a responsible decision. The patient can bring charges of negligence (an unintentional tort) when he or she has had inadequate consent, particularly if the patient sustains injury (when consent is not obtained, battery may be charged).

Obtaining informed consent protects the health care worker from legal action. The radiographer must also understand that communicating effectively with the patient is essential to alleviate his or her anxiety as well as to improve outcomes from all procedures. Display 1-8 lists the criteria for valid informed consent.

Malpractice Insurance

Precautions should be taken by radiographers to safeguard against a lawsuit. In recent years, professional (**malpractice**) liability protection has become an important kind of insurance, especially for members of the medical profession. All radiographers should carry their own malpractice insurance, even if their employer carries insurance for them. A member service ASRT provides is a resource for individual professional liability insurance (malpractice).

Malpractice is a wrongful act by a physician, lawyer, or other professional that injures a patient or client. The patient or client may file a civil lawsuit to recover damages (money) to compensate for the injury. The radiographer could be named in a lawsuit in which the legal expenses for defense are not completely covered by his employer, and he may still be liable for his own negligence. Without a malpractice insurance policy in one's own name, risk may be assumed. Professional liability insurance provides protection against claims of malpractice. It is not wise to place oneself in professional jeopardy when a professional malpractice policy can be purchased for a reasonable price. With a malpractice liability insurance policy, the insurance company assumes the risk in accordance with the policy contract.

DISPLAY 1-8

Voluntary Consent

Valid consent must be freely given, without coercion.

Incompetent Patient

Legal definition: individual who is NOT autonomous and cannot give or withhold consent (e.g., individuals who are mentally retarded, mentally ill, or comatose).

Informed Subject

Informed consent should be in writing. It should contain the following:

Explanation of procedure and its risks

Description of benefits and alternatives

An offer to answer questions about the procedure

Instructions that the patient may withdraw consent

A statement informing the patient if the protocol differs from customary procedure

Patient Able to Comprehend

Information must be written and delivered in language understandable to the patient. Questions must be answered to facilitate comprehension if material is confusing.

MEDICAL RECORDS AND DOCUMENTATION

A medical record is kept for each patient who seeks medical treatment whether he or she is an outpatient or has been admitted to the hospital for care. This record, called a *chart*, is started the moment the patient arrives or is admitted for care and is kept until he or she is dismissed or discharged from the hospital. The medical record is kept for a number of reasons:

1. To transmit information about the patient from one health care worker to another
2. To protect the patient from medical errors and duplication of treatments
3. To provide information for medical research
4. To protect the health care worker in cases of litigation
5. To provide information concerning quality of patient care for institutional evaluation teams such as The Joint Commission

The chart contains the patient's identifying data, documentation of all physician's orders, physician's consultation notes, patient progress notes, medications and treatments received, around-the-clock nurse's notes, all patient visits for outpatient or ambulatory care, laboratory and radiology reports, medical history and physical examination, admitting and discharge diagnosis, results of examinations, surgical reports, consent forms, education received by the patient, discharge planning, health care team planning, nursing care plans, and discharge summaries. All members of the health care team are expected to document the care they have rendered for the patient on this chart.

In imaging departments, a requisition from a physician contains the orders for specific procedures to be performed on patients. In addition, the requisition includes the following data: the patient's name, gender, date of birth, diagnosis, and other patient information, which the radiographer uses to verify the correct examination to be performed on the correct patient. The radiographer must assume responsibility for obtaining a medical history from the patient that is pertinent to the treatment or examination he or she is to receive in the department. This information includes the following:

1. Female patients' responses to questions concerning pregnancy and date of last menstrual period documented, if pertinent.
2. History of allergies; trauma, if pertinent; contrast media or radionuclide administered.
3. Vital signs, patient education before and after each procedure, names and credentials of the members of the health care team participating in the proce-

dure, and the diagnostic report by the physicians involved following the procedure. Many of these issues are discussed in detail in the chapters that follow.

Nurses and physicians who participate in diagnostic imaging examinations or treatments are also responsible for documentation; however, radiographers must review the documentation and bring any omissions to their attention. Any item that has not been documented on the chart is considered to be "not performed" in a court of law. All entries on a medical record must list the time and date of the procedure and be signed by the person who administered it. The credentials of the person must also be listed.

Certain documentation is specific to radiographic imaging. The radiographer is accountable for the documentation or record keeping according to departmental protocol of any radiographic images taken, including the number of images or exposures, the exposure factors, the radiographic room or equipment, and the amount of fluoroscopic time used during a procedure. The radiographer must also document any patient preparation for procedures that he makes, medications that he administers, and any adverse reactions to medications or treatments received.

Abbreviations must be approved by the institution in which the radiographer is employed. A list of acceptable abbreviations must be on record at that institution and learned by those using them. No others are acceptable.

Charting formats are also made and approved by each institution; however, the contents of the record are reviewed and either approved, disapproved, or changed according to recommendations made by the accreditation bodies inspecting the charts.

If an error is made while writing an entry into a chart, a single line may be drawn through the error, *"mistaken entry"* is written above the error, and the signature of the person making the error is signed to the error. A corrected entry may then be written. If documenting by computer, the items listed above must still be included on the chart.

Radiographic images are considered part of the patient's medical record and may be used as legal evidence in the event of a lawsuit. For this reason, all radiographic images must clearly indicate the patient's name, identification number, the name of the facility where taken, and a right or left marker correctly placed. The release of any patient medical records that include originals, copies, or electronic images requires a consent written and signed by the patient or legal guardian. A consent must be presented before any patient records are released for any reason.

CONFIDENTIALITY, PRIVACY, THE HEALTH INSURANCE PORTABILITY AND ACCOUNTABILITY ACT IN RADIOLOGIC TECHNOLOGY

In 1996, Congress recognized the need for national patient record privacy standards. For this reason, the Health Insurance Portability and Accountability Act of 1996 (HIPAA) was enacted. The law included provisions designed to save money for health care businesses by encouraging electronic transactions, but it also required new safeguards to protect the security and confidentiality of information.

In November 1999, the Department of Health and Human Services (DHHS) published proposed regulations to guarantee patients new rights and protections against the misuse or disclosure of their health records. In December 2000, DHHS issued the final rule, which took effect on April 14, 2001. Most covered entities had 2 full years—until April 14, 2003—to comply with the final rule's provisions. All medical records and other individually identifiable health information, whether electronic, on paper, or oral, are covered by the final rule.

The radiographer must abide by the same rules concerning confidentiality, security, and privacy of patient information with computerized records as with previous systems. Written consent by the patient is the only legitimate reason to obtain and pass on confidential material. The student radiographer must familiarize himself with the potential abuses of the new technology so that he will not unknowingly violate the law.

HEALTH CARE DELIVERY

In the recent past, the rising cost of health care became a major concern of the medical community and of the nation. This gave rise to major changes in the health care delivery system in the United States and has become a major political concern. The belief was that the exorbitant cost of health care and its continued rising cost did not necessarily improve the quality of patient care. Based on this belief, many restraints were placed on the institutions and the practitioners of health care. These changes are complex, and it is not within the scope of this text to discuss them at length. However, a very brief outline of the current methods of health care delivery follows.

Medicare: Covers persons 65 years of age and older, permanently disabled workers and their dependents, and persons with end-stage renal disease. There are 2 parts to Medicare:

Medicare, Part A: covers acute hospital care and home health care service and requires enrollees to pay an $840.00 deductible for hospitalization.

Medicare, Part B: covers physician services, outpatient hospital care, laboratory testing, durable medical equipment, and special services. This service requires a $100.00 deductible and a premium monthly. This premium is in the process of being increased and changed and will not be listed in this text.

All persons paid by Social Security are automatically enrolled in Part A of Medicare. Part B is optional. Medicare does not cover long-term care and limits other aspects of health care and promotion of health. This encourages elders to enroll in private health care plans called Medigap insurance if they can afford to do so.

Medicaid: This is a federally funded and state-administered program that provides medical care for families with dependent older adults, children, or otherwise disabled persons with incomes below the federal poverty level. It also provides maternal and child care for the poor.

Prospective Payment System (PPS): Instituted by Medicare, this system uses financial incentives to decrease total charges by reimbursing for medical treatment based upon diagnosis-related groups (DRGs). This is a method of grouping for payment dependent upon diagnosis. That is, every person with the same diagnosis receives the same financial payment for treatment. The DRGs have resulted in a great deal of controversy in medical circles.

Managed Care Organizations (MCOs): Are divided into two groups that supervise patient care services; they are Health Maintenance Organizations (HMOs) and Preferred Provider Organizations (PPOs). HMOs are group insurance plans that charge each person insured under their plan a preset fee for care and health care service. This fee is paid by the participant regardless of whether they utilize the HMO's services or not. The HMO attempts to perform preventative health care by education, periodic health care screening (i.e., immunizations, mammograms, physical examinations), and other preventative methods to reduce the cost of medical care. This type of financial management is called capitation. PPOs gather a group of health care providers who are guaranteed a group of consumers of health care (patients) based on their promise of discounting their fees. The patient is guaranteed health care at lower cost provided they use the PPO provided.

Point of Service Plans: A primary care provider is selected from a group of providers. The primary care physician then acts as a gatekeeper for the patient and authorizes any referrals the patient may require, thus reducing unnecessary referrals.

Physician Hospital Organizations: evolved as a result of financial concerns of hospitals and physician practices. The PHO creates a corporate structure between a hospital and a group of its physicians; they contract with a managed care organization to negotiate fees for services for their self-insured employees (Chitty, 2005).

There is a growing demand for evidence that care provided by health care providers is of high quality as well as cost-effective. Regulatory bodies such as The Joint Commission and organizations for consumers of health care have been established. These organizations examine the readmission of patients to hospitals within 30 days of discharge, wound infection rates, pressure ulcers acquired in hospitals, documentation, and many other factors that indicate quality of care.

Because of these regulatory bodies, protocols for managing care have been derived. These protocols are known as *guidelines or standards* for managing patient care. *Critical pathways* for diagnoses and procedures to treat particular illness have also been developed. Following the course of these pathways is one of several methods used to examine quality of patient care. All of these methods examine and assess morbidity and mortality rates, admissions per year for chronic illness, complications, and patient satisfaction.

In spite of efforts to control the cost of medical care, it continues to be extremely expensive, and there are many who are unable to afford medical insurance or preventative health care of any kind. When there is a medical crisis, these people are left to seek care in city emergency facilities throughout the country. The emergency may be treated; however, there is no follow-up care for these patients.

SUMMARY

Radiologic technology has evolved to meet the criteria of a profession by requiring extended education and clinical practice. It has a theoretical body of knowledge and leads to defined skills, abilities, and action. It also provides a specific service, and its members have a degree of decision-making autonomy when working within their scope of practice.

There are several educational avenues to obtain a career in radiologic technology. Each category has defined educational requirements and responsibilities that are expected to be fulfilled and continuing education requirements that are necessary to renew the radiographer's license.

The professional radiographer is expected to join and participate in professional organizations. Such participation allows one to keep informed of technological changes and alterations in professional standards. The strength of the profession is also promoted in this manner as well as prevention of infringement from groups that desire to assume parts of the professional responsibilities of the radiographer.

The practicing radiographer interacts with members of the health care team on a daily basis. It is advantageous to recognize the educational background and duties of these team members so that a harmonious working relationship with them can be built on professional knowledge and respect. The health care professionals with whom the radiographer will work most frequently are the physician, the nurse, the pharmacist, occupational and physical therapists, and the respiratory therapist.

If radiologic technology has been selected as a profession, the student must be aware of and willing to accept the ethical and legal constraints that govern practice as a member of this profession. The *Code of Ethics* and *The Practice Standards* of this profession must be understood and these principles maintained. The rights of the patient must be understood, and each patient must be treated as a human being with dignity and worth.

All professional work performed must be within the scope of the radiographer's practice at all times. It must be understood that to do otherwise is a violation of the law. The radiographer must also follow the policies concerning unusual occurrence and accident reports of the institution or health care facility in which he works. Any patient injured during a procedure must not be discharged without the consent of the physician from the radiographic imaging department.

Documentation and maintenance of medical records constitute an important aspect of health care. These records transmit information to other health care workers, protect the patient from errors, provide information for medical research, protect the radiographer and others in cases of litigation, and provide information concerning the quality of patient care for institutional evaluation.

The radiographer is believed to be a competent professional. As such, he is expected to act in a responsible and safe manner when caring for patients. It is his obligation to communicate effectively with other members of the health care team and document patient care correctly and completely. He must also respect the patient's right to refuse treatment.

CHAPTER 1 TEST

1. List the 8 criteria of a profession and explain how radiologic technology meets these criteria.
2. Name two major professional organizations in radiologic technology.
3. What is the purpose of the Practice Standards in Radiography?
4. The practice standards are divided into three sections. Name and define the sections.
5. What document represents the application of moral principles and moral values for radiologic technology?
6. Match the following:
   a. The right to make decisions concerning one's own life
   b. The intent is good, although a bad result may be foreseen
   c. Equal treatment and equal benefits
   d. Honesty to patients
   e. Duty to refrain from inflicting harm

   1. Nonmaleficence
   2. Autonomy
   3. Truthfulness
   4. Justice
   5. Double effect
7. The radiographer who mistakenly administers an incorrect drug to a patient may be guilty of a
   a. Tort
   b. Negligence
   c. Crime
   d. Battery
8. As a radiographer, you refuse to work with a patient because you do not care for persons of the patient's religion. You are guilty of violating
   a. The law
   b. The ethics of your profession
   c. You own moral values
   d. Both a and b
9. Explain the documentation for which you as a radiographer will be accountable in your department when you participate in a procedure.
10. Professional ethics may be defined as
    a. A set of principles that govern a course of action
    b. Standards of any professional person
    c. The same as not violating the law
    d. A set of rules and regulations made up by the department in which you work
11. Which of the following is an example of privileged (confidential) information?
    a. Your friend buys a new car and asks you not to tell anyone about it yet.
    b. A colleague discusses his stock market holdings with you.

c. You assist with a diagnostic study and a large adherent mass is discovered in the colon.
d. A fellow student is told that he has the highest grades in the class.
12. After completing a radiologic technology program, you are employed at the local community hospital in the diagnostic imaging department. You are approached by a colleague who asks you to become a member of the local chapter of your professional organization. You know that you will be expected to pay yearly dues. Which would be your best response to your colleague?
    a. You explain that you have just begun your first job and money is in short supply at this time.
    b. You laugh and say, "No thanks, I've had all of the organization I can take for a while."
    c. You join in 1 or 2 years when your financial status improves.
    d. You join at once because you feel that it is an obligation to be a member of your professional organization.
13. Information about a patient's condition or prognosis
    a. May be freely discussed with close relatives
    b. Must always remain confidential
    c. Should always be open discussion, since "a well-known fact is no secret"
    d. Should be discussed only on a co-worker/interdepartmental basis
14. If you are unable to solve a professional ethical dilemma, you must present the problem to
    a. Your attorney
    b. The ethics committee of the institution for which you work
    c. Your colleagues
    d. Your peers
15. As a radiographer you are assigned to a diagnostic imaging procedure for which you have had no education. Your best course of action when this occurs would be
    a. To proceed as best you can
    b. To ask a colleague for directions and then proceed
    c. To explain to your superior that you have never worked with this procedure and do not feel competent to perform the procedure without education
    d. To state that you are ill, and retreat
16. If you offer your services at the scene of an accident, you are protected from litigation by the Good Samaritan law.
    a. True
    b. False

17. If a patient requests to take his or her radiographic images to another institution for consultation, you must remember
    a. That the patient must present a signed request before the records can be released
    b. That only the original radiographic images can be released
    c. That only copies of the original radiographic images can be released
18. An unconscious child is brought to the emergency suite in your hospital for a diagnostic radiograph. There is no parent or legal guardian with the child. You will proceed with the procedure and will be functioning under the rule of implied consent.
    a. True
    b. False
19. Explain the value of personal malpractice insurance for the radiographer.
20. List three areas in which the radiographer may infringe upon patient rights.
21. List three responsibilities of the patient.
22. Match the following:
    a. Covers the acute hospital care and home health care of persons 65 years of age and older
    b. Provides medical care for children and disabled persons
    c. Groups for payment dependent upon medical diagnosis
    d. Attempts to decrease medical care costs by means of preventative medical care
    e. Has primary care physicians who act as gatekeepers for patient care

    1. DRG
    2. Point of Service plans
    3. Medicare
    4. HMOs
    5. Medicaid

Patient Assessment and Communication in Imaging

STUDENT LEARNING OUTCOMES

After completing the chapter, the student will be able to:

1. Explain the basic physical and emotional needs of the person seeking health care and the effect of stress on health.
2. Define and explain critical thinking and describe its place in the profession of radiologic technology.
3. Define the affective, cognitive, and psychomotor domain as it applies to learning.
4. Explain the method used to make an accurate assessment of the patient's needs in the imaging department and explain the rationale for using this method.
5. List the expectations that the patient may have of the radiographer assigned to his or her care.
6. Define therapeutic communication and demonstrate its techniques.
7. Explain the history-taking process for imaging and list the requirements for its successful completion.
8. Explain the problem-solving process in patient teaching.
9. Describe the special needs of the terminally ill or the grieving patient as they present in imaging.
10. Define advance directives for medical care and differentiate between the various types of advance care documents.

KEY TERMS

Advance directives: Directions given by a person while in a healthy state concerning wishes at time of death

Adverse effects: Unfavorable happenings

Aggravating or alleviating factors: That which makes a problem better or worse

Analyzing: To break down into parts for study; to dissect

Anticipatory grieving: Mourning death or loss before the event occurs

Anxiety: A troubled state of mind; distress or nervousness

Assessment: Evaluation of a patient using skills in history taking to achieve a particular goal

Associated manifestations: What else occurs during an episode

Attitudes: A manner of feeling or thinking; opinions

Auditory: Must be heard

Basic needs: Needs one cannot live without; i.e., air, food, shelter, etc

Belief: Certainty or confidence in the trustworthiness of another

Biases: Prejudices

Body image: How one imagines himself or herself to appear physically

Chronology: The arrangement of events in time

Clinical portion: Instruction in the patient care area; i.e., learning in the institution with direct patient care

Cognitively: Mental activities related to thinking, learning, and memory that result in learning

Continuum: Uninterrupted; continuing on an enduring line

Creativity: The power to invent something new or original

Critical thinking: Assessing one's thinking in order to make it more clear, more accurate, or more defensible

Culture: A set of beliefs and values common to a particular group of people

Didactic: The instructional phase of learning; i.e., classroom instruction

Dissonance: A lack of harmony or agreement

KEY TERMS (Continued)

Do-not-resuscitate (DNR): An order on the patient's chart and signed by the patient's physician that orders the staff not to perform CPR or call the emergency team if the patient expires

Ethnicity: A common history and origin

Evaluate: To make a judgement as to the value of something; to size up

Explain: To render understandable

Explore: To investigate or discover

Feedback: A response that indicates that the message delivered was correctly or incorrectly perceived

"Full code": For persons who wish to have full cardiopulmonary resuscitation if they stop breathing; this is also called "code blue"

Global: Complete; worldwide

Habit: Customary performance or practice

Health: A condition of feeling physically and mentally sound or whole

Identity: The personal characteristics by which one is able to be recognized or recognizes oneself

Infer: To arrive at a conclusion based upon evidence gathered

Informed consent forms: Approval of a medical procedure after being informed of all possible unfavorable consequences

Inquiry: To put to question; to examine

Interpret: To explain or to make understandable

Introspection: Looking into one's own mind to analyze thoughts

Kinesthetic: Perceived through movement; through action of muscles

Linear: Easy to comprehend because it is basic or logical

Localization: To determine the exact area of origin

Lower-level thinking: Using only habit and recall as one thinks

"No code": The same as a DNR order; a written medical order must follow this request in order for the patient to be allowed to expire without emergency assistance

Nontherapeutic relationship: An association with another person that is unpleasant or unsatisfactory

Nonverbal: Unspoken

Objective: Concrete evidence; based on facts that exist; i.e. the patient's chart

Objectives or outcome criteria: Goals; what is planned to achieve

Onset: Time of beginning

Paralanguage: Tone of voice, gestures, and facial expressions that accompany speech

Physiologic needs: Needs that allow our bodies to function; food, air, water

Problem solving: Using critical thinking to assess complex situations and formulating a method of solution to the problem

Psychomotor: Relating to physical movement

Rapport: A sense of harmony or agreement

Recall: To remember or to bring back to mind

Reflect: To think carefully and consider at length

Regressive behavior: To return to a former state of being; usually worse behavior, possibly infantile or childlike

Self-actualizing needs: Needs that enrich our existence; i.e. music, literature, creative work

Self-concept: That which one believes about him or herself

Self-esteem: A sense of one's own worth

Significant others: Those with whom one is in intimate contact

Stress: Pressure or weight placed upon oneself that creates strain

Subjective: Based on judgment by an individual; personal opinion

Therapeutic communication: Speaking and listening in a manner that makes the receiver of the talk feel improved or restored

Therapeutic: Healing; curative

Trauma: Tissue damage related to an injury or mental trauma related to shocking developments

Validate: To confirm; to justify or establish as true

Values: Measures of the worth or worthiness of qualities

Visual: Able to be seen with one's eyes

The student radiographer is obliged to learn to assess the needs of his patient and, having made this **assessment**, formulate a plan of care that best fits the individual. The plan is implemented and, finally, evaluated. In order to follow the steps in the assessment process, the radiographer must have an understanding of basic human needs and the expectations the patient brings to the imaging department when presenting for diagnosis or care.

Skills in **critical thinking, problem solving, therapeutic communication** and patient education are all part of the requirements of the professional radiographer. These skills must be learned as well as the ability to relate to persons who may be terminally ill or are in the process of grieving. This requires sensitivity and understanding. In order to be successful, the radiographer must be able to appreciate his own feelings about loss and death and have an understanding of the phases of the grieving process.

■ HEALTH-ILLNESS CONTINUUM

All persons seek to maintain a high level of health and a feeling of well-being. **Health** can be defined as the status of an organism functioning without any evidence of disease or disfigurement. Unfortunately a perfect state of health is rarely achieved; therefore, health is seen as on a **continuum** (Fig. 2-1). We are all in various places on this continuum depending upon our state of physical and mental health.

Stress in its various forms affects an individual's ability to maintain his health status at a high level. Stressors may take many forms from a simple change in living area or beginning a new job, to a major life change such as diagnosis of a potentially terminal illness or loosing a significant person in one's life. Any change in life requires adaptation to that change with its accompanying stressors.

All persons have **basic needs** that must be met. When basic needs are met, one aspires to higher needs. An individual who is in a state of prolonged stress eventually finds himself unable to meet his basic needs and illness may result.

Abraham Maslow, a renowned psychologist, visualized humans as governed by a hierarchy of needs, each of which he viewed as a "building block" in a pyramidal structure. At the base of the pyramid are the basic **physiologic needs;** at the top is **self-actualization,** which is the end result of growth of the human spirit.

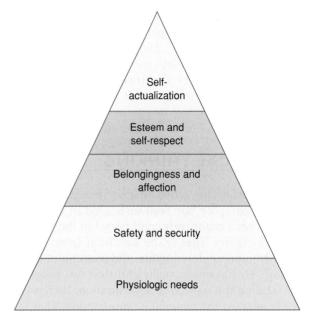

FIGURE 2-2 Drawing of Maslow's Hierarchy of Needs (From Smeltzer SC, Bare BG. *Brunnar & Suddarth's Textbook of Medical-Surgical Nursing,* 9th ed. Philadelphia: Lippincott Williams & Wilkins, 2000).

At the lowest end are the basic needs to maintain our bodies (Fig. 2-2).

Persons whose state of mental and physical health is at the most positive end of the health-illness continuum have their basic needs met and have no stressful events affecting their well-being. They are able to begin to pursue higher goals. When illness—whether physical or emotional—overtakes a person, he or she loses his or her state of well-being and no longer perceives himself or herself as one whose basic needs for food, water, air, shelter, love, belonging, and self-esteem are being met. Illness may mean the loss of ability to maintain social and economic status. The individual's place in his or her social group is threatened. As illness progresses, the awareness of unmet basic needs increases, and a feeling of great anxiety overwhelms the ill person.

When the radiographer meets the patient, he or she is often in a state of **anxiety.** Persons who are in need of imaging procedures may present themselves for diagnosis and treatment after a long period of feeling unwell. Others may come to the department immediately after a serious accident has destroyed, or threatens to destroy, their state of well-being. These situations result in a state of severe stress. When one's level of wellness has been compromised, **regressive behavior** may result. A person in such a state has difficulty communicating effectively. He or she may resort to aggressive demands, or may withdraw in silence and not be able to make his or her needs known at all.

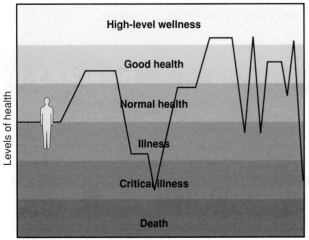

FIGURE 2-1 Drawing of health-illness continuum.

When the radiographer is assigned to care for any individual, he must be able to determine that person's state of health or illness. He must understand that the fulfillment of the patient's most basic needs may have been compromised by the stress of illness or **trauma.** Stressful life events may result in unpleasant patient behavior.

CRITICAL THINKING

Prior to performing actual imaging procedures, the student radiographer has been instructed in a classroom and has been **cognitively** conditioned to the profession of radiography. That is, he has been informed with regards to principles, insights, and concepts of the profession. He has intellectually absorbed this knowledge.

During this aspect of his education, he has effectively adapted the material he has learned. That is, he is now able to explain why the material he has learned is important to his professional growth, and, finally, through the **didactic** education, he is able to progress to the **psychomotor** aspect of his education. That is, he is able to physically perform skills that he has learned.

CALL OUT!

Learning requires cognitive, affective, and psychomotor skills!

As the student progresses from the didactic to the actual **clinical portion** of his education, he must begin to apply the knowledge he has acquired to actual patient care. Each patient care procedure requires a different application of the student's skill and knowledge. Being able to complete each assignment in a timely and efficient manner, while meeting the unique needs of each patient, is criteria for an excellent radiographer. Achieving this goal requires use of **critical thinking** skills.

Critical thinking can be defined as an analytical inquiry into any issue presented. If one is not assessing his manner of thought, he is not thinking critically. Critical thinking requires the following:

- Ability to **interpret**
- Ability to **evaluate**
- Ability to **infer**
- Ability to **explain**
- Ability to **reflect**

The ability to think critically requires a great amount of effort and self-knowledge and must be learned in a step-by-step manner. The student must examine his past methods of thinking and be aware of the limits of his knowledge, his biases, and his prejudices. Life experiences must be reviewed as they have contributed to the present manner of one's thinking abilities. After this self-examination, the student must be willing to expand and change his previous patterns of thinking. This change in thinking patterns will allow for expansion and **creativity** in the thought processes. The critical thinker is an inquisitive thinker who is tolerant of the views of others. Professional maturity comes with increased technical skill and growth in critical thinking skills.

As the radiography student begins to work with patients, he must proceed through levels of thinking. He will begin to grow personally, as well as professionally, and continue to expand technical abilities. This must be done as one's thinking methods grow from the simple to the complex.

Modes of Thinking

Thinking comprises several levels: recall, habit, inquiry, and creativity. Recall and habit make up the lower levels of thinking. Inquiry and creativity are the higher modes. Mastering the ability to analyze how one thinks is another crucial skill in critical thinking. Display 2-1 briefly defines the modes of thinking.

DISPLAY 2-1

Modes of Thinking

Recall: ability to bring to mind a large body of facts quickly.

Habit: becoming accustomed to performing a skill without deep thought because of repetition.

Inquiry: to process information thoughtfully and be willing and able to recognize, explore, and challenge assumptions to make sense of complex ideas. Includes the ability to analyze, infer, explain, and reflect upon one's work.

Creativity: ability to conceive of alternative methods of performing tasks or accomplishing a procedure that is more efficient or less traumatic. Creativity must always work within the standards of safe and ethical practice; demands accountability.

The creative radiographer does not abandon standards of practice in his field. "Minds indifferent to standards and disciplined judgment tend to judge inexactly, inaccurately, prejudicially" (Paul, 1995, p. 198).

Knowing How One Thinks

The ability to understand how one thinks may be the most difficult aspect of critical thinking. **Introspection** is a requirement. One must think while thinking. Honesty with oneself is also necessary. The following questions must be asked:

- Am I remaining in the lower levels of thinking most of the time by using only **recall** and **habit** to solve problems?
- Do I rarely (or never) move beyond these lower levels of thinking into the realm of **inquiry** by **exploring, validating,** and **analyzing** the problems before me?
- Am I combining (interpreting) thoughts, ideas, and concepts to find better solutions to problems?
- Am I creating new approaches to solve difficult patient care problems?
- Am I carefully evaluating my work?

Becoming a critical thinker takes practice and time. The successful radiographer takes the concepts presented above and applies them to each patient care problem. If a habit of higher-level thinking has been developed, then creating successful solutions to problems becomes second nature.

The ability to recall what has been learned in the classroom and performing imaging skills from habit are necessary but not sufficient skills for a professional radiographer. The **lower-level thinking** processes must be combined with the higher modes of thinking to safely care for the patient.

PROBLEM SOLVING AND PATIENT ASSESSMENT

Every patient and every diagnostic procedure presents problems ranging from simple to complex. When the radiography student obtains a patient care assignment, he must decide how to perform the assignment quickly, efficiently, and as comfortably as possible for the patient. This requires going through the problem-solving process before beginning the task. The beginning student should write down the problem-solving process. As proficiency is attained, it may become a mental process. However the process is conducted, critical thinking is necessary to achieve a satisfactory outcome. The ability to recall scientific principles of the procedure and habits cultivated in performing various skills are also needed. Problem solving requires

data collection, data analysis, planning, implementation, and evaluation.

> ### CALL OUT!
> Problem solving requirements:
> - Data collection
> - Data analysis
> - Planning
> - Implementation
> - Evaluation

Data Collection

There are basically two types of data: **subjective** and **objective.** Subjective data include anything that the patient, or a **significant other** who accompanies the patient, might say that is pertinent to the patient's care.

For instance, the patient might say, "The last time I had an x-ray, they gave me a medicine in my vein that made me itch all over," or "I can't lie flat because I can't breathe in that position." Either of these statements would be significant subjective data and needs to be part of the radiographer's data base. Anything that the patient or an accompanying significant other says that may affect the patient's care is to become part of the subjective data base.

Objective data include anything that the radiographer sees, hears, smells, feels, or reads on the patient's chart or anything reported about the patient by another health care worker that may affect the patient or the procedure to be performed.

Data Analysis

This part of the assessment process integrates all segments of critical thinking. The radiographer lists all subjective and objective data and then begins to analyze it. He then decides what data are relevant to the assignment and considers any problems and potential problems. The method required to perform the procedure demands recall. Problems and potential problems are listed in order of priority beginning with what is most significant to the procedure.

Example

The radiographer is assigned to take radiographic images of the pelvis of an 84-year-old female who may have a pelvic fracture. The patient is summoned from the waiting area. She is on a gurney. The radiographer greets the patient and inquires about her well-being.

The patient says, "I'm very hard of hearing, you'll have to speak louder." The radiographer positions himself closer to the patient and raises his voice and asks the patient again how she is feeling. She responds,

"I was very well until last evening when I fell as I was getting out of bed. Now I have a lot of pain in my right leg." The patient is then moved to the examining room. During the preceding brief interaction, the radiographer has managed to gather the following data:

> The patient is an elderly female (objective data).
> The patient is hearing impaired (subjective data).
> The patient has pain in her right leg (subjective data).

The radiographer continues his assessment of the patient in the examining room. From the data gathered, a list of problems and potential problems that may occur is formulated. By considering potential problems, the radiographer initially avoids possible difficulties. The problem list might include the following in order of priority:

> Pain and a potential for increasing the patient's pain during the procedure (moving the patient may cause further pain).
> Immobility (the patient is unable to move by herself and requires assistance for safety and to obtain adequate exposures).
> Potential for impairment of skin integrity (elderly persons have fragile skin that is easily damaged).
> Potential for further injury (if the patient is not moved carefully, the injury may be extended).
> Hearing impairment (it will be necessary to speak distinctly so the patient can hear directions).

After completing the data collection, a goal is set for successful completion of the procedure and a plan for achieving the goal is made. This process requires recall of theoretical principles concerning movement restrictions of a patient with pelvic injury. Established protocols and guidelines are reviewed. Inquiry and creativity are needed to plan how to obtain the most effective radiographic images of the patient's pelvis without causing her further pain or an extension of her injury.

Patient involvement in goal setting and formulating a plan to achieve the goal is essential. A patient who is not made part of the care planning is not able to cooperate in achieving the desired goal. Collaborating with the patient in planning his or her care instills in the patient a feeling of responsibility for a successful outcome.

After goal setting and planning care, **objectives** or **outcome criteria** for attaining the goal are formulated.

Example

- *Goal: the images will clearly demonstrate the patient's medical problem.*

Objectives or outcome criteria:

- The patient will be free of pain during the procedure.
- The patient's skin integrity will not be impaired.

- The patient's condition will remain stable during the procedure.

Planning and Implementation

After the data are analyzed and a goal is set with objectives for achieving that goal, a plan is written for achieving that goal. The plan is then implemented. Planning requires the use of all modes of thinking; theoretical concepts learned from classroom instruction are recalled. Practical experience previously gained allows reliable habits to develop that enable selection of correct exposure factors for each patient assignment. Inquiry is used to analyze the data and assess potential areas where errors may affect a safe and successful outcome. Creativity is necessary to devise a method of performing the procedure given the problems listed.

Implementation of the plan depends on the patient's problems and the need for assistance to achieve the desired goal safely. The radiographer must rely on his creativity to solve problems not anticipated during this phase. Patient safety and comfort during the implementation of the plan must always be the priority. The equipment is assessed to determine safe and satisfactory performance.

Example

- Instruct the patient concerning what is to be accomplished.
- Obtain assistance to move the patient onto the imaging table avoiding pain and further injury.
- Provide adequate radiation protection for the patient and others present.
- Prepare for imaging exposures.
- Make images.
- Process and assess images. Evaluate to assure quality.
- Return the patient safely to her room.
- Document procedure according to established guidelines.

Evaluation

Following implementation of the plan, evaluation is necessary. As a beginning student, the radiographer will be expected to perform this phase of care in writing or with an instructor's assistance. A self-assessment of the student's performance is made as well as an assessment based on quality performance standards. The student evaluates his performance and plans methods of improving his performance.

One must never cease learning from the patient regardless of how many years of experience he possesses. Each patient care situation differs in some ways from all others encountered; therefore, all patient care experiences are learning experiences.

Images are the tangible evidence of successful attainment of goals. However, the condition of the patient after the procedure must also be considered. In evaluating the procedure and patient care given, the following questions may be asked:

- *Were the patient's needs met?*
- *Was the patient's safety maintained during the procedure?*
- *Was the patient's skin intact at the end of the procedure?*
- *Did the patient complain of pain as the procedure was implemented?*
- *What problems arose that were not anticipated?*
- *What can be done differently in the future to improve the work or reduce patient discomfort?*
- *Were higher-level critical thinking skills used to successfully complete the procedure?*
- *Was documentation done in the manner required?*

A critical analysis of each patient care procedure must be made upon completion. Imaging quality is certainly the goal; however, if the patient's safety was jeopardized or if the patient was subjected to a great amount of pain as the plan was implemented, the outcome of the procedure was less than perfect. Honest inquiry is the key to evaluation. The radiography student will not achieve the optimum level of success with each procedure, but the ability to recognize errors and modify subsequent procedures accordingly is mandatory.

CULTURAL DIVERSITY IN PATIENT CARE

Culture is defined as "the socially inherited characteristics of a group of people that are transmitted from one generation to the next" (Fejos, 1959). A group from a particular culture usually shares the same **ethnicity;** in other words, "the group's sense of identification associated with its common social and cultural heritage. It is the characteristics a group may have in common. These characteristics include nationality, race, language, religious faith, food preferences, and folklore and many traits relevant to physical appearance. There are more than 106 ethnic groups and 170 native American tribes in North America" (Thermstrom, 1980). In the year 2000, it was believed that 33 percent of the population of the United States was made up of ethnically diverse people. At the publication of this text, it will have increased, and it is believed that by the year 2050, it will have increased to 50 percent. Implications of this influx of varying peoples into the health care system are significant. The radiographer will be implicated as a patient's culture and ethnicity will play a major role in his assessment of the patient. The patient

who has been reared and educated in the United States will have an understanding of the Western health care delivery system. Those from other countries may have little or no understanding of this system and may wish to return to their own traditions in health care. Critical thinking will be demanded as the patient is assessed and his care planned. Aspects of this assessment will include the following:

Culture: What are the customs and values of this patient that may affect my treatment of this patient?
Sociological: What is the patient's economic status, his educational background, and his family structure?
Psychological: How will the patient's self-concept and sexual identity affect my plan of care?
Physiological and biological: Are there anatomical or racial aspects of this patient that may affect my plan of care? Are there disease factors to consider?

All of these aspects of cultural and ethnic diversity are a part of the radiographer's assessment and plan of care. They will be discussed in various chapters of this text in some detail.

PATIENT EXPECTATIONS

The patient also has expectations of health care professionals. The patient expects to find an articulate, concerned, clean, and well-groomed professional to care for him or her. While in the imaging department, the patient also expects to be the focus of concern, to the exclusion of any personal concerns the health care professional may have at the moment.

As the world grows smaller, radiographers must expect to find persons from all parts of the world presenting themselves for health care. With ethnically diverse patients comes a host of beliefs and expectations concerning health and illness and methods of treatment. The radiographer must convey understanding and sensitivity for each patient's differences. If a sense of understanding is not conveyed, the patient may be left with a feeling of **dissonance** and feel that the health care they have received was not **therapeutic.**

The radiographer must consider the patient's ethnicity and cultural beliefs as he makes the initial assessment and care plan. Each person must be treated as an individual with dignity and worth. Sociocultural needs must be incorporated into each patient care plan. The radiographer's care of his patients must be free of any effect of his personal feelings of prejudice against a particular group whose beliefs are not shared.

COMMUNICATION

All members of the health care team must learn to communicate clearly and therapeutically with their patients. They must be able to convey messages in an organized and logical manner. Any problem of communication, whether major or minor, has an impact on the patient's health care. If a patient leaves a health care situation feeling confused or misunderstood, he or she may choose not to continue care that is necessary to his or her health. On the other hand, the patient who leaves feeling that he or she has been treated with dignity and respect will probably continue needed treatment.

Most patients' feelings about health care, whether positive or negative, are the result of communication between the health care worker and the patient. The radiographer must receive, interpret, implement, and give directions in his daily work routine. He must also offer consolation and reassurance while caring for his patient. For these reasons, being able to communicate effectively is as important as knowing the correct use of the complex equipment in the department.

Becoming a successful communicator requires developing skills in listening, observing, speaking, and writing. The student may feel that since he can hear, see, talk, write, and use a computer that he is already skilled in the art of communication. This is not necessarily the case. The ability to accept others with an open mind and to interact with people in a perceptive manner is based on learned attitudes and self-understanding.

CALL OUT!

Skills in listening, observing, speaking, and writing are required of the successful communicator!

Effective communication requires a degree of self-knowledge. Awareness of personal limitations and understanding of one's feelings, values, and attitudes that might lead to bias or discrimination in interactions with others are also important. Attitudes are a set of beliefs that one holds toward issues or persons that cause him or her to respond in a predetermined manner. These predetermined behaviors may not be acceptable to another person from a different background.

Human beings are born free of **attitudes, beliefs, values,** and **biases.** However, from the first day of life, these begin to develop as a result of exposure to a particular group of people called significant others. Significant others may be the mother, father, other relatives in the home, or persons who assume the role of parents. As the child grows and matures, this is the group with whom he or she is in daily contact. Their environment, religious beliefs, morals, food preferences, and preferences for other people become the child's own.

As the person grows older, friends and mates are sought from this pool of like-minded individuals. This is done to maintain the balance or harmony essential to a peaceful existence.

This need for harmony eventually affects every aspect of a person's manner of perceiving and reacting to the world, and no two people see the world in exactly the same way. For this reason, everyone reacts not to a particular event, but to a personal perception of that event. That perception is the result of learned attitudes. The radiographer must understand this and expect his patients to feel differently from the way he does about many things. For instance, a patient who is experiencing pain may react with a stoicism learned from past experiences. This might be difficult for the radiographer to understand as he may be used to a more open expression of discomfort.

The radiographer must use his newly learned skills of critical thinking to assess how he thinks about those with whom he relates. In order to become a skilled and thoughtful communicator, he needs to make an honest analysis of himself and his learned beliefs and biases.

Self-Concept and Self-Esteem

How we feel about and would describe ourselves may be defined as **self-concept.** It is made up of the attitudes of our significant others toward us as we interact with them over time. Elements of self-concept are:

- **Body image**
- **Self-esteem**
- Role
- **Identity**

Self-concept evolves over a lifetime and is made up of body image, self-esteem, the roles played throughout life, and identity. All of these are interrelated yet separate issues that make up who one is and how one sees himself.

Body image plays an important role in how one sees himself. If one's body reflects an appearance that is acceptable to the society in which he lives, it is a strong beginning for a satisfactory self-concept. If one's body does not fit the picture of size, masculinity or femininity, or other appearances expected in a particular society, it is difficult to overcome as self-concept develops. Changes in one's body due to injury or illness also affect body image. This type of change is an especially difficult adjustment for the adolescent or the elderly person.

Self-esteem is often confused with self-concept and is directly related to self-concept. Self-esteem is our evaluation of ourselves based upon the positive or negative returns received from personal behavior as life progresses. A child who has parents who give praise and approval during his or her childhood has a good start toward having a high self-esteem. The child who is criticized and not valued during childhood will develop negative feelings about him-or herself and will have low self-esteem.

The roles played throughout life also affect self-concept. Most persons play many roles as life evolves: that is, the role of student; member of a profession; an intimacy role with a significant other or spouse; perhaps a parent. A person who identifies as having successfully played his or her roles will have enhanced self-concept and high self-esteem.

Identity is the last element of self-concept. This is also the way in which we see ourselves; however, one's identity rarely changes over time. If one sees himself as a strong, competent person, it is difficult to alter that identity in one's own mind. One's sex is also an important aspect of our identity.

Understanding personal feelings and attitudes, their natural evolution, and how present personal self-concept has developed is the beginning of self-acceptance. These attitudes and feelings vary with the cultural and ethnic background of the individual. If the student radiographer enters his chosen profession after having completed a thorough self-evaluation and has the ability to accept himself as a person of worth, he will have fewer obstacles to overcome when beginning to relate to others in a therapeutic manner.

Nonverbal Communication

There is more to communication than the spoken word. The unspoken, or **nonverbal** aspects of communication can be defined as all stimuli other than the spoken word involved in communication. To understand nonverbal communication, one must depend on what one sees the patient doing as he or she speaks, what one hears in speech other than the spoken words, what is felt if the patient is being touched during the communication, and how the patient smells if one is close to the patient. The unspoken messages can often indicate how the patient feels more quickly than any words spoken. Nonverbal communication functions in the following ways:

- It may repeat or stress the spoken message.
- The face or body movement may be in agreement with what is said, or it may contradict what is being said.
- It may accent the spoken word.
- An emphasis on words spoken loudly or softly may occur.
- How loudly or softly the message is delivered may be significant.
- It may regulate the spoken word.
- A receiver may nod his head or look interested in the spoken word and therefore encourage further communication.

- It may substitute for verbal communication.
- It may appear with a frown, nod, or smile.

The perceptive health care worker can learn a great deal about a patient by other forms of nonverbal communication. For instance, the manner in which a person moves his or her body and face may say a great deal. The set of one's jaw may determine anger. The patient who does not look the receiver in the eye may feel insecure or mistrustful. Body carriage may indicate the patient's self-concept and mental status. Nonverbal cues may also suggest social and economic status. Clothing worn and posture or the manner in which a person enters a room or addresses those in the room are often indicators of status.

The radiographer must make certain that the verbal and nonverbal messages he or she sends match. If the patient suspects that the radiographer is not sincere in the interaction, his anxiety may increase. The work being done on a patient may force movement into the patient's personal space. This may result in feelings of discomfort for the patient as well as for the health care worker. Informing the patient before entering his personal space may alleviate anxiety.

The patient who comes to the imaging department for a difficult procedure may be fearful but may not wish to express this verbally. The sensitive radiographer will be able to detect the patient's nonverbal expression of fear and anxiety. By using therapeutic communication techniques, he will be able to establish a trusting relationship with the patient. This allows the patient to express his or her feelings, thereby reducing fear and anxiety.

Cultural Diversity in Communication

In order not to offend or be offended, misunderstand or be misunderstood, the radiographer must be aware of cultural differences in verbal and nonverbal communication. In some cultures, it is considered courteous to place one's body close to the body of another person during communication. In the United States, people are very protective of the space close to their bodies and might be offended if a person with whom they are not on very friendly terms invades this "personal space."

Nonverbal symbols such as a nod, meaning "yes," or a shake of the head, meaning "no," do not mean the same thing in all cultures. Symbols also have different meanings to different age groups. People of one age group may not understand the symbols of another. A safe rule when communicating with a patient is to use speech instead of symbols if there is any possibility of being misunderstood. Another common cause of cultural misunderstanding is the use of humor. Although humor is often an effective communication tool, it must not be used if there is a possibility of it being misunderstood.

Humor can be an effective means of releasing tension or conveying a difficult message, but it should not be used in life-threatening situations, when there is a possibility of legal action, or when there may be a cultural misunderstanding. Also, a patient's age may affect a common understanding of humor. If there is any doubt concerning the appropriateness of humor, it should not be used.

Gender Factors

The radiographer must be aware that the manner of communication will vary depending upon the sex of the patient. The male radiographer and the female radiographer may tend to deliver and receive messages in an altered manner based simply on their sex. Men tend to be reticent in their expression of feelings. Women feel comfortable in discussion rather than in activity as a means of interaction. Whatever the sex of the patient or the radiographer, it is necessary to avoid sexual innuendoes and denigration of or use of sex as a means of humor.

The radiographer must also be sensitive to the issue of gender in his professional interactions with co-workers. A nonbiased and nonjudgmental attitude in manner and speech concerning the differences in sexes and avoidance of sexual innuendoes and a flirtatious manner will prevent many uncomfortable interpersonal or legal problems in relationships with co-workers or patients.

Other Factors That Affect Communication

The rate at which one speaks, the volume of the voice, fluency, and vocal patterns are combined into one category called **paralanguage**. Paralanguage has to do with the sound of speech rather than the content. The correct pauses and inflections are extremely important if communication is to be understood. For example, if one speaks without proper inflection, a question will not sound like a question, or if words run together, they are difficult to sort out. Poor knowledge of correct grammatical usage may also make it difficult to understand what is being said.

A radiographer's first obligation is to know the material to be communicated to a patient so the message is correctly transmitted. Prior to beginning any communication, the radiographer must assess the following:

Age and sex of the patient
Educational background
Social and economic levels
Culture and ethnicity
Physical ability and disabilities

Following this assessment, the radiographer must adapt his communication in a manner that can be understood by the patient. If the patient is accompanied by another person or persons, one must be certain that the patient receives and understands the communication.

Feedback

To be certain that the transmitted message has been correctly received, it is necessary to obtain **feedback**. In interactions between the radiographer and the patient, it is effective to have the patient repeat the directions that have been given, or simply observe the patient to be certain that he or she is doing as instructed. If the patient understands the message, he will respond in the manner anticipated. If the patient does not respond correctly, it is the radiographer's responsibility to restate the message in a manner that is understood.

Developing Harmonious Working Relationships

The most important responsibility the radiographer has is to develop a harmonious working relationship with his patient and other members of the health care team. Although interactions with the patient are often brief, the patient should be made to feel that he or she is a partner in the examination process. Indeed, the patient is the most important member of the health care team and should be made to feel that he or she is sharing in the process.

Harmonious relationships are also of importance with other members of the health care team. Friction between co-workers is felt by the patient and makes for a poorly functioning department. If the patient is made to feel that he or she is an unimportant object being passed through the imaging department in order to get the job done, he or she will leave with a feeling of discontent.

An atmosphere of discontent is created primarily through communication and is called a **nontherapeutic relationship.** This can occur between radiographer and patient or between the radiographer and his co-workers. There are a series of communication techniques that, if cultivated, will assist the radiographer in becoming a therapeutic member of the health care team. Useful therapeutic communication techniques are listed in Display 2-2.

Establishing Communication Guidelines

Many relationships between the radiographer and his patient are brief, and it is essential to make the best use of the time. Establishing guidelines for the interaction is essential. Guidelines should include introducing oneself to the patient; giving an explanation of the examination or treatment to be performed; and giving an explanation of what is expected of the patient and what the patient can expect from the imaging staff. Delivery of instructions to the patient should be clear, concise, and nonthreatening in manner. This requires careful, organized

---

DISPLAY 2-2

Therapeutic Communication Techniques

- Establishing guidelines
- Reducing distance
- Listening
- Using silence
- Responding to the underlying message
- Restating the main idea

- Reflecting the main idea
- Seeking and providing clarification
- Making observation
- Exploring
- Validating
- Focusing

---

thought. If the patient understands the message, he or she will be able to comply with the plan. Successful communication requires critical thought on the part of the radiographer.

Reducing Distance

Physical distance between the patient and the radiographer must be reduced in order for communication to be effective. Proximity makes the patient feel included and involved. Physical barriers and a noisy environment are to be avoided. The patient must be faced directly, and eye contact when speaking and being spoken to is essential. Crossed arms or legs by the radiographer convey a lack of receptiveness. Performance of other tasks while speaking to the patient indicates disinterest in the patient.

Listening

Listening in a therapeutic manner requires that the radiographer overcome his personal biases. In order to do this, one must think critically about his biases and learn to dismiss them and assume a totally nonjudgmental attitude as he is listening to his patient. To compare or interpret what the speaker is saying, one must listen without anticipating one's own responses. The goal must be to gather accurate information and to understand the feeling and meaning of the message the patient is trying to convey.

Using Silence

Use of short periods of silence as one listens to the patient allows the patient to arrange his thoughts and consider what he wants to say. These periods also give the radiographer an opportunity to assess the patient's nonverbal communication as well as his own.

Responding to the Underlying Message

When a patient expresses a feeling of frustration, anger, joy, or relief, it is helpful if there is a response that lets him know that his feelings about the situation have been understood. An example of this type of response might be as follows:

> PATIENT: *I'm really discouraged. I'm not sure that being so sick following these treatments is worth it.*
> RADIOGRAPHER: *You are feeling disheartened because you're sick after these treatments, and you aren't sure they're making you better.*

Restating the Main Idea

Restating or repeating the main idea expressed by the patient is a useful communication technique. It validates the radiographer's interpretation of the message and also informs the patient that he or she is being heard. Consider the following:

> PATIENT: *I am having a lot of pain in my left hip, and I might need help getting up on the examining table.*
> RADIOGRAPHER: *You think that you'll need help getting up on the table because of pain?*
> PATIENT: *Yes. Will you please help me?*

Reflecting the Main Idea

Reflecting or directing back to the patient the main idea of what he or she stated is another useful technique. It keeps the patient as the focus of the communication and allows the patient to explore his or her own feelings about the matter. In this instance, the radiographer helps the patient make his or her own decision. For example:

> PATIENT: *Do you think that I really need this procedure? It's really expensive, and I'm not sure it will help.*
> RADIOGRAPHER: *Do you feel that you should refuse this procedure?*

Seeking and Providing Clarification

Seeking clarification is another useful therapeutic technique one might use. It indicates to the patient that the radiographer is listening to what is being said but is not sure he has fully understood the message. In such a situation, the radiographer should simply state that he has not clearly heard the message. The radiographer may clarify directions by using different terminology. For instance:

>RADIOGRAPHER: *In preparation for this procedure, you must drink this full flask of fluid.*
>PATIENT: *How much of this do I have to drink?*
>RADIOGRAPHER: *Before we begin the procedure, you must drink all of the fluid.*

Making Observations

Making observations or verbalizing the perceived feeling of another person is a useful communication technique. For example, the radiographer might say, "You seem to be very tense, Mr. Smith. Are you concerned about this examination?"

Exploring

The radiographer must direct questions relating to the problems of the patient. When the patient relates information about him or herself, it may be helpful to pursue the problem by exploring further. An example of this technique might be:

>PATIENT: *Every time I receive that type of injection, I feel very strange.*
>RADIOGRAPHER: *Can you tell me what it feels like when you have this type of injection?*

Validating

When speaking to a patient, the radiographer may wish to verify what the patient has reported. This is called validating the message.

>RADIOGRAPHER: *Mr. Angelo, you are saying that you have difficulty breathing when you are lying flat?*
>PATIENT: *Yes, I must be in a sitting position in order to breathe well.*

These are examples of techniques that may be used to communicate with the patient in a therapeutic man-

ner. The guiding principle of therapeutic communication is to keep the communication focused on the patient by asking open-ended questions; that is, questions that allow the patient to expand his or her answers to questions. Avoid "what" and "why" types of questions or questions that require only a yes-or-no response. It is important for the conversation to be focused on the patient. The radiographer's verbal responses should be kept to a minimum, and the communication should always be redirected to the patient. For example:

>PATIENT: *Do you have children at home, Mr. Smith?*
>RADIOGRAPHER: *Yes, I have two children. And you?*

> 📢 **CALL OUT!**
>
> Respond to the feeling and the meaning of the patient's verbal expression!

Blocks to Therapeutic Communication

Several factors actually block or destroy the possibility of creating a therapeutic atmosphere in communication. Rapid speech, complex medical terminology, and distracting environments such as a noisy waiting room or crowded hallway are serious barriers to communication. Radiographers should deliver messages to the patient in a quiet area of the department in a simple and direct manner and make sure that the patient understands English. If this is not the case, an interpreter of the appropriate language must be provided.

Obtaining incomplete answers or failing to explore the patient's description of a problem can also be detrimental to communication. The radiographer must listen to what the patient is saying. If the message is not clear, the radiographer must explore by further questioning until certain that the message is understood. Failure to do this may result in harm to the patient.

Using nontherapeutic communication techniques may also block communication. Some of the common nontherapeutic communication techniques are listed in Display 2-3.

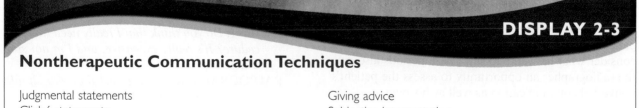

DISPLAY 2-3

Nontherapeutic Communication Techniques

Judgmental statements	Giving advice
Cliché statements	Subjective interpretation
False reassurance	Disagreeing
Defending	Probing
Changing the subject	Demanding an explanation

Judgmental statements place the patient in the position of feeling that he or she must gain the approval of the health care worker in order to receive care. These statements can be as simple as saying, "that's good," or "that's bad." They may also take the form of cliché statements such as, "We have to take the bad with the good, you know." Another nontherapeutic communication is false reassurance to the patient who expresses fear or anxiety by making a comment such as, "Now don't you worry. Everything will be just fine."

Defending is another block to therapeutic communication. This type of communication rejects the patient's opinion and prevents the patient from continuing to communicate. For instance:

PATIENT: *I'm not sure Dr. Jay knows what to do for me.*

RADIOGRAPHER: *Dr. Jay is an experienced physician, and he has taken care of many people with problems just like yours.*

This type of nontherapeutic response ends the communication with the patient feeling rejected and unworthy. A better response would have been if the radiographer simply restated the patient's comments and allowed him to complete his expression of concern.

Changing the subject while the patient is speaking is a nonverbal means of informing the patient that what he or she is saying is unimportant. The radiographer must also avoid giving advice, offering subjective interpretations of a patient's statements, disagreeing, probing, or demanding explanations. All of these responses interfere with therapeutic communication.

Obtaining a Patient History

The goal of a patient history is to obtain necessary information to perform a safe and comfortable examination or treatment. Frequently, the radiographer may not need to take a complete health history as that has been accomplished by the patient's physician or nurse prior to the patient's presentation in the imaging department.

On many occasions, the radiographer must often obtain information from the patient that is personal and confidential. Obtaining this information accurately demands sensitivity and critical thinking on the radiographer's part. As the interviewer, the radiographer will be asking direct, personal questions of a relative stranger. During the history-taking process, the radiographer must convey a professional image to ensure the patient's confidence.

Rules to follow to complete a successful patient history are:

- Provide an atmosphere that is private and as quiet as possible.

- Establish **rapport** with the patient by approaching the patient in a respectful but friendly manner.
- Ask the patient how he or she prefers to be addressed; i.e., Mr., Mrs., first name.
- Inform the patient why the information is needed.
- Inform the patient that the information will be shared only with persons necessarily involved in his/her medical care.
- Use open- and closed-ended questions as necessary to elicit information concerning the patient's medical condition; for example:
  - Closed-ended question: RADIOGRAPHER: *What is your age, Mr. Gleam?* PATIENT: *I am 35 years old.*
  - Open-ended question: RADIOGRAPHER: *Can you tell me what makes your pain worse, Mr. Gleam?* PATIENT: *It hurts all of the time. If I turn on my left side, the pain stops for a while, but when I'm on my back, it is much worse.*

Information of utmost importance in imaging is as follows:

- For female patients of childbearing age: last menstrual period and possibility of pregnancy.
- Confirmation with the patient of the imaging examination to be performed.

The radiographer must gather the information necessary for a successful examination. To compile a complete history, the radiographer must listen, observe, reply, and question in an organized and analytical manner. The items necessary in a complete history must include the following:

- **Localization** of problem (Where is the problem or area of pain?)
- **Chronology** (When and for how long has the problem been present?)
- Quality (How severe is the problem or pain?)
- **Onset** (When did the problem begin?)
- **Aggravating** or **alleviating factors** (What makes the pain or problem worse or better?)
- **Associated manifestations** (What else happens during the pain episodes?)

Samples of structured interview questions are presented in each chapter of this text that deals with a particular body system.

▌ PATIENT EDUCATION

A patient who comes to the imaging department for treatment or diagnosis has a right to expect that he or she will be instructed in the procedure he or she is to receive and that the care or instruction following the procedure is complete. The radiographer is often the health care worker who must provide this education. Instruction must include the following:

- A detailed description of the preparation necessary for the procedure or examination
- A description of the purpose and the mechanics of the procedure and what will be expected of the patient; for instance, frequent position changes, medications to be taken or injected, and any contrast agent to be administered
- The approximate amount of time the procedure will take
- An explanation of any unusual equipment that will be used during the examination
- The follow-up care necessary when the procedure or examination is complete

The patient who is hospitalized prior to imaging procedures receives pre-examination preparation from the nurse assigned to his or her care. The radiographer's obligation as a member of the health care team is to communicate the preparation needs for imaging procedures in his or her department to other members of the health care team who will be preparing the patient. The member of the health care team who usually prepares hospitalized patients for imaging examinations is the nursing staff.

The radiographer must be certain that the nurses who prepare the patient have explicit and current preparation instructions for each procedure to be performed. He must also plan the scheduling of imaging procedures with other members of the health care team so that the examinations are performed in a logical sequence that meets the patient's health care needs and accomplishes the diagnostic goals in the most time- and cost-efficient manner.

The possible **adverse effects** of a procedure should be addressed by the patient's physician before the patient is left in the radiographer's care. The radiographer is responsible for determining the extent of the patient's knowledge of the procedure and his or her understanding of what is to occur. The techniques of therapeutic communication can be used to explore this with the patient. If the patient does not completely understand the purpose of the procedure or has concerns about it, the radiographer should not begin the examination until the patient's concerns have been addressed by the technologist/supervisor or in some cases by the patient's physician. **Informed consent forms** must be correctly signed if they are required. If a patient refuses an examination, the patient's physician must be notified.

CALL OUT!

If the patient questions an examination or procedure, do not begin until the problem is resolved by the patient and the department supervisor/technologist.

Establishing a Plan for Patient Teaching

Assessment skills, critical thinking skills, problem-solving skills, and therapeutic communication skills are required to establish the patient's need for instruction and the method to be used. Patient assessment should include:

- The patient's previous experience with the procedure to be performed
- Knowledge of the preparation needed for the procedure
- The patient's age, culture, ethnicity, and educational level
- The patient's health status
- The patient's anxiety level and ability to assimilate instruction

Every person has a different learning style that must be considered. The styles of learning are as follows:

1. **Global** *versus* **linear:** Some people look at the entire picture and the details (global). Others look at each component of the material before looking at the whole (linear).
2. **Visual:** Material must be presented as a graphic design or in pictures.
3. **Auditory:** Learning is by verbal explanation alone.
4. **Kinesthetic:** Learning is by demonstration and followed by return demonstration.

The radiographer must plan a method of evaluation to be certain that the patient has understood his instruction. This may be done by obtaining verbal or written feedback or by a return demonstration. The plan is then implemented and evaluated.

When an examination or procedure is complete, the radiographer must reinforce to the patient what was initially taught concerning follow-up treatment or care. The patient may be anxious and somewhat forgetful of previous instruction. Written instruction and verbal instruction are beneficial.

LOSS AND GRIEF

Grief is a normal response to the loss of a loved one, a prized possession, social status, a bodily function, or body part. It is also to be expected when a person is

Phases of the Grieving Process

Phase 1: Denial

The patient who is facing imminent death or loss often responds by not accepting the truth. This is a defense mechanism that allows the person receiving the loss to become accustomed to the idea. The physician is the person who must inform the patient of approaching death or loss. If questioned by the patient, the radiographer may respond in a reflective manner.

Phase 2: Anger

The patient may become angry preceding death or disfigurement. He may hurl criticism and abuse at family members or at health care workers as he feels that he has been done a serious injustice and hopeless rage is his only defense. In this instance, the radiographer who is the object of this type of anger should be matter-of-fact and understanding. Releasing anger is therapeutic for the patient and should be permitted.

Phase 3: Bargaining

The patient feels that if he becomes the "good and submissive patient" he may be spared or miraculously cured. During this phase, the patient may seek alternative modes of treatment, some of which may be unusual or even nontherapeutic.

Phase 4: Depression

The patient accepts the impending loss and begins to mourn for his or her past life and all that will be lost. The patient may be very silent and unresponsive at this time. Quiet support is the best response of the health worker during this period.

Phase 5: Acceptance

The patient accepts the loss and loses interest in all outside occurrences. He becomes interested only in the immediate surroundings and the support of persons near him. The patient deals with pain and begins to disengage from life. The health care worker should be quietly supportive and allow the patient to discuss whatever he wishes.

faced with the possibility of imminent death. This is called **anticipatory grieving.** Unfortunately, the process of grieving is often a long and difficult one. One may never fully recover from a serious loss, but will learn to live without the person or object of that loss.

How one manages the process of grieving depends largely on cultural, ethnic, religious, and economic factors as well as on the value placed on the loss. Grief reactions are often more severe for children and the elderly, especially if they have lost a person on whom they have depended.

In all health care professions, exposure to the loss and grief of others is common. Radiologic technology is no exception. Before being exposed to persons who are in various stages of the grieving process, the student must examine his own feelings and attitude concerning death and loss. It is not unusual for a health care worker to be filled with emotion when caring for a person who has suffered a tremendous loss; however, these emotions must not prevent one from caring for the grieving patient. If the radiographer feels that he may have difficulty in this aspect of patient care, it may be wise to seek counseling or discuss these fears with a respected colleague.

Scholars have presented many concepts and theories that may be used to facilitate understanding of persons who are grieving. Each theory identifies phases in the process of grieving. One must remember that grieving is a human process and, as such, does not follow an

orderly sequence. The grieving person may go from one phase of grief to another and then return to a previous phase. He or she may even be in more than one phase of grief at a time.

Dr. Elizabeth Kubler-Ross (1969) summarized the process of grieving in a concise manner. Remember that the picture of the grieving person presented in this text is general and varies with each individual. The radiographer's ability to care for the grieving patient may be enhanced by some understanding of the grieving process. The phases as described by Dr. Kubler-Ross are listed in Display 2-4.

During the phase of acceptance, if the patient is facing permanent disability, this is the time that he or she makes the first attempt at rehabilitation. He or she faces the reality that it is necessary to make the most of life. This does not mean that the disability is forgotten or totally accepted. The disabled person may have a longer grieving period than the person suffering the loss of a loved one because of the constant reminder that he or she is no longer the same person as before.

The radiographer caring for this patient must remember this and be sensitive in his care. The rehabilitating patient must be allowed to direct his own care as much as possible. The radiographer must stand by to assist, rather than taking the lead. A matter-of-fact approach in the disabled patient's care is recommended with compliance to the patient's request for assistance.

When caring for a person who has suffered a serious loss, the radiographer must be supportive and allow the patient to retain hope for attaining his or her short-term or long-term goals. If the patient wishes to discuss his problem, he should be allowed to do so. All patients have the right to be treated as persons with dignity and worth until they have taken their last breath. Depriving patients of hope or treating them as if their reason for living is no longer valid is a violation of patient rights.

Grief is a normal human reaction to loss. If the person or object of loss was of vital importance in the individual's life, the process of grieving may not be resolved completely. In some situations, the grieving process becomes maladaptive. This may happen when a person cannot adequately express grief or has a feeling of guilt concerning the relationship with the deceased. When the loss results in social dysfunction and mental illness, the grieving person must seek or be taken to a counselor or psychiatrist for assistance in resolving the grief.

PATIENT RIGHTS RELATED TO END-OF-LIFE ISSUES

The science of medical care has advanced to the point at which life can be maintained by mechanical means almost indefinitely, or at least long after the quality of life has deteriorated. This may not be in the patient's best interest and would not be the patient's wish if he was able to make this decision. The public's wishes to make its own determination in this matter were resolved when the Patient Self-Determination Act (PSDA) was made law in 1990. PSDA establishes guidelines concerning patients' wishes when confronted with serious illness. It creates clear understanding of the patient's desires if he has an illness that cannot be cured or if the illness renders him so infirm that his life is without quality.

Advance directives are legal documents that are formulated by a competent person that provide written information concerning the patient's desires if the patient is unable to make the decision on his or her own. All health care institutions are required to provide written information to all patients informing them of their right to make an advance health care directive and to inquire if such a directive is already established. The patient's admission records should state whether such directives exist. These directives dictate preferences for the type of medical care and the extent of

treatment desired. These directives become effective if the patient is unable to make his or her own health care decisions. There are three instruments through which the patient's wishes are dictated. They are as follows:

A living will: Expresses the patient's wishes concerning their future medical care. These may be altered by a competent patient at any time. Each state has different rulings concerning changes in a living will by an incompetent patient.

Directive to physician: A physician is appointed by a person to serve as his proxy on a prescribed form. The physician verifies that the patient is competent at the time of signing. This is much like a living will.

Durable Power of Attorney for Health Care (DPAHC): Unlike the two previous documents, this document appoints a person other than the physician to act as the patient's agent and make health care decisions if the patient is unable to do so. The patient may alter this document if competent to do so. No physician certification is required.

When copies of these documents have been completed, they should be copied and given to the agent appointed and included in the patient's hospital chart.

The radiographer may find a **do-not-resuscitate (DNR)** order on his patient's chart. This may also be called a "no code" order. A DNR order is often included as part of the patient's advance health care directives; however, the radiographer must have a written medical order to follow this request. Each institution has its own policy concerning these orders, and the radiographer must understand his facility's policy.

There are some persons who do not wish to have a **"no code"** inclusion in their desires for end-of-life care. In this case, there will often be an order for a **"full code"** that indicates full cardiopulmonary resuscitation. This is referred to as a "code blue" in most institutions.

All patients are entitled to pain control despite the nature of their illness. This includes persons who are at the end of life. The objective of pain control for a dying patient is to block pain at a level that does not suppress consciousness. Pain medication should be administered at a level that permits a plateau level of control. This maintains the patient's comfort and prevents the agony and exhaustion that comes with severe pain.

SUMMARY

All human beings have basic needs. Threats to basic human needs create stress, and stress may lead to illness. The patient who seeks medical care does so

because his or her basic needs are no longer being met due to illness. The radiographer must understand that a person in poor health may relate to him in an unpleasant manner. If this is understood, he will be able to care for the patient in a sensitive and caring manner regardless of patient behavior.

The successful radiographer has learned the skills of critical thinking. These skills require a great deal of practice and introspection. To think in a critical manner requires the ability to interpret, analyze, evaluate, infer, explain, and reflect. These are all aspects of the higher levels of thinking and are required in daily professional life.

Each patient care assignment involves critical thinking and problem solving. Both lower and higher modes of thinking are called for in this process. The steps in the problem-solving process are data collection, analysis, planning, implementation, and evaluation. Consideration of racial, cultural, and ethnic differences of each patient must be included in each problem-solving process.

Communication is central to all health care situations. The radiographer must be able to communicate in a therapeutic manner with his patients. The ability to communicate effectively begins with self-understanding and development of a positive self-concept. Recognizing one's own biases and attitudes and how they came to be is the beginning of developing a positive self-concept.

In order to formulate a safe and effective plan of care, the radiographer is required to obtain a patient history. History-taking requires acquiring deeply personal information about the patient. Completing this in a sensitive manner demands that the radiographer present a professional and respectful image in a private atmosphere. Determining when it is appropriate to use open-ended or closed-ended questions during the history-taking process requires the use of critical-thinking skills.

Patient education before procedures is an obligation of the radiographer. He must assess his patient's level of knowledge and his cultural differences prior to making an instructional plan. Teaching must be designed according to each individual's need. Plan assessment can be done by obtaining a return demonstration or by requesting verbal or written feedback.

A patient who is suffering from loss of a body part or body function or who is grieving for another type of personal loss must have special consideration. Assessment of the grieving patient's needs and communication with him in an understanding manner are essential.

The radiographer must respect the patient's right to make choices concerning his or her own health care. The student radiographer must familiarize himself with the various health care directives and the terminology used in these documents.

CHAPTER 2 TEST

1. All persons have basic needs that must be met. Match the situations listed below with the basic need that is not being satisfied:
   a. A patient is waiting alone on a gurney in a corridor. Everyone rushes by without offering explanations or communicating.
   b. For this imaging procedure, no food was allowed after dinner the previous evening. The examination is scheduled for 8 a.m.; however, it is now 11 a.m. and the patient is still waiting for care.
   c. A middle-aged patient who is having a lower gastrointestinal (GI) series has an involuntary evacuation of the barium on the examination table.

   1. Physiologic need
   2. Safety and security need
   3. Love and belonging need
   4. Self-esteem need
   5. Self-actualization need

   d. A young mother is studying music in her leisure time.
   e. A child is taken from her parents into the imaging department for examination. The parents are told to wait outside.

2. Define critical thinking and list and define the modes of thinking.

3. An elderly woman loses her spouse of 40 years. Shortly after his death, she becomes ill and requires a surgical procedure. One might consider that her illness might be related to:
   a. Relief
   b. Fear
   c. Stress
   d. Hope

4. The student radiographer is preparing for an anatomy examination. He is certain that the instructor will ask him to identify the bones of the skull. What type of answer will this question demand?
   a. Synthesis
   b. Analysis

c. Recall
d. Inquiry
e. Habit

5. Learning the profession of radiologic technology requires _____, _____, and _____ skills.

6. A return demonstration of an imaging examination by the radiologic technology student requires:
a. Synthesis
b. Inquiry
c. Affective skill
d. Psychomotor skill

7. A radiologic technologist who has been working in his profession for a number of years is assigned to perform an imaging examination that he has performed many times. The modes of thinking that will take precedence in this instance will be:
a. Habit
b. Recall
c. Inquiry
d. Creativity

8. How a patient feels about his health care experience is strongly related to:
a. The expense of the procedure
b. The time of the visit
c. The knowledge level of the health care worker
d. The communication skills of the health care worker caring for him
e. The diagnosis

9. Sadie South has just been informed that she has been accepted into the radiologic technology program at Utopia University. She is very pleased about this, but she begins to worry about her ability to succeed in the program. She is concerned about her manner of speaking, her ability to help others, and her appearance. One might say that Ms. South has:
a. Low self-esteem
b. An identity crisis
c. Depression
d. A grief reaction
e. Poor critical thinking skill

10. List the requirements of the problem-solving process.

11. Mr. Ritch enters the imaging department for an examination. He informs the radiographer that he is having severe back pain and is short of breath. This data would be listed as:
a. Objective data
b. Acceptance
c. Validating
d. Subjective data
e. Irrelevant to the problem

12. When setting a goal for accomplishing an assignment, the radiographer must include the following:
a. Objective data
b. Subjective data
c. The patient
d. The health care team
e. All of those listed above

13. List the questions one might ask when evaluating his work with a patient.

14. Define culture and ethnicity.

15. When assessing a patient, the aspects of this assessment must include:
a. The patient's culture
b. The patient's economic background
c. The patient's psychological status
d. The patient's physiological background
e. All of those listed above

16. You are taking the history of a male patient before placing him on the examining table. He tells you that he has difficulty moving from a sitting to a standing position. The radiographer says, "You feel that you need help to stand?" This therapeutic communication technique is called:
a. Exploring
b. Silence
c. Making an observation
d. Verbalizing the implied
e. Validating

17. The concerns of the radiographer preparing to take a history on a patient must include:
a. Privacy and a quiet environment
b. Ensuring confidentiality
c. A professional demeanor and appearance
d. Establishment of rapport with the patient
e. All of those listed above

18. The process of grieving, though painful and difficult, is normal and cannot be avoided in the case of a significant personal loss.
a. True
b. False

19. Mr. Leo Lee was diagnosed with cancer 6 weeks ago and told that the disease was incurable. He has decided to seek treatment in another country that promises instant cure with natural herbs. One might conclude that Mr. Lee is in which stage of the grieving process?
a. Denial
b. Anger
c. Bargaining
d. Acceptance
e. Depression

20. List the skills required of a successful communicator.

21. Mary Nilworth is scheduled for a magnetic resonance imaging procedure. She tells the radiographer

that she is afraid that she may not be able to tolerate this examination. The radiographer states, "Don't worry, it will be simple and over quickly." This is an example of:

a. Verbalizing the implied and is therapeutic
b. Reflecting and is therapeutic
c. Changing the subject and is nontherapeutic
d. False reassurance and is nontherapeutic

22. When the radiographer is required to instruct a patient concerning an imaging examination to be performed, he must assess which of the following:

a. The patient's address
b. The patient's health status
c. The patient's marital status
d. The patient's mode of transportation

23. Define the following: a living will; durable power of attorney for health care.

24. Pain control is not within the radiographer's scope of practice; therefore, he does not need to be concerned about it.

a. True
b. False

Patient Care and Safety

STUDENT LEARNING OUTCOMES

After studying this chapter, the student will be able to:

1. Give clear verbal instructions to an ambulatory patient concerning the correct manner of dressing and undressing for a radiographic procedure.
2. Correctly assess a patient's need for assistance to complete a radiographic procedure safely.
3. Demonstrate the correct method of moving and positioning a patient to prevent injury to the patient or the radiographer.
4. Demonstrate the correct method of assisting a disabled patient with dressing or undressing for a radiographic procedure.
5. List the safety measures that must be taken when transferring a patient from a hospital room to the radiographic imaging department.
6. Describe steps that must be taken as the radiographer to protect the patient's integumentary system from injury.
7. Explain the criteria to be used when immobilization of a patient is necessary.
8. List the types of immobilizers available, and demonstrate the correct method of applying each one.
9. List the precautions to be taken if a patient is in traction or wearing a cast.
10. Demonstrate the correct manner of assisting a patient with a bedpan or urinal.
11. Explain the responsibilities of a radiographer concerning radiation safety.
12. List the departmental safety measures that must be taken to prevent and control fires, patient falls, poisoning or injury from hazardous materials, and burns as well as the measures to evacuate patients in case of a disaster.

KEY TERMS

Ambulatory: Walking, or able to walk

Atrophy: Decrease in the size of the organ, tissue, or muscle

Decubitus ulcer: A pressure sore or ulcer

Dyspnea: Labored or difficult breathing

Immobilizer: Velcro straps that are used on a patient's limbs or waist to prevent a patient from injuring him or herself or others

Ischemia: Deficiency of blood in a body part due to functional constriction or actual obstruction of a blood vessel

Tissue necrosis: Localized death of tissue due to injury or lack of oxygen

Ulceration: An area of tissue necrosis that penetrates below the epidermis; excavation of the surface of any body organ

Approaching the profession and patients in a courteous and tactful manner can put the patients at ease and decrease their level of embarrassment so that the procedure can be performed in a smooth and timely manner. The radiographer sets the tone for the entire exchange when a patient arrives as an outpatient. The radiographer is responsible for protecting him of herself and the patient from injury in every way possible. Health care workers are often injured while moving and lifting patients, but almost all of these injuries are preventable if the correct body mechanics and rules of safety are used. Patients are also victims of injuries caused by being improperly moved or lifted. Most of these injuries can also be prevented.

Moving patients from the radiographic table to a gurney or wheelchair, or from a hospital bed to a gurney or wheelchair, requires some forethought regarding the safety of the patient as well as to the body mechanics used. Special care with the ancillary equipment must be taken when moving it with a patient during transport. A patient's integumentary system must be protected from damage. This is of particular concern when the patient is unable to move by his or her own power.

Occasionally, a patient may have to be immobilized for his or her own safety during a radiographic procedure. Not only must the institution-specific rules concerning **immobilizers** be learned, but also the correct use of these devices must be carefully learned to protect the patient from harm.

The need for a bedpan or urinal may be a requirement that a patient may find embarrassing but unavoidable. As a professional, the radiographer will be able to put the patient at ease and proceed with tact and confidence that will facilitate the procedure to a swift conclusion. The different styles of bedpans require some knowledge as to the correct placement under the patient. An understanding of how a bedpan feels underneath a patient and the embarrassment that the patient experiences will help the radiographer empathize with the patient.

Adhering to rules of radiation safety, preventing and controlling fires, using and disposing of hazardous chemicals correctly, and observing other rules of patient and departmental safety are important parts of the radiographer's education.

CARE OF PATIENT'S BELONGINGS

A patient who comes to the radiology department as an outpatient is frequently required to remove all or some items of clothing and to put on a patient gown before an examination procedure or treatment can be performed. It is usually the radiographer who receives the patient and determines which items of clothing are to be removed. The patient's discomfort or embarrassment can be decreased if the situation is approached in a courteous and professional manner.

The patient should be taken to the specific dressing area and shown how to close the dressing room door or draw the curtain of the cubicle while undressing. Clearly explain that he or she is to put on the examining gown and point out where to go for the examination once prepared. (Remember that not everyone knows that some types of examining gowns open at the back rather than at the front; this information should be part of the explanation.) Doing this takes only a few moments, and it will make the patient feel more comfortable.

The patient should be given hangers for clothing. If it is permissible to leave clothing in the dressing room, explain this to the patient. If the patient cannot leave the clothing, show him or her what to do with it. Purses, jewelry, and other valuables should be treated with special care so that they will not be lost or stolen.

Many patients wear jewelry or carry a purse or other valuable items to the radiology department. The dressing rooms in most departments are not safe places to leave these items, and the patient may feel justifiably uneasy about leaving them there. Again, consider the patient's concern and explain what must be done with personal items to keep them safe.

Metal items such as necklaces, rings, and watches are not to be worn for many diagnostic procedures and must be removed before the procedure can begin. An envelope or other container large enough to accommodate all such items should be offered to the patient. Identifying information should be written on a receipt, and all items should be tagged and placed in the designated safety area. This procedure will prevent losses that may result in inconvenience and expense to both the patient and the department.

Do not place value on a patient's belongings. An item that may seem insignificant to others may be the patient's most treasured belonging. Every article of clothing or jewelry and the personal effects that a patient brings to the diagnostic imaging department should be treated with care.

BODY MECHANICS

Constant abuse of the spine from moving and lifting patients is the leading cause of injury to health care personnel in all health care institutions. Following the correct rules of body mechanics will reduce the amount of fatigue and chance of injury. Rules of body mechanics are based on the laws of gravity.

Gravity is the force that pulls objects toward the center of the earth. Any movement requires an expenditure of energy to overcome the force of gravity. When an object is balanced, it is firm and stable. If it is off balance, it will fall because of the pull of gravity. The center of gravity is the point at which the mass of any body is centered. When a person is standing, the center of gravity is at the center of the pelvis.

Safe body mechanics require good posture. Good posture means that the body is in alignment with all the parts in balance. This permits the musculoskeletal system (the bones and joints) to work at maximal efficiency with minimal amount of strain on joints, tendons, ligaments, and muscles. Good posture also aids other body systems to work efficiently. For instance, if the chest is held up and out (the musculoskeletal system), then the lungs (the respiratory system) can work at maximal efficiency.

Rules for correct upright posture are as follows:

- Hold chest up and slightly forward with the waist extended. This allows the lungs to expand properly and fill to capacity.
- Hold head erect with the chin held in. This puts the spine in proper alignment, and there is no curve in the neck.
- Stand with the feet parallel and at right angles to the lower legs. The feet should be 4 to 8 inches apart. Keep body weight equally distributed on both feet.
- Keep the knees slightly bent; they act as shock absorbers for the body.
- Keep the buttocks in and the abdomen up and in. This prevents strain on the back and abdominal muscles.

The forces of weight and friction must be overcome when moving and lifting objects. Keep the heaviest part of the object close to the body. If this is not possible, one or more persons should assist with moving or lifting the load.

The force of friction opposes movement. When moving or transferring a patient, reduce friction to the minimum to facilitate movement. This can be done by reducing the surface area to be moved or, in the case of a patient, by using some of the patient's own strength to assist with the move, if possible. If the patient is unable to assist, reduce friction by placing the patient's arms across the chest to reduce the surface area. The surface over which the patient must be moved must be dry and smooth. Pulling rather than pushing also reduces friction when moving a heavy object or person. A sliding board or pull sheet placed under an immobile patient also reduces friction. Directions for the use of these items are presented later in this chapter.

To avoid self-injury when moving heavy objects, remember to keep the body's line of balance closest to the center of the load. Rules for picking up or lifting heavy objects are:

- When picking up an object from the floor, bend the knees and lower the body. Do not bend from the waist (Fig. 3-1)
- The biceps are the strongest arm muscles and are effective when pulling; therefore, pull heavy items or patients rather than push them.
- When assisting a patient to move, balance the weight over both feet. Stand close to the patient, flex the gluteal muscles, and bend the knees to support the load. Use arm and leg muscles to assist in the move.
- Always protect the spine. Rather than twisting the body to move a load, change the foot position instead. Always keep the body balanced over the feet, which should be spread to provide a firm base of support.
- Make certain the floor area is clear of all objects.

CALL OUT!

To prevent lower back injury, always keep the center of gravity, the knees flexed, and the weight over both feet. Do not bend at the waist or twist with the body.

MOVING AND TRANSFERRING PATIENTS

The radiographer may be called upon to transfer or assist in transferring a patient from a hospital room to the diagnostic imaging department. Several precautions must be taken when moving a patient from the hospital room to the imaging department. They are as follows:

1. Establish the correct identity of the patient. Approach the patient and identify yourself and the reason for being there. Ask to see their identification wristband. This is extremely important, as many times the patient has been transferred to another room since the radiology request was submitted.

2. Request pertinent information concerning the patient's ability to comply with the physical demands of the procedure while at the nurses' station.

3. Request information concerning the patient's ability to **ambulate** and any restriction or precautions to be taken concerning the patient's mobility.

4. Move the patient to the imaging department according to the necessary restrictions after greeting and identifying him or her and providing an explanation of what is to occur.

CALL OUT!

Never move a patient without enough assistance to prevent injury to yourself and/or the patient.

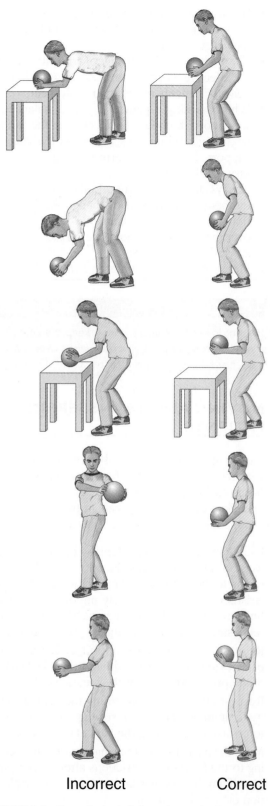

Incorrect   Correct

FIGURE 3-1 Keep the body balanced over the feet to provide a broad base of support.

When the procedure is completed, return the patient to the hospital room using the following procedure:

1. Stop at the appropriate nurses' station, return the chart, and inform the unit personnel that the patient is being returned to the room. Request help if it is needed at this time.

2. Return the patient to the room, help the patient get into bed, and make him or her comfortable and safe. Place the patient's bed in the position that is closest to the floor with the side rails raised and the call button within reach in case the patient needs assistance.

Assessing the Patient's Mobility

Before beginning to move a patient, critical thinking and problem-solving skills must be used to plan the most effective manner of accomplishing the task. The expected outcome of this plan will be to accomplish the move without causing additional pain or injury to the patient. Use interviewing and assessment skills to complete this.

Look for the following during patient assessment:

1. *Deviations from correct body alignment.* Deviations in normal physiologic body alignment may result from the following: poor posture, trauma, muscle damage, dysfunction of the nervous system, malnutrition, fatigue, or emotional disturbance. Support blocks or pillows, which are used to assist the patient during the procedure, must be available.

2. *Immobility or limitations in range of joint motion.* Any stiffness, instability, swelling, inflammation, pain, limitation of movement, or **atrophy** of muscle mass surrounding each joint must be noted and considered in the plan of care.

3. *The ability to walk.* Gait includes rhythm, speed, cadence, and any characteristic of walking that may result in a problem with balance, posture, or independence of movement. Before beginning the move, the amount of assistance needed to safely complete the move and procedure must be planned.

4. *Respiratory, cardiovascular, metabolic, and musculoskeletal problems.* Obvious respiratory or cardiovascular symptoms that impair circulation and signal potential problems in positioning must be planned for. Metabolic problems such as diabetes mellitus or rheumatoid arthritis may be discovered during the interview process and planned for as necessary (symptoms and care of patients with medical problems are discussed in Chapter 8).

Other assessment considerations are:

1. *The patient's general condition.* How well or how poorly is he or she functioning?
2. *Range of motion and weight-bearing ability.* Has the patient had a surgical procedure that restricts motion or limits weight bearing until it is healed?
3. *The patient's strength and endurance.* Will the patient become fatigued and be unable to complete the transfer with only stand-by assistance?
4. *The patient's ability to maintain balance.* Can the patient sit or stand for as long as the procedure requires?
5. *The patient's ability to understand what is expected during the transfer.* Is he or she responsive and alert?
6. *The patient's acceptance of the move.* Does the patient fear or resent the transfer? Will the transfer increase the pain? Does the patient feel that the move is unnecessary?
7. *The patient's medication history.* Has the patient received a sedative, hypnotic, or other psychoactive drug in the past 2 or 3 hours? Will any medication that he or she has taken affect the ability to move safely?

Before going to the patient, a consultation with the nurse in charge of the patient is recommended so that the patient's condition and limitations can be understood. If assistants are needed, they must be on hand. A patient must never be moved without adequate assistance; to do so may cause injury to the patient or the radiographer. The radiographer must decide how the patient can be transferred safely and comfortably, whether by gurney or by wheelchair. Hospital patients are seldom allowed to walk to and from the diagnostic imaging department for reasons of safety. Someone must always be at the patient's side as he or she moves. The following rules should be observed during a move:

1. Give only the assistance that the patient needs for comfort and safety.
2. Always transfer a patient across the shortest distance.
3. Lock all wheels on beds, gurneys, and wheelchairs before the move begins.

4. Generally, it is better to move a patient toward his or her stronger side while assisting on the patient's weaker side.
5. The patient should wear shoes for standing transfers, not slippery socks.
6. Inform the patient of the plan for moving and encourage him or her to help.
7. Give the patient short, simple commands and help the patient to accomplish the move.

Methods of Moving Patients

There are essentially three ways of transferring patients: by gurney, by wheelchair, and by ambulation.

By Gurney

When a patient is moved from a gurney to a radiographic table, or the reverse, great care must be taken to prevent injury. If the patient is unconscious or unable to cooperate in the move, the patient's spine, head, and extremities must be well supported. Convenient and safe ways to do this are by using a sliding board or a sheet to slide the patient from one surface to another.

Sheet Transfer

To place a sheet under a patient, use a heavy draw sheet or a full bed sheet that is folded in half. Have one person stand on each side of the table or bed at the patient's side. Turn the patient onto his or her side toward the distal side of the bed or table. Place the sheet on the table or bed with the fold against the patient's back (Fig. 3-2A). Roll the top half of the sheet as close to the patient's back as possible (Fig. 3-2B). Inform the patient that he or she will be turned onto the side toward the opposite side and will be moving over the rolled sheet. Then turn the patient across the sheet roll and have the assistant straighten the sheet on the distal side (Fig. 3-2C). Return the patient to a supine position, and the transfer may begin.

If the patient is an adult, three or four people should participate in the maneuver. One person stands at the patient's head to guide and support it during the move, with another at the side of the surface to which the patient will be moved, and a third person at the side of the surface on which the patient is lying. If there are four people, two may stand at each side. The sheet is rolled at the side of the patient so that it can easily be grasped, close to the patient's body. In unison (usually on the count of three), the team transfers the patient to the other surface. Extra care over the metal parts of the radiographic table's metal edges should be taken as well as assuring that the tube housing is positioned out of the way.

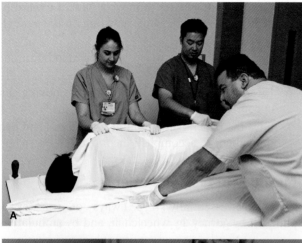

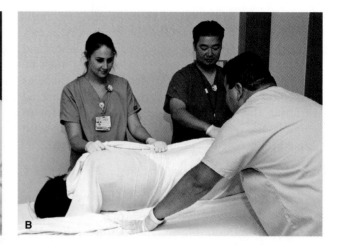

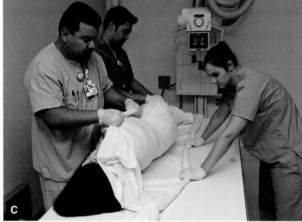

FIGURE 3-2 (**A**) Place the sheet on the table with the fold against the patient's back. (**B**) Take the top half of the sheet and roll it against the patient. (**C**) After the patient is rolled to the opposite side, the rolled half of the sheet is straightened out.

Sliding Board Transfer

The sliding board (also called a smooth mover and a "smoothie") is a glossy, plasticized board approximately 5 feet 10 inches in length and about 2 feet 6 inches wide. This item facilitates moving patients from one surface to another, usually from a gurney to an examining table. The sliding board usually requires fewer personnel to make the move than the sheet transfer because it creates a firm bridge between the two surfaces over which the patient can be easily moved. The sliding board transfer procedure is as follows:

1. Obtain the sliding board and spray it with antistatic spray if necessary.
2. Obtain the assistance of one other person if the patient is of average size and weight; if the patient is large, three people may be necessary to move the patient safely.
3. Move the patient to the edge of the gurney. One person should hold the sheet that the patient is laying on over the top of the patient to keep the patient from possibly rolling off the gurney.
4. Move the gurney up against the radiographic table and lock the wheels of the gurney.

5. Assist the patient to turn onto his or her side, away from the radiographic table, and place the sliding board under the sheet upon which the patient was lying.
6. Create a bridge with the board between the edge of the radiographic table and the edge of the gurney (Fig. 3-3A).
7. Place the sheet over the board, and allow the patient to roll back onto the board.
8. With one person at the side of the radiographic table and the other at the side of the gurney, slide the patient over the board and onto the radiographic table (Fig. 3-3B).
9. Assist the patient to roll toward the distal side of the radiographic table, keeping the patient secure by holding onto the sheet on which he or she was lying. The person standing on the side of the gurney should remove the sliding board from under the patient (Fig. 3-3C).
10. Remove the gurney and perform the radiographic procedure.
11. When the procedure is completed, the patient can be transferred back to the gurney by repeating the steps above.

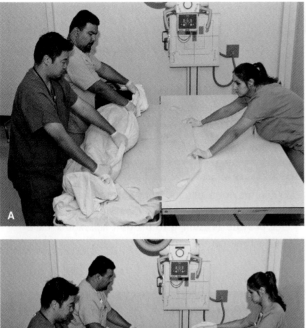

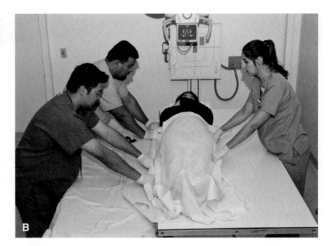

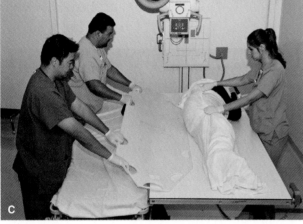

FIGURE 3-3 (**A**) Create a bridge with the board between the table and the gurney. (**B**) Roll the sheet close to the patient and slide the patient onto the table. (**C**) Remove the sliding board while safely securing the patient.

12. Once the patient is back on the gurney, place a pillow under the patient's head, if this is permitted, and put the side rails of the gurney up. Place a soft immobilizer over the patient. The patient may then be transferred.

13. When the move is complete, discard the soiled linen that was used on the radiographic table, and clean the sliding board and the table with a disinfectant spray.

14. After washing hands, place clean linen on the table.

🔊))) CALL OUT!

Always obtain enough assistance to move a patient, even with a smooth mover. This is for the safety of both the patient and the radiographer.

▌ USE OF IMMOBILIZERS

The ethical and legal restrictions concerning use of **immobilizers** (often called restraints) in patient care are discussed in Chapter 1. The radiographer must remember that immobilizers must be ordered by the physician in charge of the patient's care and applied in compliance with institutional policy.

The Joint Commission states that immobilizers should be used only after less restrictive measures have been attempted and have proved ineffective in protecting the patient. Remember this and use critical thinking skills to avoid the use of immobilizers if at all possible. Immobilizers are defined as any manual method or physical or mechanical device, material, or equipment attached or adjacent to the person's body that the person cannot remove easily that restricts freedom of movement or normal access to one's body (Omnibus Reconciliation Act, 1989).

The most effective method of avoiding the need to restrain an adult patient is the use of therapeutic communication to explore the patient's fears. If a patient seems fearful or is striking out or moving in an unsafe manner, assure the patient that the procedure will be carried out quickly and in a manner that keeps him or her as comfortable as possible. If this does not reassure the patient, other less restrictive devices, such as soft, Velcro straps (Fig. 3-5A), sandbags (Fig. 3-5B and 3-5C), and sponges may be used to remind the patient to refrain from moving. If immobilizers are to be used, be

Wheelchair Transfer

If a patient must be moved from a bed or radiographic table to a wheelchair, or the reverse, he or she must be helped. Never allow a patient to get off a table or onto a wheelchair without some assistance. The patient is often not as strong as he or she thinks. The sudden movement may cause dizziness, and the patient may fall.

If the patient has been in a supine position and is to be helped to a sitting position, have the patient turn to the side with knees flexed. Then stand in front of the patient with one arm under the shoulder and the other across the knees.

1. If the patient can assist, instruct him or her to push up with the upper arm when told to do so (Fig. 3-4A).

2. On the count of three, move or help the patient to a sitting position at the edge of the table. Before helping the patient to stand, allow him or her to sit for a moment and regain a sense of balance. While the patient is "dangling," place nonskid slippers on the patient's feet.

3. If the patient needs minimal assistance to get off the table, stand at the patient's side and take the patient's arm to help.

4. If the radiographic table is high, never allow a patient to step down without providing a secure stepping stool. Always stay at the patient's side to assist. A telescoping radiographic table must be placed in the lower position before a patient is assisted to move off of it.

5. The wheelchair must be close enough so that the patient can be seated in the chair with one pivot (Fig. 3-4B). Have the foot supports of the chair up and the wheels locked.

6. The footrests on the wheelchair should then be put down and the wheels unlocked. A safety belt should be put across an unsteady patient.

🔊 CALL OUT!

When moving a patient from hospital bed to wheelchair, always place nonskid slippers on the patient's feet, provide assistance to prevent falls, and secure the seatbelt on the wheelchair.

⚠ WARNING!

Before allowing a patient to get out of a wheelchair, raise the foot supports out of the way. Many patients step on these, causing the wheelchair to flip over, which causes injury to the patient!

Once placed on the radiographic table, cover the patient with a protective sheet. Do not allow the patient to become chilled.

A patient who has received a narcotic, hypnotic, or other type of psychoactive medication; a confused, disoriented, unconscious, or head-injured person; or a child must never be left alone on a radiographic table or gurney. If the patient's behavior cannot be predicted or if the patient is in a wheelchair; observe him or her carefully. A soft immobilizer belt should be placed over any patient on a gurney or in a wheelchair. The side rails of the gurney must always be up.

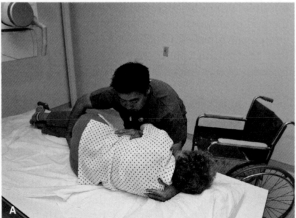
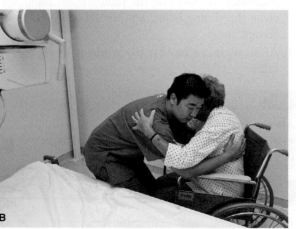

FIGURE 3-4 (**A**) Stand in from of the patient and place an arm under her shoulders and over across her knees. Assist to a sitting position. (**B**) Wheel the wheelchair close to the table pivot and help the patient sit in the chair.

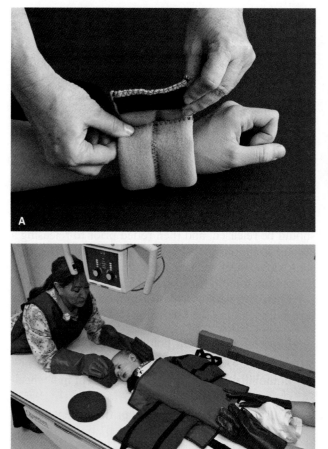

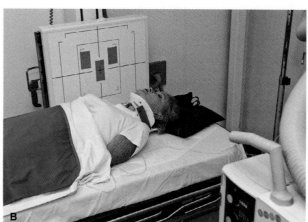

FIGURE 3-5 (**A**) A Velcro strap being placed snuggly but not tightly. (**B**) Sandbags will help remind the adult patient to remain still. (**C**) Sandbags will also assist in immobilizing the infant while holding the shield in place.

certain that they are being used to protect the patient's safety and that their use is the only alternative.

There are various types of immobilizing devices that may be used for adult patients. Immobilizers for use with children are discussed in Chapter 10. Reasons for application of immobilizers in the care of an adult patient include the following:

1. To control movement of an extremity when an intravenous infusion or diagnostic catheter is in place
2. To remind a patient who is sedated and having difficulty remembering to remain in a particular position
3. To prevent a patient who is unconscious, delirious, cognitively impaired, or confused from falling from a radiographic table or a gurney; from removing a tube or dressing that may be life sustaining; or from injuring him or herself by impact with diagnostic imaging equipment

When caring for a patient who has been immobilized, explain the reason for using immobilizers to the patient and to anyone who may accompany the patient. After immobilizers are applied, do not leave the patient unattended, and inform the patient that he or she is not alone and is not being punished. Also explain that the immobilizers are only temporary and that as soon as the procedure is finished, the immobilizer will be removed.

A calm, reassuring manner often soothes an agitated or confused patient who has been immobilized. A patient in this state needs repeated orientation as well as a quiet and quick explanation to complete the procedure. Return the patient to the hospital room or wherever he or she is to be taken on completion of the radiographs.

Always apply immobilizers carefully and in the manner prescribed by the manufacturer of the device. The type of immobilizer to be used is dictated by need. As explained in Chapter 1, all radiographers must document application of immobilizers. The following are rules for application of immobilizers:

1. The patient must be allowed as much mobility as is safely possible.
2. The areas of the body where immobilizers are applied must be padded to prevent injury to the skin beneath the device.
3. Normal anatomic position must be maintained.
4. Knots that will not become tighter with movement must be used (a half-knot is recommended; Fig. 3-6).
5. The immobilizer must be easy to remove quickly, if this is necessary.

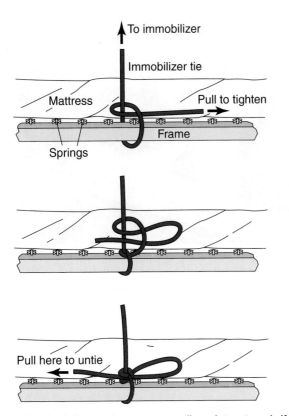

FIGURE 3-6 Following this sequence will result in tying a half-bow knot. The knot will remain secure until the free end is pulled.

6. Neither circulation nor respiration must be impaired by the immobilizer.

7. If leg immobilizers are necessary, wrist immobilizers must also be applied to prevent the patient from either unfastening the device or, in an attempt to leave the radiographic table or gurney, accidentally hanging him or herself.

Although the radiographer is not usually the health care worker who monitors the patient in immobilizers for long periods of time, it should be known that immobilizers may need to be removed and the joints affected by the immobilizer be put through range of motion exercises. Only one immobilizer at a time should be released, and then retied prior to releasing a second immobilizer. Always tie the immobilizer to a stationary object such as the gurney frame or side of the radiographic table (if possible).

There are various types of immobilizers that may be used, including the following:

1. Limb holders or four-point restrains (Fig. 3-7A)
2. Ankle or wrist immobilizers (Fig. 3-7B)
3. Immobilizing vest for keeping a patient in a wheelchair
4. Waist immobilizer, which keeps the patient safe on an examining table or in a bed, but allows the patient to change position (Fig. 3-7C)

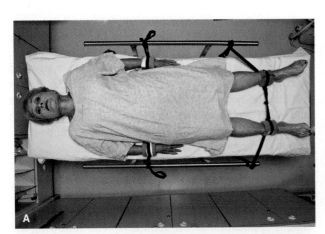

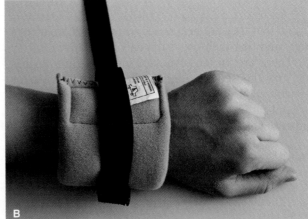

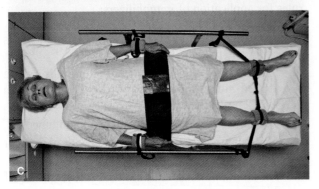

FIGURE 3-7 (**A**) Limb holders (four-point restraints). (**B**) Wrist immobilizer. (**C**) Waist immobilizer.

At times, a patient who is aggressive and delusional may need to have waist as well as four-point immobilizers that are stronger than those shown in Figures 3-7A and B. Immobilizers of this type also have locks. If this type of immobilizer is necessary, one or more security officers should be called to assist with application. A radiographer, with only the assistance of one other radiographer, must never attempt to apply immobilizers to an extremely aggressive or combative patient. Persons who have been trained to deal with this type of patient problem must do this. When this type of immobilization is necessary, the rules of immobilizer application still apply.

POSITIONING THE PATIENT FOR DIAGNOSTIC IMAGING EXAMINATIONS

When a patient must spend a long period of time in the diagnostic imaging department, it is the radiographer's duty to assist the patient to maintain his or her body in normal alignment for comfort and to maintain normal physiologic functioning. There are several protective positions that the body may assume or be assisted to assume for comfort. There are also several positions that the patient may be requested to assume to facilitate diagnosis or treatment. These positions are likely to be used in the radiology department for various procedures:

Supine or dorsal recumbent position: Patient is flat on the back. The feet and the neck will need to be protected when the patient is lying in this position. A pillow may be placed under the head to tilt it forward. The feet should be supported to prevent plantar flexion or footdrop (Fig. 3-8A).

Lateral recumbent position: Patient is on the right or the left side with both knees flexed. This position relieves pressure on most bony prominences. The patient may be supported with pillows or sandbags to maintain the position (Fig. 3-8B).

Prone position: Patient lies face down. A small pillow should support the head to prevent flexion of the cervical spine. The patient maybe moved down on the table so that the feet drop over the edge, or a pillow may be placed under the lower legs at the ankles to prevent footdrop (Fig. 3-8C).

High Fowler position: Patient semi-sits with head raised at an angle of 45 to 90 degrees off the table. This position is used for patient in respiratory distress (Fig. 3-8D).

Semi-Fowler position: Patient's head is raised at an angle of 15 to 30 degrees off the table. The arms must be supported to prevent pull on the shoulders, and the feet must be supported to prevent plantar flexion or footdrop. Pillows or blocks under knees must be removed after a brief time (15 to 20 minutes) to prevent circulatory impairment (Fig. 3-8E).

Sims position: Patient lies on either left or right side with the forward arm flexed and the posterior arm extended behind the body. The body is inclined slightly forward with the top knee bent sharply and the bottom knee slightly bent. This position is frequently used for diagnostic imaging of the lower bowel as an aid in inserting the enema tip (Fig. 3-8F).

Trendelenburg position: The table or bed is inclined with the patient's head lower than the rest of the body. Patients are occasionally placed in this position during diagnostic imaging procedures and for promotion of venous return in patients with inadequate peripheral perfusion caused by disease (Fig. 3-8G).

Patients in respiratory distress or who have COPD must not be left in a prone, supine, or Sims' position for more than brief periods of time to avoid becoming increasingly **dyspneic**.

ASSISTING THE PATIENT TO DRESS AND UNDRESS

The patient may arrive in the diagnostic imaging department alone if he or she comes from outside the hospital. The patient may need assistance in removing clothing. This may be necessary if the patient is in a cast or a brace, is very young, or is in too weakened a condition to help him or herself. The patient may have a contracture of an extremity or poor eyesight. Whatever the problem, if the radiographer senses that the patient will have difficulty undressing if left alone, then assistance should be offered and given as needed.

If a trauma patient is brought to the diagnostic imaging department from the emergency unit, removing the clothing in the conventional manner may cause further injury or pain. It may be necessary to cut away garments that interfere with acceptable radiographs; however, clothing must not be cut without the patient's consent except in extreme emergencies. If the patient is unable to give consent, a family member should do so in writing for protection.

If clothing must be cut off, try to cut into a seam if at all possible. The clothes should not be automatically thrown in the trash. They should be offered to the patient and placed with the patient's other belongs.

If the patient is very young and is accompanied by a familiar adult, he or she will be more relaxed and cooperative if the adult helps him to dress and undress. Explain to the adult how the child should be dressed

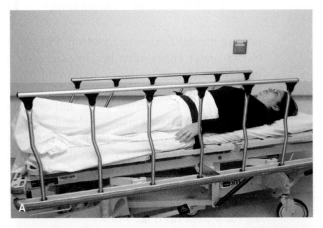

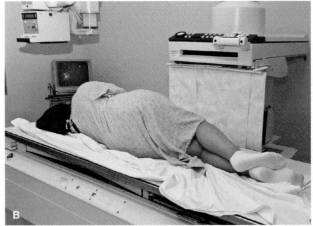

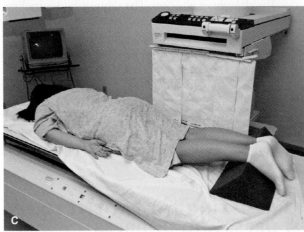

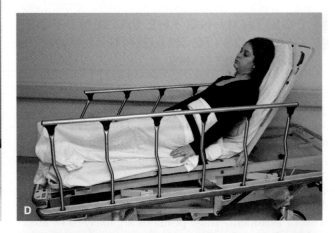

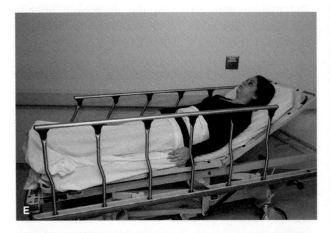

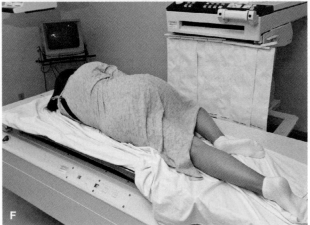

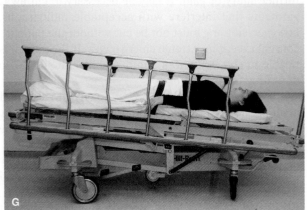

FIGURE 3-8 (**A**) Supine position. (**B**) Lateral position. (**C**) Prone position. (**D**) High Fowler position. (**E**) Semi-Fowler position. (**F**) Sims position. (**G**) Trendelenburg position.

58

for the procedure, arrange a meeting place, and leave them alone.

If a patient with a disability of the lower extremities must have assistance, the clothing should be removed from the top part of the body first.

1. Place a long examining gown on the patient. Instruct him to loosen belt buckles, buttons, or hooks around the waist and slip the trousers over the hips. If the patient cannot do this, reach under the gown and pull the trousers down over the hips.

2. Have the patient sit down. Squat down in front of the patient and gently pull the clothing over the legs and feet to remove it. If the patient is not able to help, call for an assistant.

Some dresses may be removed in the same way. If this method is not practical, however, and the dress must be pulled over the woman's head, proceed as follows:

1. Place a draw sheet over the patient and then help her to remove her slip and brassiere.

2. Help her to put on an examining gown and then remove the draw sheet.

The following are steps to re-dress a patient with a paralyzed leg, a leg injury, a cast, or a brace:

1. Slide the clothing (pants or skirt) over the feet or legs as far as the hips while the patient is sitting and still wearing an examining gown.

2. Have the patient stand and pull the clothing over the hips if he or she can tolerate it.

3. If the patient is not able to pull the clothing over the hips alone, have an assistant raise the patient off the chair so that you may slip the clothing over the hips and waist.

4. Remove the patient's arms from the sleeves of the gown. Have the patient hold the gown over his or her chest, and carefully pull the shirt over the head, or put it on one sleeve at a time.

5. When the outside items of clothing are on the patient, remove the gown from under the clothes.

THE DISABLED PATIENT

If the patient is on a gurney or the radiographic table and the patient's clothing must be changed, this can most easily be accomplished with the patient in the supine position.

1. Cover the patient with a draw sheet and have an examining gown ready. Explain what is to be done and ask the patient to help if he or she is able. If the patient is paralyzed or unconscious, summon help before beginning the procedure.

2. Remove the clothing from the less affected side first and then remove the clothing from the more affected side and place the clean gown on that side, making sure to keep the patient covered with the draw sheet.

3. Next place the clean gown on the unaffected side and tie the gown at the back, if practical.

4. If the patient is wearing an article of clothing that must be pulled over the head, roll the garment up above the waist. Then remove the garment up above the waist. Next, remove the patient's arms from the clothing, first from the unaffected side and then from the affected side.

5. Neatly, gently lift the clothing over the patient's head. One person alone should not attempt to undress a disabled patient; to do so may cause further injury or discomfort.

6. To remove trousers, loosen buckles and buttons and have the patient raise his buttocks as the trousers are slipped over his hips. If the patient is unable to help, have an assistant stand at the opposite side of the table. After the trousers have been loosened, have the assistant pull the patient toward him or her, and then slide the trousers off one side of the hip. Next, draw the patient toward the opposite side and have the assistant slide the trousers off the other hip.

7. Slip the trousers below the knees and off.

8. Fold the clothing and place it in a paper bag on which the patient's name has been printed. If a relative or a friend accompanies the patient, ask that person to keep the patient's clothing. If the patient is alone, the radiographer is responsible for caring for the clothing.

When a patient's gown becomes wet or soiled in the radiology department, it is the duty of the radiographer to change it. If a patient is allowed to remain in a wet or soiled gown, the skin may become damaged, or he or she may become chilled.

When changing the gown of a patient who has an injury or is paralyzed on one side, remove the gown from the unaffected side first. Then, with the patient covered by the soiled gown, place the clean gown first on the affected side and then on the unaffected side. Pull the soiled gown from under the clean one.

Always make sure that the patient is covered during the process.

> ### 🔊 CALL OUT!
> When changing a disabled patient's gown, allow enough material to work with by removing the unaffected side first or by placing the gown on the affected side first.

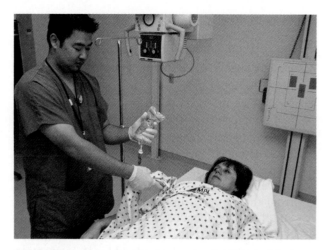

FIGURE 3-9 *Place the clean gown over the IV container.*

THE PATIENT WITH AN INTRAVENOUS INFUSION

Frequently, patients are taken to the diagnostic imaging department with an IV infusion in place.

1. If the patient's gown must be changed, slip the clothing off the unaffected side first.
2. Carefully slide the sleeve of the unaffected side over the IV tubing and catheter, then over the container of fluid. For this step, the container must be removed from the stand.
3. When replacing the soiled gown with a clean one, first place the sleeve on the affected side over the container of fluid, then over the tubing and onto the arm with the venous catheter in place (Fig. 3-9). Rehang the bottle of fluid and complete the change.
4. When moving the arm of a patient who has an IV catheter in place, support the arm firmly so that the catheter does not become dislodged. Remember to keep the bottle of fluid above the infusion site to prevent blood from flowing into the tubing.

If the intravenous infusion is being controlled by a pump and the patient's gown becomes wet or soiled and must be changed, do not attempt to disengage the IV tubing from the pump. In this case:

1. Remove the gown from the unaffected arm, and place the soiled gown to one side of the table until the nurse in charge of monitoring the infusion can remove it.
2. Replace the soiled gown with a clean gown over the unaffected side and the chest only.

SKIN CARE

The radiographer is responsible for the care of the patient's skin or integumentary system while in the diagnostic imaging department. Skin breakdown can occur in a brief period of time (1 to 2 hours) and result in a **decubitus ulcer** that may take weeks or months to heal. Mechanical factors that may predispose the skin to breakdown are immobility, pressure, and shearing force.

Immobilizing a patient in one position for an extended period of time creates pressure on the skin that bears the patient's weight. This, in turn, restricts capillary blood flow to that area and can result in **tissue necrosis.**

Moving a patient to or from a diagnostic imaging table too rapidly or without adequately protecting the patient's skin may damage the external skin or underlying tissues as they are pulled over each other creating a shearing force. This, too, may lead to tissue necrosis.

Another factor that contributes to skin breakdown is friction caused by movement back and forth on a rough or uneven surface such as a wrinkled bed sheet. Allowing a patient to lie on a damp sheet or remain in a wet gown may lead to skin damage. Similarly, urine and fecal material that remain on the skin act as an irritant and are damaging to the skin.

Early signs that indicate imminent skin breakdown are blanching and a feeling of coldness over pressure areas. This condition is called **ischemia.** Ischemia is followed by heat and redness in the area as the blood rushes to the traumatized spot in an attempt to provide nourishment to the skin. This process is called *reactive hyperemia.* If, at the time of reactive hyperemia, the pressure on the threatened area is not relieved, the tissues begin to necrose, and a small **ulceration** soon becomes visible. Ischemia and reactive hyperemia are difficult to observe in patients who are dark-skinned. In these cases, the skin must be felt to assess any threat of damage. A shearing injury to the skin may cause it to appear bluish and bruised. If such an area is not cared for, necrosis and ulceration will occur.

Persons who are most prone to skin breakdown are the malnourished, the elderly, and the chronically ill. A patient who is elderly and in poor health may have dehydrated skin, an accumulation of fluid in the tissues (edema), increased or decreased skin temperature, or a loss of subcutaneous fat that acts to protect the skin. Any of these factors can contribute to skin breakdown, and the radiographer must be particularly cautious when moving or caring for this type of patient.

Preventing Decubitus Ulcers

Protection of the integumentary system must always be a consideration when caring for patients in the diagnostic imaging department. The tables on which the patients must be placed for care are hard, and often the surface is unprotected. The areas most susceptible to **decubitus ulcers** are the scapulae, the sacrum, the trochanters, the knees, and the heels of the feet.

The patient who is on the imaging table for a long period of time should be allowed to change position occasionally to keep pressure off the hips, knees, and heels. This can be done by placing a pillow or soft blanket under the patient or by turning him or her to a different position whenever possible. This is done in the usual hospital situation every 2 hours. If the patient is lying on a hard surface, such as the radiographic table, it should be done every 30 minutes. If a patient is perspiring profusely or is incontinent of urine or feces, make certain that he or she is kept clean and dry, and take precautions when moving the patient to prevent skin abrasions.

Special precautions should be taken to protect the patient's feet and lower legs during a position change or transfer. Shoes should protect the feet, and care should be taken to prevent bruising while the move is made. Circulatory impairment in the lower extremities is common, and the slightest bump may be the beginning of ulceration.

CAST CARE AND TRACTION

Radiographic exposures of fractures that have been casted are often needed to determine correct positioning of musculoskeletal tissues. Casts may be made of plaster, fiberglass, plastic, or cast-tape materials. The material used depends on the type of injury, the length of time needed for immobilization, and the physician's preference.

The radiographer will often care for the patient who has a newly applied cast. Some of the materials used, particularly plaster, contain water and can accidentally be compressed. Compression of a cast may produce pressure on the patient's skin under the cast, and this, in turn, may lead to the formation of a decubitus ulcer at the site of cast compression. A cast that becomes too tight may cause circulatory impairment or nerve compression. To prevent these complications, the radiographer must be able to assess the patient for circulatory or neurologic impairment and must learn to move a cast with care.

When moving a patient who is wearing a cast, slide an opened, flattened hand under the cast. Avoid grasping the cast with fingers, since this may cause indentations if the cast material is sill damp. A cast must be supported at the joints when it is moved. A casted extremity must be moved as a unit with flat hands supporting it at the joints (Fig. 3-10). When moving a patient who has an abduction bar placed between the legs of a spica cast, it is imperative that the abduction bar not be used as a moving or turning device.

To position a patient who is in a cast, positioning sponges or sandbags must be on hand so that the cast can be well supported. A recently casted limb usually should be kept elevated. If a cast is allowed to put pres-

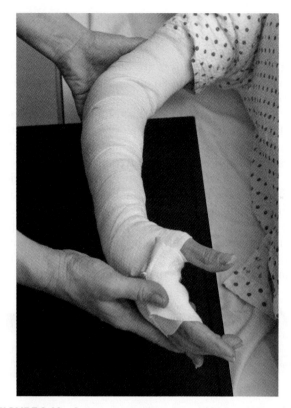

FIGURE 3-10 Support a casted or wrapped limb at both joints when moving it.

sure on the skin in any area, it may impede circulation or damage underlying nerves.

A patient with a cast who is in the diagnostic imaging department for any length of time should be assessed for signs of impaired circulation or nerve compression every 15 minutes. A cast applied to an arm may cause a circulatory disturbance in the hand; a leg or body cast may affect circulation in the feet, toes, or lower leg. Signs of impaired circulation or nerve compression that may be easily detected are as follows:

- *Pain*: Sudden pain or pain that increases with passive motion may indicate nerve damage.
- *Coldness*: Fingers or toes distal to a cast should feel warm.
- *Numbness*: A cast that is too tight may cause numbness, another sign of nerve damage.
- *Burning or tingling of fingers or toes*: These symptoms may indicate circulatory impairment.
- *Swelling*: Indicative of edema, swelling may result in circulatory impairment or nerve compression.
- *Skin color changes (to a pale or bluish color)*: Skin should remain pink and warm. In dark-skinned persons, temperature and comparison with the normal extremity are evaluated.
- *Inability to move fingers or toes*: All fingers and toes should be able to be moved and fully extended and flexed.

- *Decrease in or absence of pulses*: These changes may indicate circulatory impairment.

If the last three changes are observed, the physician should be notified and an attempt to relieve the pressure must be made.

If the patient in a body cast or a spica cast reports difficult respirations or nausea or is vomiting, notify the physician because this may indicate abdominal distress that requires immediate treatment.

Radiographic images of patients who are in traction will require the use of the portable unit. When working with a patient in a traction device, the traction apparatus must never be removed or pulled on. To do so may cause a reduced fracture to become misaligned. Enlist the help of another radiographer or a nurse to obtain the images without endangering the patient's well-being.

> ⚠️ **WARNING!**
>
> Never remove or move a traction bar from a patient while performing radiographic procedures.

ASSISTING THE PATIENT WITH A BEDPAN OR URINAL

A patient may spend several hours in the diagnostic imaging department; often the patient is not able to postpone urination or defecation. He or she may be embarrassed about making the request and will wait until the last possible moment to do so. When a patient makes such a request, the radiographer should respond quickly yet treat it in a matter-of-fact manner.

1. If possible, help the patient to reach the lavatory near the examining room; this is the most desirable way to handle the situation. However, do not allow the patient to go to the toilet without assistance. Help the patient put on slippers or shoes, and wrap the draw sheet around him or her if no robe is available. Help the patient off the radiographic table or out of the wheelchair and lead the patient to the lavatory. The patient may have been fasting or may have been given drugs that make him or her very unsteady; therefore, it is not safe to leave the patient unattended.

2. If the patient can help him or herself in the lavatory, close the door and tell the patient that assistance is just outside the door waiting if help is needed. Each lavatory should be equipped with an emergency call button, and its use should be explained to the patient. If there is no emergency call button, check on the patient at frequent intervals to be certain that his or her condition is stable.

3. After the patient has finished using the lavatory, help him or her to wash hands if unable to do so.

4. Accompany the patient back to the examination area and cover the patient to make him or her comfortable.

5. Return to the lavatory and make certain that it is clean.

6. The radiographer must wash his or her hands.

The Bedpan

The patient who is unable to get to the lavatory must be offered a bedpan or urinal. In the diagnostic imaging department, clean bedpans and urinals are usually stored in a specific place. Most departments stock disposable units.

There are two types of bedpans. The standard bedpan is made of metal or plastic and is approximately 4 inches high. Most patients can use this type. However, a patient may have a fracture or another disability that makes it impossible to use a pan of this height. For these patients, the fracture pan is used. All diagnostic departments should have these pans available (Fig. 3-11).

1. Before assisting the patient, obtain tissue and a bedpan with a towel to cover it. Close the examining room door, or screen the patient to ensure privacy. Always place a sheet over the patient while helping her onto the bedpan. Put on clean, disposable gloves.

2. Approach the patient and place the bedpan at the end of the table. If the patient is able to move, place one hand under the lower back and ask the patient to raise the hips.

3. Place the pan under the hips (Fig. 3-12). Be sure the patient is covered with a sheet. If the patient is unable to sit up, assist the patient to a sitting

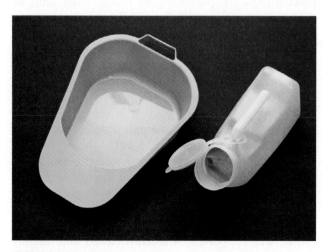

FIGURE 3-11   A fracture bedpan and a male urinal.

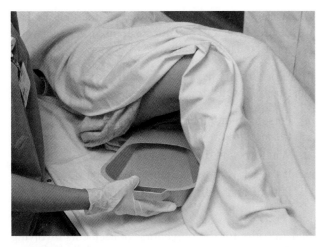

FIGURE 3-12 Place one hand under the patient's lower back, and ask the patient to raise the hips so that the bedpan may be placed under the patient.

position. Do not leave a patient sitting on a bedpan—he or she is poorly balanced and may fall.

4. Place the toilet tissue where the patient can reach it. Let the patient be alone as much as possible by turning around and facing away from the patient, or if the patient is able to sit by him or herself, step away from the patient to provide privacy.

5. When the patient has finished using the bedpan, put on clean, disposable gloves and help the patient off the pan. Have the patient lie back, place one hand under the lumbar spine and have the patient raise the hips.

6. Remove the pan, cover it, and empty it in the lavatory. Rinse it with clean cold water (dump the water into the toilet, not the sink) and then discard the disposable bedpan in the trash receptacle.

7. Offer the patient a wet paper towel or washcloth to wash the hands and a dry towel to dry them.

8. The radiographer must then remove his or her gloves as described in Chapter 4 and wash the hands thoroughly.

If a patient is unable to assist in getting onto and off a bedpan, do not attempt to help him or her alone. Enlist the aid of another team member. Have that person stand at the opposite side of the table. With the assistance of the second radiographer, turn the patient to a side-lying position. Place the pan against the patient's hips, then turn the patient back to a supine position while holding the pan in place. Be certain that the hips are in good alignment on the pan. Place pillows under the patient's shoulders and head and stay nearby. When the patient has finished using the pan, put on clean gloves and reverse the procedure to remove the pan. Be sure to secure the pan before rolling the patient as it will tip and spill the contents as the patient rolls to the side.

If the patient is not able to clean the perineal area, the radiographer will have to do this. Wear clean disposable gloves.

1. Take several thicknesses of tissue and fold them into a pad. Wipe the patient's perineum from front to back and drop the tissue into the pan. If necessary, repeat the procedure until the perineum is clean and dry.

2. Cover the pan to take it to the bathroom and empty it. If the bedpan is disposable, and the patient will not be staying in the department long enough to use it a second time, the pan may be discarded.

3. Remove the gloves and wash hands correctly.

If a patient has difficulty in moving or adjusting to the height of a regular bedpan, follow the procedure using the fracture pan. The end with the lip is the back of the pan and goes under the patient's buttocks.

> 🔊 **CALL OUT!**
>
> Wipe the perineal area from front to back to prevent a possible urinary tract infection.

The Male Urinal

The male urinal is made of plastic and is shaped so it can be used by a patient who is supine, lying on the right or left side, or in Fowler position. The urinal may be offered to the male patient who is unable to get off of the gurney or examining table to go to the lavatory.

1. If the patient is able to help himself, simply hand him an aseptic urinal and allow him to use it, providing privacy whenever possible.

2. When he has finished, put on clean, disposable gloves, remove the urinal, empty it, and rinse it with cold water. If the urinal is disposable and the patient will not be staying in the diagnostic imaging department long enough to use the urinal a second time, the urinal may be discarded.

3. Offer the patient a washcloth with which to cleanse his hands.

4. Remove the clean glove and wash hands.

If a patient is unable to assist himself in using the urinal, the radiographer must position the urinal for him.

1. Put on clean, disposable gloves; raise the cover sheet sufficiently to permit adequate visibility, but do not expose the patient unduly.

2. Spread the patient's legs and put the urinal between them.

3. Put the penis into the urinal far enough so that it does not slip out, and hold the urinal in place by the handle until the patient finishes voiding.

4. Remove the urinal, empty it, discard it, remove the gloves, and wash the hands.

■ DEPARTMENTAL SAFETY

Prevention of patient and personnel injury is the responsibility of all health care workers. It is the responsibility of the radiographer to practice safety in all aspects of work. This includes fire and electrical safety, prevention of patient or staff falls, prevention of poisoning, and safe disposal of hazardous waste and toxic chemicals.

Institutional, local, state, and federal agencies regulate safety in health care institutions, and there are safety committees in all JCAHO-accredited health care agencies. Fire departments in all cities routinely evaluate the fire safety of health care and community institutions. Poison control centers advise health care institutions if poisoning is possible. The Nuclear Regulatory Commission enforces radiation safety and nuclear medicine standards, and the Environmental Protection Agency establishes guidelines for the disposal of radioactive waste.

Fire Safety

The radiographer has an obligation to learn the fire containment guidelines in any institution in which he or she is employed. The following are essential:

1. The telephone number of the institution for reporting a fire; the number must be posted in a clearly visible location next to the telephone
2. The agency's fire drill and fire evacuation plan
3. The location of the fire alarms
4. The routes of evacuation in case of fire
5. The locations of fire extinguishers and the correct type of extinguisher for each type of fire

   Carbon dioxide extinguisher: grease or electrical fire
   Soda and acid water extinguisher: paper and wood fire
   Dry chemical extinguisher: rubbish or wood fire
   Antifreeze or water: rubbish, wood, grease, or anesthetic fire

6. A fire must be reported before an attempt is made to extinguish it, regardless of the size.
7. Hallways must be kept free of unnecessary equipment and furniture.
8. Fire hoses must be kept clear at all times.
9. Fire extinguishers must be inspected at regular intervals. Fire drills must be regularly scheduled for agency personnel.

10. Warning signs must be posted stating that, in case of fire, elevators are not to be used and stairways must be used instead.

If fire occurs, the correct procedure for patient safety must be followed:

1. Persons in imminent danger are to be moved out of the area first.
2. Windows and doors are to be closed.
3. If oxygen is in use, it must be turned off.
4. Patient and staff evacuation procedures must be followed.

General rules for the prevention of accidents involving electrical equipment should include the following:

1. Use only grounded electrical plugs (three pronged) inserted into a ground outlet.
2. Do not use electrical equipment when hands or feet are wet or when standing in water because water conducts electricity.
3. When removing an electrical plug from an outlet, grasp the plug at its base. Do not pull on the electrical cord.
4. Electrical cords must be unkinked and unfrayed; if they are kinked or frayed, don't use them.
5. Any electrical equipment must be in sound working order to be used for patient care. If it is not, the equipment must be returned to the manufacturer or to the area designated for repair service.
6. All electrical equipment must be tested before it is used for patient care.
7. Report any shock experienced; do not use equipment if a patient reports that it gives a tingling feeling or a shock.
8. Do not use a piece of electrical equipment that has not been explained.
9. To prevent falls, do not use extension cords that are not rounded and secured to the floor with electric tape.

Prevention of Falls

Patient falls are one of the most common hospital accidents. The radiographer must always be on guard to prevent falls. No patients should be allowed to get out of a wheelchair or off a gurney or radiographic table without assistance from the radiographer or designee.

The patients most prone to falls are the frail elderly, persons with neurologic deficits, persons who are weak and debilitated due to prolonged illness or lengthy preparations for procedures, persons with head trauma, persons with sensory deprivations, persons who have been medicated with sedating or psychoactive drugs, and confused patients. Adhere to the following rules to prevent falls:

1. Learn the condition of the patient and determine whether he or she is safely able to enter, remain in, or leave the diagnostic imaging department without assistance.
2. Keep floors clear of objects that may obstruct pathways.
3. Keep equipment such as gurneys, portable radiographic machines, and wheelchairs in areas where they do not obstruct passageways.
4. Side rails must always be up when a patient is on a gurney.
5. A wheelchair must be locked if a patient is in it; a soft restraint may be needed if the patient is not reliable and may try to get up without assistance.

Poisoning and Disposition of Hazardous Waste Materials

The number of the nearest Poison Control Center must be posted near department telephones. As the radiographer, the following must be adhered to:

1. Any toxic chemical or agent that may poison patients or staff must be clearly labeled as such.
2. These substances must be stored in a safe area as designated.
3. Emergency instructions to be followed in case of poisoning must be conspicuously posted in the diagnostic imaging department.
4. Chemicals must remain in their own containers and marked as toxic substances.
5. Chemical and toxic substances must be disposed of according to federal mandates and institutional policy.
6. Restrictions for disposal of hazardous materials must be posted in a conspicuous area and followed by all in the department.
7. Contrast agents and other drugs must be kept in a safe storage area where access to them is not available to anyone not designated to use them.
8. All containers of hazardous substances must be clearly marked with the name of the substance, a hazard warning, and the name and address of the manufacturer.
9. Hazardous substances may be labeled with a color code that designates the hazard category, for instance health, flammability, or reactivity.

The radiographer must read and fully understand all hazard warnings before using any product, and follow the guidelines as stated on the label. If there is no label, or if the label is unclear, the product should not be used.

If an accidental spill of a hazardous substance occurs, first aid guidelines are as follows:

Eye contact. Flush eyes with water for 15 minutes or until irritation subsides. Consult a physician immediately.
Skin contact. Remove any affected clothing; wash skin thoroughly with gentle soap and water.
Inhalation. Remove from exposure; if breathing has stopped, begin CPR; call emergency number and a physician.
Ingestion. Do not induce vomiting; call emergency number and Poison Control Center.

Diagnostic imaging personnel must understand the potential hazards of scalds or burns that may occur in their department. Although the radiographer does not commonly deal with heating pads and hydrotherapy, they do present potential hazards and must be handled safely.

Hot beverages must be kept away from children. Coffee and tea equipment used in staff lounges must be kept in safe working order and deactivated when empty or not in use. If a patient is offered a hot beverage, it should be at a temperature that will not scald him or her if it is accidentally spilled.

Radiation Safety

It is the responsibility of a radiographer to protect patients and personnel from radiation exposure. While the benefit of rapid medical diagnosis by exposure of the patient to radiation outweighs the associated risks, radiation exposure must be kept to a consistently low level.

Ionizing radiation in excessive amounts or in amounts higher than the accepted level in a brief time period can result in either illness to the recipient or a potential genetic disturbance to the descendants of the recipient. Other factors that can increase the risk of suffering the adverse effects of ionizing radiation are the patient's age at exposure, sensitivity of exposed cells, and the size and area of the body exposed. The very young, the very old, and pregnant women are the most vulnerable to adverse effects of radiation.

The goal of the radiographer must be to limit the amount of ionizing radiation acceptable limits in the patient, others in the vicinity, and personnel. To do this, the following precautions must be taken:

1. Maintain exposure to a level *as low as reasonably achievable* (ALARA).
2. Minimize the length of time the patient or others in the vicinity are placed in the path of the x-ray beam.
3. Maximize the distance between the source of the ionizing radiation and the person exposed to it.
4. Maximize the shielding from exposure of the patient and others in the vicinity of the radiation.

Time. Use the shortest exposure time possible. Remember that radiation dosage increases with fluoroscopic imaging.

Distance. The closer a person is to the radiation beam, the greater the exposure. The larger the field of radiation, the greater the risks of scattering the ionizing radiation and the greater the exposure risk. Increasing distance from the source greatly reduces the exposure risk of the radiographer and others in the vicinity.

Shielding. Shielding persons who are unable to reduce their exposure either by limiting time or increasing distance is the third alternative for protection from ionizing radiation. Shielding is done by setting up a protective barrier, usually lead or an equivalent, between the source of the ionizing radiation and the subject involved, whether the patient or others in the vicinity. There are primary and secondary barriers. Primary barriers are usually made of lead or similar material; they are designed to withstand being struck by the beam exiting the x-ray tube without allowing passage of ionizing radiation. Secondary barriers are designed to prevent passage of scatter and leakage, rather than direct radiation.

The radiographer's obligation is to ascertain that all persons who are involved in or in the vicinity of a radiographic procedure are provided with appropriate protective apparel to shield them from ionizing radiation. This includes the patient, the physician, nurses, observers, and radiographer. Shielding can include a lead apron, lead gloves, a gonadal shield, a thyroid shield, and lead goggles (Fig. 3-13).

Use of gonadal shielding to protect male and female reproductive organs (ovaries and testes) is of vital importance. This is of particular importance when the patient is a child or an adult of childbearing age. There are several types of gonadal shields, including flat and molded contact shields.

The radiographer must use his or her technical expertise to minimize patient exposure to radiation. This includes beam limitation, technique selection, filtration, intensifying screens, and grids. Explanations of these techniques are beyond the scope of this text; their use is discussed in detail in other radiologic technology courses.

The radiographer has the responsibility to understand the technical aspects of the profession so that the number of repeat radiographs necessary to achieve the diagnostic purpose is minimized. The need to frequently repeat exposures should be cause to put critical thinking skills to work to assess and solve the problems that are being encountered. Assess communication with the patient as well as the skills necessary to properly position the patient and set the

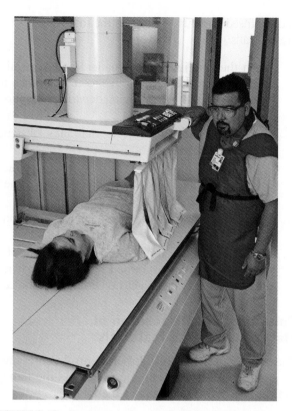

FIGURE 3-13   Lead apron, thyroid shield, lead goggles, and radiation monitor should all be worn while in the room when the beam is energized.

proper technical factors to achieve a diagnostic radiograph on the first attempt.

Estimates of patient exposure to ionizing radiation must be made available in the radiographic imaging department. These estimates denote the amount of radiation an average patient undergoing a given procedure would expect based on standard technique charts. The amount of exposure actually received is less than compared with these estimates. All radiographic imaging equipment must also be inspected for radiation safety at regularly scheduled times.

Lead aprons and other protective apparel must be inspected periodically for quality control purposes. This apparel must be hung carefully over a wide bar or on special hangers when not in use. To fold or drop them may jeopardize their integrity.

The radiographer and any health care worker who works in constant contact with ionizing radiation must be monitored to assess the amount of exposure to it. This may be done by wearing a radiation-monitoring badge sensitive to low radiation doses. A specialized company processes the badge on a monthly or quarterly basis. The results are then returned to the institution and must be made available to all occupational persons who wear the badge.

Special precautions must be taken to prevent exposing pregnant patients and pregnant health care workers to ionizing radiation. This is particularly true during the early weeks of pregnancy, when particular fetal tissues are especially sensitive to radiation. This is why it is critical to ask the female patient if there is any possibility of her being pregnant and also when her last menstrual period was. Pregnant workers who "declare" themselves to be pregnant are double badged, and rotations in the department are varied so as to limit the amount of exposure to radiation. The occupational

dose limit for a fetus must not exceed 0.5 rem during the entire gestation. The exposure must be limited to no more than 0.05 rems in any month.

To minimize radiation exposure, the radiographer should not hold the patient during a procedure on a routine basis. Sand bags and positioning sponges should be used if possible. If this is not feasible, then a relative or a person who is not working regularly in radiography should be requested to assist.

SUMMARY

When an outpatient arrives in the diagnostic imaging department, it is often necessary for that patient to undress entirely or partially for the diagnostic examination or treatment. Always show the patient where and how to do so in a sensitive manner to spare the patient embarrassment.

It is the responsibility of the radiographer to provide the patient with a safe place for personal belongings. Remember that the patient may treasure an article of clothing or jewelry that may not seem valuable. Everything that belongs to the patient must be treated as if it were of value.

Correct body mechanics must always be used. When moving or lifting in the workplace, keep the weight close to the body and maintain a firm base of body support. This is accomplished by having the feet slightly spread out and knees flexed. Twist or bend the body at the waist when lifting a heavy load. Weight should be pulled, not pushed. Use arm and leg muscles, not the spine for lifting.

The three ways of moving patients are by gurney, by wheelchair, or by ambulation. When moving and lifting patients, assess the patient and resolve potential problems before beginning the transfer. The plan for moving the patient should be explained, and the patient's help should be enlisted before beginning. Always notify the ward personnel when taking a patient to or from his or her hospital room. The use of enough assistants and equipment such as a smooth mover facilitates the move and protects personnel and the patient from possible injury.

When a patient is on the radiographic table or on a gurney in the diagnostic imaging department, his or her body must be in good alignment. If the patient is moved to a particular position for an examination, restore correct body alignment as soon as possible.

There are times when immobilizers must be used for the safety of the adult patient. When immobilizers are required, apply them according to the manufacture's directions and the policy of the institution. Do not immobilize a patient without an order by a physician. When a patient is immobilized, attend to him or

her at all times and release the immobilizers at least every 2 hours. Follow the correct manner of documenting immobilization use.

Take care to prevent the patient's skin from being damaged while being cared for in the diagnostic imaging department. This can be done by preventing injury that may come from immobility, pressure, shearing force, or friction. Patients most susceptible to skin breakdown are the malnourished, the elderly, and the chronically ill. Take special care to protect these patients from injuries to their integumentary system, because they may result in a decubitus ulcer that can take months to heal. Also, take extra precautions when caring for a patient who is wearing a cast or who is in traction. Observe the patient's extremities for evidence of neurocirculatory impairment, which may result from the pressure of a cast on the skin. Some symptoms of neurocirculatory impairment that are easily detected are pain, coldness, numbness, burning or tingling of fingers or toes, swelling, color changes of the skin, and an inability to move fingers or toes. If these symptoms are noted, change the patient's position and report the problem to the physician immediately. Do not release a traction apparatus while taking a radiographic image. If the procedure cannot be completed because of the traction bar, request assistance from the nurse in charge of the patient.

If a patient is unable to undress alone, offer assistance. Give assistance in a matter-of-fact manner that does not violate the patient's privacy. Patients must be kept clean and dry while in the diagnostic imaging department. It is the radiographer's duty to change the disabled patient's gown and covering if they become wet or soiled. Do this in a prescribed manner to ensure privacy, safety, and comfort.

Some examinations in the imaging department are long and tedious. They often stimulate peristalsis and a need to defecate or urinate. Meeting these needs cannot be postponed. Be prepared to assist with either the bedpan or urinal if necessary and do it in a way that ensures the patient as much privacy as possible. Infection control measures must be taken when assisting a patient with a bedpan or urinal. These items must be used for one patient only and then disposed of in the proper waste receptacle. Put on clean, disposable gloves when assisting with the patient's elimination needs and wash thoroughly after removing the gloves. The patient must not be left unattended while on a bedpan, gurney, or diagnostic imaging table. Patients must never be allowed to get on or off an examining table or out of a wheelchair without assistance. They must also be carefully attended on trips to the lavatory and in a dressing area after an examination or treatment.

The radiographer must be constantly on guard to protect patients and other staff members from accidents in hospitals. Most falls and injuries to patients can be prevented if the radiographer is knowledgeable about the patient's condition and comfort. The radiog-

rapher must understand the precautions to take routinely to prevent fire and the correct procedures to follow if a fire occurs. Prevention of accidents due to faulty electrical equipment or poisoning and the correct use and disposal of hazardous materials are also the radiographer's professional obligation.

Unnecessary exposure to radiation to the patient and personnel is the responsibility of the radiographer. Excessive amounts of radiation from improper technical factors or from repeat exposures have an adverse affect on living tissue. The very young, the very old, and pregnant women are particularly susceptible to adverse affects of ionizing radiation. Precautions to prevent excessive exposure involve knowledge, technical expertise, and constant vigilance.

CHAPTER 3 TEST

1. When admitting a patient to the diagnostic imaging department, what should be done? (Circle all that apply)
   a. Take the patient to the dressing area and explain in some detail how he or she should dress for the procedure.
   b. Give the patient directions concerning how to care for valuables brought to the department.
   c. Assist any patient who appears to need assistance with preparation for an examination.

2. The most effective means of reducing friction when moving a patient is by:
   a. Placing the patient's arms across the chest and using a pull sheet
   b. Pushing rather than pulling the patient
   c. Rolling the patient to a prone position
   d. Asking the patient to cooperate

3. When transporting a patient back to the hospital room, some safety measures to be used are (circle all that apply):
   a. Place the side rails up, the bed in "low" position, and the call bell at hand.
   b. Inform the nurse in charge of the patient that the patient has been returned to the room.
   c. Give the patient something to eat or drink.
   d. Be sure that the TV is in place for the patient's viewing.

4. Which procedures must be observed when assisting a patient with a bedpan (circle all that apply):
   a. Respect the patient's privacy.
   b. Seek assistance for an immobile patient.
   c. Wear clean gloves to remove the bedpan.
   d. Make sure to offer tissue to the patient and a towel to clean his or her hands.

5. Contributing factors to skin breakdown are (circle all that apply):
   a. Turning the patient every 1 to 2 hours
   b. Friction and pressure
   c. Frequent diagnostic imaging procedures
   d. A wet environment

6. If a patient who has a cast in place complains of pain that is sudden in onset and increases in intensity when the affected limb is moved, what should be done? (Circle all that apply.)
   a. Complete the procedure and discharge the patient.
   b. Elevate the affected limb.
   c. Notify a physician immediately.
   d. Find a nurse to administer pain medication.

7. When caring for a patient who has a new cast applied to an extremity, what must be remembered? (Circle all that apply.)
   a. Hold the cast firmly at a position between the joints when moving it.
   b. Observe for signs of impaired circulation.
   c. Support the cast with bolsters and sandbags where needed.
   d. The extremity is now almost impervious to pain and can be twisted as needed for the image.

8. When caring for a patient who is disabled and is difficult to move, it is best to:
   a. Keep the patient as quiet as possible.
   b. Work quickly.
   c. Obtain as much help as necessary to avoid injury to the patient and to the radiographer.
   d. Move the patient by gurney.

9. When moving a heavy object, you should _____ the weight, not _____ it.

10. Patients most prone to falls are (circle all that apply):
    a. The frail elderly
    b. The person who is confused

c. Persons who have been given a psychoactive drug

d. Persons with sensory deficits

11. When moving a patient into an unnatural position for a radiographic examination, the patient should maintain that position:

a. Until he or she asks to be moved

b. Until the radiograph has been processed and approved by the radiologist

c. Only for the time it takes to make the exposure

12. Match the following:

a. Fowler position

b. Supine position

c. Semi-Fowler position

d. Trendelenburg position

e. Sims position

i. Patient on side with forward arm flexed and top knee flexed

ii. Semi-sitting position with head raised 45 to 60 degrees

iii. Patient laying flat on back

iv. Patient on back with head lower than extremities

v. Patient on back with head raised 15 to 30 degrees

13. Name the two convenient and safe methods of moving a patient from a radiographic table to a gurney.

14. Describe three legitimate reasons for application of immobilizers to an adult patient.

15. List four signs of circulatory impairment if a patient is wearing a cast.

16. What are three methods of reducing a patient's exposure to ionizing radiation?

17. The leading cause of work-related injuries in the field of health care is:

a. Bumping into misplaced equipment

b. Overexposure to radiation

c. Infection owing to poor hand-washing techniques

d. Abuse of the spine when moving and lifting patients

Infection Control

STUDENT LEARNING OUTCOMES

After studying this chapter, the student will be able to:

1. Define the basic terminology used in the practice of infection control.

2. List and describe the known microorganisms that may cause infection.

3. Explain the rise in antibiotic-resistant diseases and the emergence of previously unknown or unrecognized diseases.

4. Describe and demonstrate the methods of controlling infection in health care settings.

5. Discuss the modes of transmission of HIV, all forms of viral hepatitis, methicillin-resistant *Staphylococcus aureus*, vancomycin-resistant *S. aureus*, vancomycin-resistant *Enterococcus*, *Clostridium difficile*, extended spectrum beta-lactamase, and tuberculosis and the methods of preventing their spread in health care settings.

6. List the regulatory agencies that set and maintain the guidelines for safety in health care and the community at large.

7. Define the two tiers of isolation precautions as outlined by the Centers for Disease Control and Prevention (CDC), and describe the precautions required in each tier.

8. Demonstrate the isolation precautions used in each tier of isolation precautions, as required by the CDC and other regulating bodies.

9. Explain the actions the radiographer should take if exposed to blood or body substances or other potentially infectious material or a sharp injury occurs in the course of his work.

KEY TERMS

Antimicrobial drugs: Drugs that tend to destroy microbes or prevent their multiplication

Antibiotics: Soluble substances derived from a mold or bacterium that kills or inhibits growth of other microorganisms

Arthropod vector: In the family arthropoda that includes spiders, mites, ticks, mosquitoes, etc.; can transmit infection to man or animals

Attenuated vaccine: A weakened or dilute solution of microbes

Bacteria: Colorless, minute, one-celled organisms with a typical nucleus

Broad-spectrum antimicrobial drug: A drug effective against a wide variety of different microorganisms

Carrier: A person or animal that harbors a particular infectious agent and does not have clinical disease but is able to transmit the disease to others

Cilia: Mobile extensions of a cell surface

Cytomegalovirus infections: A group of viruses in the Herpesviridae family

Encephalopathy: A disorder of the brain

Enterotoxigenic: Referring to an organism that produces toxins specific for cells in the intestinal tract

Fecal-oral route: Disease passed from one person who has poor hand-washing hygiene to another through food touched by that person following stool elimination

Fungi: Cells that require an oxegenated environment to live; may be either yeasts or molds

Genetic predisposition: Inherited potential via the genetic transmission for a particular illness or characteristic

Helminths: Parasitic worms that may live in the human intestinal tract for long periods of time if not treated

KEY TERMS (Continued)

Immune: Free from acquiring a particular infectious disease

Immune suppressed: Persons whose immunity is prohibited for physiologic reasons

Infectious disease: A disease capable of being passed from one person to another

Nucleoid: A part of a nucleous (a nuclear inclusion body)

Parasite: An organism that lives in or on another and draws its nourishment from that on which it lives

Pathogenicity: The ability to cause disease

Percutaneous injection: Passage through the skin by needle puncture including introduction of wires and catheters

Prion: An infectious particle of nonnucleic acid composition; must mutate to become infectious

Protozoa: One-celled organisms; often parasitic and are able to move by pseudopod formation, by the action of flagella, or by cilia

Retention urinary catheters: Tubes that are placed in the urinary bladder and fixed in place for a period of time

Sterile: Free of all living microorganisms

Vascular access devices: Catheters or needles that are able to enter the blood vessels

Virulent: Extremely toxic

Viruses: Minute microbes that cannot be visualized under an ordinary microscope; the smalles microoganism known to produce disease

---

The AIDS epidemic, the increasing number of microbes resistant to **antimicrobial drugs**, and the increasing incidence of tuberculosis and various forms of hepatitis in the United States and throughout the world have forced all health care workers to be more vigilant in the practice of infection control in order to protect themselves and others from acquiring **infectious diseases**. This makes the practice of infection control measures a necessity for all who are working in, being treated in, or visiting health care settings.

The radiographer must understand the methods of isolating body substances (called Standard Precautions) and be able to correctly perform all transmission-based precautions as he works with patients. Correct cleaning of equipment, correct hand hygiene, and correct disposal of contaminated waste must be part of every procedure in imaging to guard against the spread of infection.

■ NOSOCOMIAL INFECTIONS

In spite of increasing use of infection control measures and the control or elimination of many diseases, infections in patients while they are receiving health care has increased. This is the result of increase of organisms becoming resistant to **antibiotics** and the emergence of new or here-to-for unrecognized diseases. Infections acquired in the course of medical care are called *nosocomial infections*. This term is most often applied to infections contracted in an acute care hospital; however, it also applies to infections patients receive while in extended care facilities, outpatient clinics, and behavioral health institutions. Infections contracted at birth by infants of infected mothers are also classified as nosocomial. A nosocomial infection that results from a particular treatment or therapeutic procedure is called

an *iatrogenic infection*. Although a patient acquires a particular infection while in a health care unit, he or she may not develop symptoms of the illness until leaving the health care environment. This is still considered to be a nosocomial infection. A person who enters a health care facility with an infection is said to have a *community-acquired infection.*

Everyone has microorganisms in their bodies at all times. These microorganisms are called normal flora. Infections that are caused by microorganisms that are not normal flora are called *exogenous* nosocomial infections. When a person acquires an infection in the health care setting as a result of an overgrowth of normal flora, it is called an *endogenous* nosocomial infection.

Endogenous infections are often the result of the alteration in the number of normal flora present in the body or the alteration in placement of normal flora into another body cavity. Endogenous infections may also be the result of treatment with a **broad-spectrum antimicrobial drug** that alters the number of normal flora. Many factors in health care facilities encourage nosocomial infections. Display 4-1 lists these factors.

Factors That Increase the Patient's Potential for Nosocomial Infection

People who present themselves for health care come from many social and economic environments. A variety of factors in the social and economic environment may render a person more susceptible to acquiring a nosocomial infection. Display 4-2 describes some of these factors.

The bloodstream and the urinary tract are common sites of nosocomial infections. These are often the result of long-term use of **vascular access devices (VAD)** and **retention urinary catheters.** Infections in

DISPLAY 4-1

Factors That Encourage Nosocomial Infections

Factor	Reasons for Increased Incidence
Environment	Air contaminated with infectious agents; other patients who have infectious diseases; visitors; contaminated food; contaminated instruments; hospital personnel
Therapeutic regimen	Immunosuppressive and cytotoxic drugs used to treat malignant or chronic diseases, which decrease the patient's resistance to infection; antimicrobial therapy, which may alter the normal flora of the body and encourage growth of resistant strains of microbes sometimes called hospital bacteria
Equipment	Instruments such as catheters, intravenous tubing, cannulas, respiratory therapy equipment, and gastrointestinal tubes that have not been adequately cleaned and sterilized
Contamination during medical procedures	Microbes transmitted during dressing changes, catheter insertion, or any invasive procedure may introduce infective organisms if correct technique is not used.

DISPLAY 4-2

Factors That Increase the Potential for Nosocomial Infection

Factor	Reasons for Susceptibility
Age	The very young have immature immune systems and are more susceptible to nosocomial infections. Also, as one ages, the immune system becomes less efficient and organ function declines, making infections more difficult to resist.
Heredity	Congenital and genetic factors passed on from birth make individuals more or less resistant to disease.
Nutritional status	Inadequate nutritional intake, obesity, or malnourishment as a result of illness render one increasingly susceptible to nosocomial infections.
Stress	Work-related or other stress factors increase potential for infection as levels of cortisone in the body increase related to constant tension.
Inadequate rest and exercise	Efficient elimination and circulation decline as a result of inadequate rest or exercise.
Personal habits	Smoking, excessive use of drugs and alcohol, and/or dangerous sexual practices contribute to lowering the body's defenses against nosocomial infections.
Health history	Persons with a history of poor health such as diabetes, heart disease, or chronic lung disease, or children who have not been immunized against diseases of childhood are at increased risk for acquiring a nosocomial infection.
Inadequate defenses	Broken skin; burns or trauma; or immunocompromised persons related to a medical regimen are at increased risk of acquiring a nosocomial infection.

wounds following surgical procedures and respiratory tract infections also occur frequently. Early removal of urinary catheters, intravenous catheters, and other types of invasive treatment devices is recommended whenever possible to reduce the incidence of nonosocomial infections. Meticulous care of vascular access devices and retention catheters while they are inserted is of great importance and will be discussed later in this text.

MICROORGANISMS

Infectious diseases are caused by microorganisms. Microorganisms do not fit into the plant or animal kingdom; therefore, a third kingdom was formulated by Haeckel, named the Protista kingdom. This kingdom includes **bacteria, fungi, protozoa, helminths, viruses,** and **prions.**

Four major groups of microorganisms are known to produce diseases: bacteria, fungi, viruses, parasites. Prions are present in brain cells and may mutate to become infectious disease. If a microorganism is known to produce disease, it is called a *pathogenic microorganism,* or a *pathogen.* There are also believed to be unidentified pathogens that produce newly recognized diseases. Within the known groups of microorganisms, many different species may produce infections in humans, and many are useful or, at least, not harmful. Microorganisms are used in a variety of ways: in food and drug processing to destroy waste and, frequently, as a means of effecting a positive change in the environment.

Some microorganisms that are natural flora in one area of the body produce infection if they are accidentally relocated to a site other than their natural habitat. For example, *Escherichia coli (E. coli),* which normally inhabits the human intestinal tract, does not cause disease there; however, if it gains entrance to the urinary bladder, it can cause a urinary tract infection. There are certain strains of *E. coli* that are extremely **virulent** and are not considered normal flora. This strain of *E. coli* is called an **enterotoxigenic** strain and may cause a severe cholera-like infectious disease. This disease has been linked to the *E. coli* from cattle and is spread by introduction into beef or contamination from irrigation of vegetables with contaminated water.

Often, it is the quantity of microorganisms in an area that produces infection. A small number of a particular bacterium in the body may be harmless; however, if the number increases, it may produce an infection. There are few areas of the human body that are considered **sterile.** These are the brain, blood, bone, heart, and the vascular system.

Another factor that determines the **pathogenicity** of a microorganism is its ability to find susceptible body tissue to invade. For example, the skin is a normal habitat for staphylococci; however, if this microorganism

enters the lungs, it can cause an infection. Some microorganisms are more virulent than others. This means that some microbes are more certain than others to cause disease if they enter the human body.

The human body houses *resident flora.* That is, there are colonies of bacteria living on the skin that do not result in infections. This means that there are microbes that live in the body at all times in a quantity that is usually stable. When the quantity of resident flora increases, the flora may become pathogenic. Staphylococci are resident flora on the superficial layers of the skin that, in large numbers, may cause a serious infection. Resident flora require firm friction and an effective soap and quantities of water to remove them from the skin.

Flora that are acquired by contact with an object on which they are present are called *transient flora.* Transient flora are more easily removed from the dermal layers of the skin because they are not firmly adherent. For an infection to occur, the microorganism must be able to survive and multiply in the body of the host, whether the host is human, plant, or animal. Moreover, the microorganism must be able to produce a disease, and the host must be unable to mobilize its defenses against the infectious microbes.

Bacteria

Bacteria are colorless, minute, one-celled organisms with a typical nucleus. They contain both deoxyribonucleic acid (DNA) and ribonucleic acid (RNA). DNA carries the inherited characteristics of a cell, and RNA constructs cell protein in response to the direction of DNA.

Bacteria are classified according to their shape, which may be spherical (cocci), oblong (bacilli), spiral (spirilla), or pleomorphic (lacking a definitive shape). Short rods are called *coccobacilli.* They may also be classified according to their divisional grouping as diplococci (groups of two), streptococci (chains), or staphylococci (grapelike bunches) (Fig. 4-1).

Bacteria must be stained to be seen under a microscope and are classified according to their reaction to various staining processes in the laboratory. They may be gram-positive, which means that they take the stain; gram-negative, which means that they do not take the stain; or acid-fast, which means that the bacteria are resistant to colorization by acid alcohol. Bacteria may also be classified according to their immunologic or genetic characteristics (Gladwin and Tattler, 2000).

Rickettsias, chlamydias, and mycoplasmas are gram-negative bacteria-like microbes that are smaller than bacteria and do not have all of the characteristics of bacteria. They used to be considered viruses because they are too small to be seen under normal microscopic conditions. Rickettsias and chlamydias usually live as **parasites** inside another cell. Rickettsias are transmitted from animal to animal by the bite of an infected **arthropod vector** such as a tick or flea. Typhus and Rocky Mountain

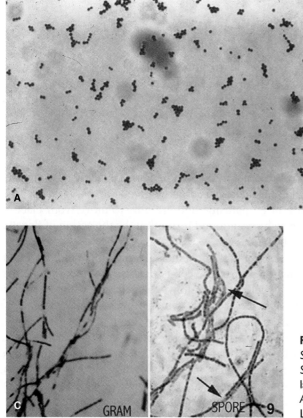

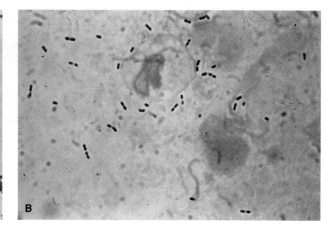

FIGURE 4-1 Forms of bacteria. (**A**) Gram-stained smear of *Staphylococcus aureus* in grapelike clusters. (**B**) Gram smear of *Streptococcus pneumoniae:* in elongated pairs. (**C**) *B. anthracis* grows as large gram-positive bacilli arranged in chains (From *Koneman's Color Atlas and Textbook of Diagnostic Microbiology,* 6th ed. Philadelphia: Lippincott Williams & Wilkins, 2006).

spotted fever are caused by rickettsias. Chlamydia is transferred by direct contact between hosts often during sexual contact. It causes infections of the urethra, bladder, or sexual organs of the host. Mycoplasmas may be parasitic or free-living and cause pneumonia and genitourinary infections in humans (Fig. 4-2).

Some forms of bacteria are able to form a protective coat or *spore* when conditions are unfavorable for survival. Bacterial spores are called *endospores.* Endospores encase the genetic material in the cell and may protect it for many years. When conditions for survival are again favorable, the endospore germinates and the bacterial cell again grows and replicates. Endospores are more difficult to destroy than are vegetating bacteria; therefore, many methods of destroying pathogenic bacteria do not affect their endospores (Fig. 4-3).

There are bacteria that survive and thrive only in an oxygen environment. These are called *aerobes.* Others are unable to live in the presence of oxygen and are called *anaerobes.* Many bacteria are opportunists and learn to adapt or thrive in any condition. They may also learn to live in the presence of antimicrobial drugs or disinfectants.

Some diseases caused by bacteria include tuberculosis, streptococcal infections of the throat, staphylococcal infections of many parts of the body, *Salmonella* poisoning, Lyme disease, gonorrhea, syphilis, and tetanus.

Fungi

Fungi are cells that require an aerobic environment to live and reproduce. Fungi exist in two forms—yeasts and molds. Yeasts are one-celled forms of fungi that reproduce by budding. Molds (also called mycelia) form multicellular colonies and reproduce by spore formation.

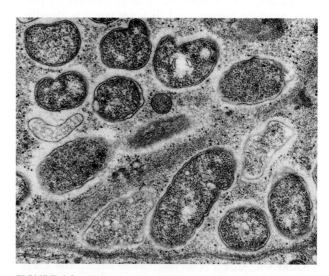

FIGURE 4-2 *Rickettsia prowazekili* in experimentally infected tick (From Benjamin DC, Kadner RJ, et al. *Essentials of Medical Microbiology.* Baltimore: Lippincott-Raven, 1996).

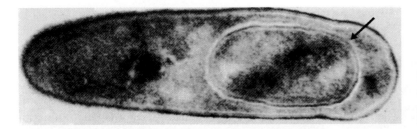

FIGURE 4-3   A bacillus with a well-defined endospore (From Burton GW, Englekirk P. *Microbiology for the Health Sciences*, 6th ed. Baltimore: Lippincott Williams & Wilkins, 2000).

There is a form of fungi that can grow as either a yeast or a mold depending on temperature and environment. It is called a *dimorphic fungus.* Another variety of fungi live in and utilize organic matter such as rotting vegetation as a source of energy and are called *saprophytes.*

Yeasts and molds can be harmful and cause a number of infectious diseases. On the other hand, molds are often extremely useful. They are a primary source of material for the production of antibiotic drugs; they produce enzymes for medical use and are used in the production of foods to flavor various cheeses. Yeasts are used commercially to produce beer and wine and to leaven bread. They are also a source of vitamins and minerals; however, some yeasts are pathogens that produce diseases in humans and animals. A commonly seen disease caused by yeast infection is *Candida albicans* (thrush). Diseases caused by dimorphic fungi are histoplasmosis, blastomycosis, and coccidioidomycosis (Fig. 4-4).

Parasites

Parasites are organisms that live on or in other organisms at the expense of the host organ. Parasites may be plant or animal, but animal parasites are those that are pathogenic to humans. A large number of parasites produce disease, and they are roughly classified as *protozoa* and *helminths.*

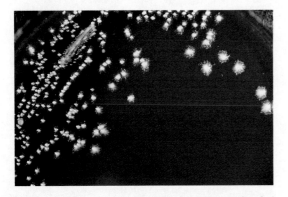

FIGURE 4-4   Colony of the yeast, *Candida albicans*, after 3 days of incubation (From *Koneman's Color Atlas and Textbook of Diagnostic Microbiology*, 6th ed. Philadelphia: Lippincott Williams & Wilkins, 2006).

Protozoa

Protozoa are more complex one-celled microorganisms than those described in the preceding paragraphs. They are often parasitic and are able to move from place to place by pseudopod formation, by the action of flagella, or by *cilia.*

Pseudopod movement is an amoeboid action in which a part of the cell is pressed forward and the rest of the cell rapidly follows. Flagella are whiplike projections on the protozoa, which move the cell by their swift movements. Cilia are smaller and more delicate hairlike projections on the exterior of the cell wall, which move swiftly and in a synchronous manner to propel the microorganism (Fig. 4-5). Many protozoa are able to form themselves into cysts, which are protected by a cyst wall in adverse conditions to prolong their existence.

Many of the diseases in humans caused by protozoa affect the gastrointestinal tract, genitourinary tract, and circulatory system. Some of the common protozoa diseases are amebiasis, giardiasis, trichomoniasis, malaria, and toxoplasmosis.

Helminths

Helminths can be simply described as parasitic worms classified as either *Platyhelminthes* (flatworms) or *Aschelminthes* (roundworms). Many of these worms can live in the human intestinal tract for long periods of time if they are not treated.

Some of the more pathogenic types of helminths migrate to the body organs, where they cause serious illness. Although some can be seen with the naked eye, an examination of their eggs is necessary to make a positive identification before initiating treatment. Common diseases caused by helminths are enterobiasis (pinworm), trichinosis, and infection with *Diphyllobothrium latum* (tapeworm) (Fig. 4-6).

Viruses

Viruses are minute microorganisms that cannot be visualized under an ordinary microscope. They are the smallest microorganisms known to produce disease in humans. The genetic material of a virus is either DNA or RNA, but never both. A *virion* is a complete infectious particle with a central **nucleoid.** The genetic material is protected by a capsid or protein coat that is composed of minute protein units called *capsomeres.* The complete

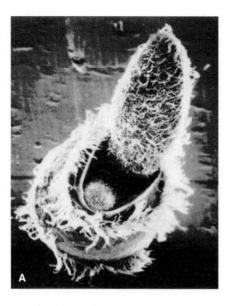

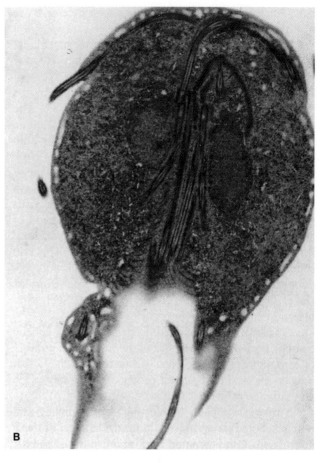

FIGURE 4-5 Protozoa. (**A**) *Didinium nasutum* with partially ingested prey. (**B**) Longitudinal section of *Giardia lamblia* by transmission electron microscopy (From Burton GW, Englekirk P. *Microbiology for the Health Sciences*, 6th ed. Baltimore: Lippincott Williams & Wilkins, 2000).

nucleocapsid with a nucleic acid core constitutes a complete virus. Some viruses are surrounded by an envelope that is composed of a lipoprotein. Viruses must invade a host cell in order to survive and reproduce.

Whatever its structure, the virus is transported by way of its capsid to a host cell that has receptor sites on its surface that are suitable to a particular virus that it invades. A virus does not invade a cell at will. It must attach itself at a membrane receptor site for which it

has a specificity; that is, specific for that particular type of host cell and no others.

Once in the cell, production of new viral particles does not take place with certainty. Other factors in the cell environment must be favorable for the multiplication to take place. There are various theories concerning what makes the environment favorable. These include, but are not limited to, poor nutritional status of the host, poor health related to heart disease or dia-

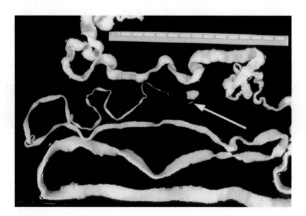

FIGURE 4-6 *Diphyllobothrium latum*, the giant adult tapeworm (From *Koneman's Color Atlas and Textbook of Diagnostic Microbiology*, 6th ed. Philadelphia: Lippincott Williams & Wilkins, 2006).

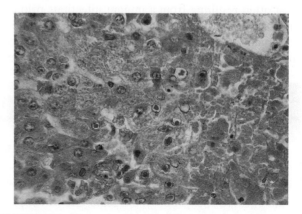

FIGURE 4-7 Herpes simplex vesicular lesion; a mature squamous epithelial cell stains pink (From *Koneman's Color Atlas and Textbook of Diagnostic Microbiology*, 6th ed. Philadelphia: Lippincott Williams & Wilkins, 2006).

betes, increased life stress for the host, or excessive use of drugs and alcohol.

To reproduce, the virus uses the genetic machinery of the host cell. When reproduction is complete, new viruses leave the original host cell. As some types of viruses leave the host cell, they destroy the cell by the rapid release of new viruses. This is called *lysis*. The second type of viral replication produces viruses that lie dormant, but very much alive and destructive, within the host cell.

Some viruses have the capacity to invade nerve ganglia and leave their genetic material in the ganglia in a latent phase after an acute infective period. The virus remains there until the body is under some type of stress such as an emotional life event or illness or until it is exposed to sunlight for a period of time. This will often induce the virus to take over nearby cells and produce more viruses, as in the case of herpes simplex (fever blisters) or herpes zoster (shingles). Such viral infections may occur repeatedly.

A virus may be classified on the basis of its genetic composition; the shape or size of the capsid; the number of capsomeres or the absence of an envelope; the host it infects; the type of disease it produces; or its target cell and immune properties (Fig. 4-7).

Viruses are capable of infecting plants, animals, and humans. Some common viral diseases that affect humans are influenza, the common cold; mumps; measles; HIV (AIDS); and hepatitis A, B, C, D, and E.

Prions

A prion is a protein that does not contain DNA or RNA. Like microorganisms, there are a number of prions present in brain cells that prevent neurologic diseases; however, they may mutate and become an infectious disease. A mutant prion may be present by **genetic predisposition** or may be the result of infection. Acquiring an infectious prion is the result of transmission from an infected animal or person. The disease most often resulting from a mutant infectious prion is Creutzfeldt-Jakob disease. This disease is transmitted to humans by eating infected meat or meat products and is known as mad cow disease. Prion diseases are known as transmissible spongiform encephalopathies (TSE). "When TSE is suspected clinically, elaborate precautions must be taken in the autopsy room and histology laboratory because the agents of these infections survive formalin fixation and are even demonstrable after tissue is embedded in paraffin blocks" (Koneman, 2006, p. 1367). There is currently research ongoing to determine if prions are contributory to Alzheimer's disease.

ELEMENTS NEEDED TO TRANSMIT INFECTION

Infection cannot be transmitted unless the following elements are present (Display 4-3):

1. *An infectious agent, which may be a bacterium, a fungus, a virus, a prion, or a parasite.* Infectious agents vary in their ability to cause disease. These characteristics are pathogenicity, virulence, invasiveness, and specificity.

   Pathogenicity refers to the causative organism's ability to cause disease.

   Virulence refers to the causative organism's ability to grow and multiply with speed.

   Invasiveness is the term used to describe the organism's ability to enter tissues.

   Specificity characterizes the organism's attraction to a particular host.

2. *A reservoir or an environment in which the pathogenic microbes can live and multiply.* The reservoir can be a human being, an animal, a plant, water, food, earth, or any combination of organic materials that support the life of a particular pathogen. Infection is prevented by removing the causative microbe from the reservoir.

3. *A portal from which to exit the reservoir.* In the case of a human reservoir, the portals of exit might be the nose, mouth, urinary tract, intestines, or an open wound from which blood or purulent exudate can escape. There can be more than one portal of exit.

DISPLAY 4-3

Elements Needed to Transmit Infection

1. An infectious agent and a reservoir of available organisms
2. An environment in which the pathogenic microbes can live and multiply
3. A portal of exit from the reservoir
4. A means of transmission
5. A portal of entry into a new host

4. *A means of transmission.* Infection is transmitted by direct or indirect contact, by droplet, by vehicle, by vector, or by airborne route. Contact is direct when a person or an animal with a disease or his blood or body fluids are touched. This contact can be by touching with the hands, by kissing, by **percutaneous injection,** or by sexual intercourse. A person who transmits disease-causing organisms but has no apparent signs or symptoms of that disease is called a **carrier.** Particular organisms require specific routes of transmission for infection to occur.

Indirect contact is defined as the transfer of pathogenic microbes by touching objects *(called fomites)* that have been contaminated by an infected person. These objects include dressings, instruments, clothing, dishes, or anything containing live infectious microorganisms.

Droplet contact involves contact with infectious secretions that come from the conjunctiva, nose, or mouth of a host or disease carrier as the person coughs, sneezes, or talks. Droplets can travel from approximately 3 to 5 feet and should not be equated with the airborne route of transmission, which is described later.

Vehicles may also transport infection. Vehicle route of transmission includes food, water, drugs, or blood contaminated with infectious microorganisms.

The *airborne route* of transmission indicates that residue from evaporated droplets of diseased microorganisms are suspended in air for long periods of time. This residue is infectious if inhaled by a susceptible host.

Vectors are insect or animal carriers of disease. They deposit the diseased microbes by stinging or biting the human host.

5. *A portal of entry into a new host.* Entry of pathogenic microorganisms into a new host can be by ingestion, by inhalation, by injection, across mucous membranes, or, in the case of a pregnant woman, across the placenta.

A human host can be any susceptible person. Persons particularly susceptible to infection are those who are poorly nourished or are fatigued. Those at greater risk are persons with chronic diseases such as diabetes mellitus or cancer. **Immune-suppressed persons** are at great risk of acquiring infections. Previous infection with a particular disease or vaccination against a particular disease can render an individual **immune** to infection.

Socioeconomic status and culture also play a role in host susceptibility. Persons living in poor environments are more likely to contact some diseases owing to poor hygienic conditions and the poor diets that they are forced to endure. Some diseases have a strong hereditary aspect, which makes them more likely to occur in particular races or families who are genetic carriers of the disease.

THE BODY'S DEFENSE AGAINST DISEASE

The human body has both mechanical and chemical methods of warding off contamination and infection. The radiographer must be aware of these defenses because this knowledge will play a role in his professional work and personal life.

THE IMMUNE SYSTEM

The body has a highly complex immune system that reacts to specific invaders that are able to bypass the nonspecific body defenses by forming antigens. Antigens are foreign or unrecognizable organic substances that invade the body and induce it to produce antibodies. An antibody is a protein substance produced by a particular white blood cell, the lymphocyte or, more specifically, the B cell. B cells work with other lymphocytes called T cells, macrophages, and neutrophils. Together, the components of this highly complex system attempt to destroy invading antigens. All antibodies are immunoglobulins (Ig), but not all immunoglobulins are antibodies. Antibodies in the bloodstream and in other body systems react against specific antigens to produce an immunity to further infection by that particular antigen.

Antibodies are also found in human tears, saliva, and colostrum. Colostrum is the fluid initially secreted by the mammary glands of the new mother. If given to the infant during breastfeeding, it protects the infant, because the infant's body is not capable of producing antibodies for itself. There are several types of immunity and various methods of acquiring immunity as described in Display 4-4.

Vaccines are administered to produce artificial immunity to a number of diseases that have been extremely pathogenic in times past. These vaccines may be made from living or dead (inactivated) microorganisms. If made from living microbes, the pathogenic microbe is rendered less pathogenic and is called an **attenuated vaccine.** A third type of vaccine called a *toxoid* is made from inactivated, nontoxic exotoxin of a pathogenic microbe.

Occasionally, antibodies function as antigens and produce diseases called *autoimmune diseases.* This occurs when substances identical with one's own tissues stimulate antibody production, and these substances react with the host's tissues in an adverse manner. In other words, one's own antibodies destroy healthy tissue. Some diseases believed to be autoimmune diseases are rheumatoid arthritis, systemic lupus erythematosus, and multiple sclerosis.

Methods of Acquiring Immunity

Type of Immunity	How Acquired
Acquired immunity	Results from active production or receipt of antibodies.
Active acquired immunity	Antibodies actually produced within a person's body; usually a long-term immunity.
Passive acquired immunity	Antibodies are received from another person or an animal; usually short-term immunity.
Natural active acquired immunity	Antibodies acquired by actually having a particular disease; re-infection may be short or long term.
Artificial active acquired immunity	Antibodies formed by vaccination that enable one to form antibodies against that particular pathogen.
Passive acquired immunity	Antibodies formed in one individual are transferred to another to protect against infection.
Natural acquired immunity	Antibodies present in a mother's blood or colostrum are passed on to the infant to protect him temporarily from some infections.
Artificial passive acquired immunity	Antibodies are transferred from an immune individual to a susceptible individual to give temporary immunity. This is usually done by administering hyperimmune serum globulin or immune serum globulin (ISG) from the blood of many immune persons.

There is ongoing research using stem cells to restore the immune systems of persons with autoimmune diseases. Stem cells are found in the bone marrow and in the peripheral blood. The stem cell is also called a precursor cell as it furnishes a continuous supply of red and white cells.

THE PROCESS OF INFECTION

Infection invades the body in a progressive manner, that is, "in stages." Although some diseases are considered to be infectious (contagious or communicable) during only one or two of their stages, in the radiographer's practice, he must deal with all diseases as if they are highly infectious at all stages, since it is difficult to be certain of the period of infectivity. Display 4-5 outlines the process of infection.

Hereditary Diseases

Some diseases are the result of alterations in a person's genetic makeup and are inherited from his or her parents or grandparents. The environment may also play a role in influencing the course of these diseases. They may result from aberrations in chromosomal makeup, monogenic (Mendelian) alterations, or other multifactorial errors as the fetus develops. Monogenic disorders are defined as a mutation of one gene that produces disease. It is not pos-

sible in this text to fully discuss these problems; however, you must be aware that such problems are seen relatively often and are diagnosed as hemophilia, diabetes mellitus, sickle cell disease, and congenital heart anomalies.

Immune Deficiency

A person whose body does not adequately defend itself against disease is said to be *immunodepressed* or *immunocompromised*. This condition may be present at birth, may be the result of malnutrition, or may be the result of medical treatment, disease, injury, or an unknown cause later in life. An immunocompromised person is unable to neutralize, destroy, or eliminate invading antigens from his or her body systems. These conditions are often chronic and untreatable. Immune deficiency results in frequent, sometimes life-threatening infections. HIV, which causes AIDS, is an example of an infection that can have disastrous consequences for the body's immune system.

INFECTIOUS DISEASES

There are an increasing number of infectious diseases that may be acquired or transmitted by health care workers. The radiographer must be aware of these and understand the precautions that must be taken to prevent the spread of these in the workplace and refrain

DISPLAY 4-5

The Process of Infection

Stage	Process
Incubation stage	The pathogen enters the body and may lie dormant for a short period, then begins to produce nonspecific symptoms of disease.
Prodromal stage	More specific symptoms of the particular disease are exhibited. The microorganisms increase, and the disease becomes highly infectious.
Full disease stage	The disease reaches its fullest extent or, in some cases, produces only vague, subclinical symptoms; however, the disease continues to be highly infectious.
Convalescent stage	The symptoms diminish and eventually disappear. Some diseases disappear, but the microbe that caused the disease goes into a latent phase. Examples of these diseases are malaria, tuberculosis, and herpes infections.

from acquiring them himself as he cares for patients. Each of these will be described briefly and methods of infection control needed to prevent their spread will be discussed later in this chapter.

Human Immunodeficiency Virus (HIV) and Acquired Immunodeficiency Syndrome (AIDS)

Because HIV and AIDS are critical health conditions that have a huge impact on health care workers, it is necessary for the radiographer to understand the underlying disease process. HIV usually results in AIDS, a disease that is currently incurable and has a high mortality rate. Before it was understood how the spread of HIV could be controlled, health care workers were insecure and, in some cases, frightened when caring for persons known to be infected with HIV or who had symptoms of AIDS. They were also concerned when caring for potential HIV-positive carriers who had not yet been identified as being infected with this virus.

HIV is a retrovirus. This means that it converts its viral material from RNA to DNA after it penetrates the host cell. Retroviruses have an enzyme complex called *reverse transcriptinase* which boosts their ability to replicate and destroy the host cell. After the host cell has been destroyed, the viruses leave and infect other cells. As retroviruses in the bloodstream increase in number, they begin to destroy the cells of the immune system. The infected cells (T4 cells) malfunction and cause the entire immune system to lose its ability to protect the body from infection.

Phases of HIV Infection

HIV enters the body after exposure through contact with the blood or body fluids of an HIV-positive person and begins an assault on the human immune system. The process of infection is divided into five phases and

not until the fifth phase is the person diagnosed as having AIDS. The Centers for Disease Control and Prevention (CDC) has established criteria for reporting persons with AIDS based on a uniformity of symptoms. The five phases are as follows:

Phase 1: HIV enters the body and replicates in the bloodstream. No signs of infection are physically present or present in the laboratory tests; however, HIV can be transmitted during this phase.

Phase 2: There is a period of illness with flu-like symptoms; lymph nodes may enlarge, and fever, a skin rash, and malaise may be present. Symptoms may be somewhat more severe with a stiff neck and seizures present. HIV diagnosis may be possible at this time, but the symptoms may be mild and ignored. The infected person may continue to transmit HIV during this time.

Phase 3: No external symptoms of HIV infection are present on an average of 1 to 10 years. The immune function of the body is declining during this phase, and the T lymphocytes (also called CD4 cells) are decreasing in number.

Phase 4: The HIV-infected person develops persistently enlarged lymph nodes; has low-grade fevers, night sweats, mouth lesions, weight loss, and rashes; fatigues easily; and develops changes in cognition and develops peripheral neuropathy.

Phase 5: The infected person becomes immunosuppressed and meets the criteria for the diagnosis of AIDS as established by the CDC. These criteria include all persons who have a CD4 T-lymphocyte count of less than 200 cells per mm. The infected person suffers from multiple opportunistic viral, protozoal, and bacterial infections and possibly cancer. Eighty to 90 percent of persons with this diagnosis die within 3 years.

An infectious disease commonly seen in persons with AIDS is *Pneumocystis carinii,* a type of pneumonia. Also seen are **cytomegalovirus infections**, *Candida,* herpes simplex, Kaposi's sarcoma (a malignant tumor of the endothelium), AIDS dementia complex (in which it is believed that nerve cells are directly attacked resulting in dementia), tuberculosis, and many other diseases. Death is usually the result of recurrent opportunistic infections. Malignant diseases may also be the cause of death.

Treatment of HIV-Infected Persons

Treatment of HIV-infected persons has changed and improved over the past few years; however, a vaccine for prevention of infection or a cure for AIDS has not been found. The goal of treatment remains the same at present—decreasing the viral load in the bloodstream. The cost of drug therapy for the HIV-infected person is great, and, because of this, persons in developing countries are often deprived of treatment. "The CD4+T-lymphocyte determinations are an integral part of medical management of HIV infected persons with CD4-T-lymphocyte counts of less than 200 cells/u/L or a CD4+ percentage of less than 14. The treatment protocol should contain these key components: prevention of transmission; preservation of immune function; prophylaxis against opportunistic infection, particularly cytomegalovirus (CMV), pneumocystic disease (PCP), and mycobacterium (MAC); early diagnosis and treatment of opportunistic infection; good physician-patient relationship, close patient follow-up, and attention to patient education; and optimizing the quality of life (psychosocial, financial and death and dying issues" (Van Slambrook, 2007).

A new problem is the increasing laxity of persons in danger of being exposed to HIV because of the success of drug therapy. This has resulted in a new increase in the number of persons acquiring HIV infection. Education in the methods of prevention of the populations throughout the world who are not infected with HIV and the education of the already infected constitute the greatest defense. Those infected with HIV must be instructed on the slow progression of the disease, the potential for infecting others, and the need to be treated to retard the disease progression. Education must include the following for all populations:

1. Avoid sexual contact with high-risk persons (prostitutes, persons who have multiple sex partners, and IV drug users).
2. Follow safe sex practices such as use of condoms.
3. Health care workers must always practice Standard Precautions and be cautious in handling needles and other items that may puncture their skin in the workplace.
4. Maintain good nutritional practices.
5. Get adequate amounts of rest and sleep.

Remember that the patient with HIV infection or with AIDS has a right to confidentiality in regard to his or her diagnosis. Maintenance of strict confidentiality is mandatory when caring for persons with a known AIDS diagnosis or with a patient who is known to have an HIV-positive blood test. In some areas of the United States, violation of the patient's right to confidentiality concerning this issue is punishable by fine and, in some cases, imprisonment. The chart of a patient containing information concerning an AIDS diagnosis or HIV-positive test must be kept in a place where it cannot be inspected by anyone other than the persons directly caring for that patient. The radiographer must not discuss the diagnosis with anyone other than the patient's immediate caregivers. Patients who are HIV-positive and are not ill feel that their livelihood or status in their family or community are threatened if this confidentiality is violated.

If the radiographer or any health care worker is accidentally exposed to HIV while working with a patient diagnosed with HIV or AIDS, he must report the incident to his superior immediately. If you receive a needle-stick or other penetrating injury while working, report the incident and follow the policy of your institution and of the state in which you reside concerning testing to determine the HIV status of the person to whose blood you were exposed.

◀)) CALL OUT!

Immediately report to your superior any accidental exposure to HIV or AIDS sustained while working with an infected person!

Viral Hepatitis

Viral hepatitis is an inflammation of the cells of the liver that is initially acute, but, in some cases, may render its victims chronic carriers of the disease. It may be caused by five separate RNA viruses: hepatitis A virus (HVA), hepatitis B virus (HVB), hepatitis C virus (HVC), hepatitis D virus (HVD), hepatitis E virus (HVE), and hepatitis G virus (HVG). Other hepatitis viruses may exist, but this has not been proved at this time.

Both hepatitis A and hepatitis E are transmitted by the **fecal-oral route**; the others are transmitted by blood or body fluid contacts. Hepatitis G is a new form of hepatitis thought to be an isolate of the same virus as HVB and HVC but with a longer incubation period usually following transfusions. Research into this form of hepatitis is ongoing. Health care workers most often contract hepatitis B from needle-stick injuries. Persons who share contaminated needles or have multiple sex partners and hemophiliacs are most susceptible to blood-to-blood methods of contracting HVB and HVC.

Hepatitis C has also become more prevalent in recent years and has become the most common blood-borne infection in the United States. This was formerly called hepatitis non-A, non-B. It is increasingly prevalent in persons who share contaminated needles and in health care workers who receive needle-stick injuries. Persons who have multiple sexual partners, IV drug users, and persons needing multiple transfusions are most apt to contract this disease. Persons with this disease frequently become chronic carriers and are at increased risk of developing chronic liver disease, cirrhosis, or liver cancer.

The onset of viral hepatitis is most often sudden with symptoms ranging from mild to severe. The resolution is most often complete. However, it may have a prolonged course that eventually becomes chronic, or the victim may become a silent carrier of the disease. HVB, HVC, and HVD can cause chronic hepatitis.

The onset of acute viral hepatitis demonstrates flu-like symptoms with a low-grade fever, muscle aches, and fatigue. After 1 or 2 weeks, the patient becomes jaundiced, and as the disease progresses, the liver becomes enlarged, and the liver cells die. If the disease does not progress, the inflammation subsides and the liver regenerates. If the inflammatory process continues, the disease may become chronic. Cirrhosis of the liver, a spontaneous relapse, or a severe fulminating hepatitis resulting in rapid cell destruction, no regeneration, and **encephalopathy** may result. If this occurs, the outcome may be fatal. The disease is communicable during the incubation period and throughout the course of the illness. Carriers may also be contagious.

Prevention is the goal when considering hepatitis A and B. There are vaccines available for prevention of both diseases. Sanitation, particularly use of effective hand hygiene, is of great importance in the prevention of HVA. Avoidance of HBV by screening blood donors and use of Standard Precautions by health care workers is mandatory. This will be discussed later in this chapter.

The incidence of HVC has been reduced by meticulous screening of blood donors and blood donated for transfusions. There are antiviral agents that are of some use in treating patients with HVC. Interferon and ribavirin have proven effective in treatment of this disease.

Tuberculosis

Tuberculosis is a recurrent, chronic disease caused by the spore-forming *Mycobacterium tuberculosis*. This disease most commonly affects the lungs, but is capable of infecting any part of the body. With the increasing immigrant population from third-world countries into the United States and the increase of HIV, tuberculosis is increasing in incidence in the United States. It is a communicable disease and must be treated as such by all health care workers.

Pulmonary tuberculosis may be asymptomatic, and most often, the onset and early states of the disease go unnoticed. Early symptoms of the disease are fatigue, loss of appetite, weight loss, and fever that occurs late in the day. A shallow cough and hemoptysis (coughing up bloody sputum) occur later in the course of the disease. As the disease advances, wheezes, rales, tracheal deviation, and pleuritic chest pain develop. The initial infection may subside as the bacteria are walled off and lie dormant for an indefinite period of time. If the host organism becomes weakened, the disease process may reappear.

Pulmonary tuberculosis is a treatable disease if it is diagnosed and treatment is begun early in its course. If left untreated, massive destruction of lung tissue and respiratory failure may result. A number of anti-infective drugs are used to treat pulmonary tuberculosis; unfortunately, there is an increasing incidence of drug-resistant bacilli. Because of drug resistance, treatment is begun with four or more medications (Fig. 4-8). Health care workers who must come in contact with patients with active tuberculosis must be fitted with a particular respirator mask. This will be discussed later in this chapter.

The radiographer must recognize that tuberculosis consists of infectious, airborne bacilli to which he may be exposed. There are several methods of preventing this disease. Tuberculin testing is required of all health care workers on a yearly basis to detect possible exposure to infected persons. This is a skin test called a PPD test. If there is a positive tuberculin reaction, a chest x-ray is done. If there is an indication of need, a prophylactic course of treatment is begun.

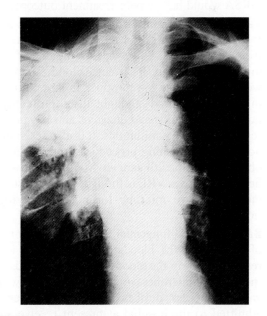

FIGURE 4-8 X-ray films of a patient with pulmonary tuberculosis (From *Koneman's Color Atlas and Textbook of Diagnostic Microbiology*, 6th ed. Philadelphia: Lippincott Williams & Wilkins, 2006).

Nosocomial Infections Related to Specific Microorganisms

The ever-increasing rate of nosocomial infections in hospitalized patients is alarming. It is the responsibility of all health care workers to strictly adhere to all infection control guideline to prevent their spread. Each year there are new microbes that become resistant to treatment with antibiotics. They will be listed and described as follows:

1. **Methicillin-resistant _Staphylococcus aureus_ (MRSA):** Shortly after penicillin was used to treat _S. aureus_ it became resistant to it. The newer semisynthetic penicillin (methicillin) was used successfully for a time to treat these infections, but the war against _S. aureus_ is being lost as it becomes resistant to this drug.

   Since _S. aureus_ is easily colonized on the skin, it must be assumed that all patients may be carriers of this microbe, and all health care workers must take precautions to prevent its spread. Persons who are transferred from nursing homes, dialysis patients, the aged and debilitated, intensive care patients, and all persons who have been hospitalized for a long period of time are most susceptible to MRSA. Some diseases produced by MRSA are decubitus ulcers, pneumonia, endocarditis, bacteremia, osteomyelitis, and septic thrombophlebitis.

2. **Vancomycin-resistant _S. aureus_ (VRSA):** Vancomycin was used successfully for a time to treat MRSA; however, it is feared that _S. aureus_ will become resistant to this drug.

   This would be a tragedy as those infected with MRSA would have a poor treatment outcome.

3. **Vancomycin-resistant _Enterococcus_ (VRE):** _Enterococcus_ is a part of the normal flora in the gastrointestinal tract; however, it is capable of causing disease when it affects blood, urine, or wounds. It is able to reproduce in large numbers in areas of the body thought to be protected by normal body fluids and enzymes and has become resistant to many antibiotics. It is also resistant to normal handwashing procedures and adheres to objects in the health care environment and is difficult to remove. VRE is thought to be the second most causative microbe for nosocomial infections.

4. **Bacteremia and fungemia:** Bacteremia is the result of bacteria in the bloodstream. Fungemia is the result of fungi in the bloodstream. Both are usually the result of microbes entering the blood by way of vascular access devices (VAD). Most persons admitted to the hospital at present receive some type of VAD during their stay. Control of infections of this type are the responsibility of all health care workers who care for patients with these in place or who insert VADS. The radiographer will care for patients with VADs in place and, at times, insert them; therefore, he must pay the strictest attention to infection control practices to prevent this type of infection. The infection control practices for this activity will be discussed later in this text.

5. **_Clostridium difficile:_** Most hospitalized patients are receiving antibiotics that may predispose them to infection with _C. difficile_ by disrupting the normal flora of the intestinal tract. This organism is emerging as a frequent cause of nosocomial infections. _C. difficile_ is a spore-forming bacteria that releases toxins into the bowel that are resistant to disinfectants and so can be easily spread from the hands of health care providers. The disease process resulting from _C. difficile_ is a **pseudomembranous colitis** and can produce profound **sepsis.** Control is achieved by using contact precautions and will be discussed later in this chapter.

6. **Extended spectrum beta-lactamase (ESBL):** Beta-lactamase infections are an ever increasing threat to treatment by antibiotic therapy. Beta-lactamase is a type of enzyme produced by some bacteria that is responsible for their resistance to beta-lactam antibiotics like penicillins, cephalosporins, cephamycins, and carbapenems. These antibiotics have a common element in their molecular structure: a four-atom ring known as a beta-lactam. The lactamase enzyme breaks that ring open, deactivating the molecule's antibacterial properties (Abraham EP, Chain E. "An enzyme from bacteria able to destroy penicillin." _Nature_ 46: p. 837). _E. coli_ and many gram-negative bacteria are resistant to treatment by most antibiotics that are the result of ESBLs.

AGENCIES CONTROLLING INSTITUTIONAL, PATIENT, AND WORKPLACE SAFETY

There are international, federal, state, and local agencies that control safe practices for the general public and for all accredited health care institutions, including the various extended care facilities. As health care in the United States changes, more emphasis is being placed on transferring patients from acute care institutions to extended care facilities and into their own homes for care as soon as it is safe to do so. This increases the burden of overseeing the safety of both the patient and the health care worker. Institutions now being overseen by some or all of the regulatory agencies are acute care hospitals, skilled and intermediate care nursing facilities, inpatient rehabilitation centers, inpatient chemical dependency centers,

DISPLAY 4-6

Institutions That Control Safety of Patients, Workers, and the General Public

The Joint Commission: Sets requirements for hospital safety, infection control practices, and patient care standards (Quality Assurance, QA) that must be met if the institution or agency is to receive accreditation

The Occupational Safety and Health Administration (OSHA): A federal agency that protects workers and students from work-related injuries and illnesses, inspects work sites, and makes and enforces regulations concerning workplace safety

Centers for Disease Control and Prevention (CDC): Performs research and compiles statistical data concerning infectious diseases; develops immunization guidelines and administers OSHA and OSHA'S research institute, the National Institute of Occupational Safety Health (NIOSH)

United States Public Health Service: Investigates and controls communicable diseases, controls carriers of communicable diseases from foreign countries, prevents spread of endemic diseases, and controls manufacture and sale of biologic products

Food and Drug Administration (FDA): The United States Public Health Service branch responsible for protecting the public from false drug claims and regulates the manufacture and sale of medications; requires pre-clinical tests for toxicity of new drugs on animals and the testing of medications clinically on humans in three phases before marketing

World Health Organization (WHO): Works under the auspices of the United Nations to reduce famine and disease throughout the world. Compiles information concerning infectious diseases from all countries and compiles this information into reports for every country

United Nations Children's Fund: Helps children, especially children in developing countries, to avoid malnutrition and disease; also assists with educational programs for deprived children

The U.S. Department of Health and Human Services (DHHS): Specifies and notifies agents to destroy various types of medical waste

The U.S. Environmental Protection Agency (EPA): Specifies destruction practices for waste from patients with contagious highly communicable diseases

Nuclear Control Agency (NCA): Controls disposal of nuclear waste

---

inpatient behavioral health hospitals, and home health care agencies. Display 4-6 lists the agencies that control institutional, patient, and workplace safety in the United States and throughout the world.

INFECTION CONTROL PRACTICES IN HEALTH CARE SETTINGS

Controlling infection or breaking the cycle of infection is the duty of all health care workers. Medical aseptic practices and use of Standard Precautions must become routine for the radiographer. He must also learn the use of transmission-based precautions that are used for patients in hospitals if they are suspected of having an infection with a transmissable pathogen that may be transmitted by droplet, airborne, or contact route.

People who are ill are particularly susceptible to infection. It is the duty of the radiographer to practice strict medical asepsis at all times in his practice. There is a difference between medical asepsis and surgical asepsis. *Medical asepsis* means, insofar as possible, microorganisms have been eliminated through the use of soap, water, friction, and various chemical disinfectants. *Surgical asepsis* means that microorganisms and their spores have been completely destroyed by means of heat or by a chemical process. It is not practical or necessary to practice surgical asepsis at all times, but one must always adhere to the practice of strict medical asepsis.

Most health care institutions now require all students and staff involved in patient care to be immunized or to show proof of immunization—to hepatitis B, rubella, rubeola, poliomyelitis, diphtheria, and tuberculosis. Some institutions require varicella titers for health care workers.

Dress in the Workplace

Fingernails must be short. Cracked or broken nails and chipped nail polish harbor microorganisms that are difficult to remove. Shoes must have closed, hard toes.

Jewelry, such as rings with stones, must not be worn. A plain wedding band and a wristwatch are the only pieces of jewelry that are acceptable for the health care worker to wear in the patient care setting.

Always wear freshly laundered, washable clothing when working with patients. Uniforms or scrubs are recommended because they will not be worn for other purposes. Short sleeves are recommended because cuffs of uniforms are easily contaminated. If a laboratory coat is worn to protect clothing, button or zip it closed and remove it when not in the work area.

Laboratory coats, scrubs, and uniforms must be washed daily with hot water and detergent. Chlorine bleach is recommended for clothes that have become heavily contaminated. A protective gown must be worn when working with any patient who may soil one's clothing or if it is possible that blood or body fluids will contaminate clothing. On some occasions, the radiographer may need to wear a moisture-proof apron along with a gown. (Gowns for isolation patients are discussed later in this chapter.)

Hair

Hair follicles and filaments also harbor microorganisms. Hair is a major source of staphylococcal contamination. For these reasons, hair must be worn short or in a style that keeps it up and away from your clothing and the patient. Hair should be shampooed frequently.

Hand Hygiene

Microbes are most commonly spread from one person to another by human hands. It follows that the best means of preventing the spread of microorganisms continues to be hand hygiene. According to CDC guidelines, the term *hand hygiene* applies to either handwashing with plain soap and water, use of antiseptic handrubs, including alcohol-based products, or surgical hand antisepsis (CDC, 2002).

Correct hand-washing procedure before and after handling supplies used for patient care and before and after each patient contact is required. Hand hygiene is required even if gloves have been worn for a procedure as there may be small punctures in the gloves. Treat all blood and body substances as if they contain disease-producing microorganisms and dispose of them correctly. Then wash your hands. Cover any exposed break in your skin with a waterproof protective covering. If there is an open or weeping wound on the hands, the radiographer must not work with patients until it has healed.

The radiographer should follow a specific hand-washing technique that is accepted as medically aseptic when working with patients (Fig. 4–9 A–C). This technique must not be confused with the surgical aseptic scrub procedure described later in this text. The medically aseptic hand-washing procedure is as follows:

1. Approach the sink. Do not lean against the sink or allow clothing to touch the sink because it is considered to be contaminated. Remove any jewelry except for a wedding band.
2. Turn on the tap. A sink with foot or knee control is most desirable but is not always available. If the faucet is turned on by hand, use a paper towel to touch the handles and then discard the towel.
3. Regulate the water to a comfortable warm temperature.
4. Regulate the flow of water so that it does not splash from the sink to one's clothing.
5. During the entire procedure, keep hands and forearms lower than the elbows. The water will drain by gravity from the area of least contamination to the area of greatest contamination.
6. Wet hands and soap them well. A liquid soap is the most convenient.
7. With a firm, circular, scrubbing motion, wash your palms, the backs of your hands, each finger, between the fingers, and finally the knuckles. Wash to at least one inch above the area of contamination. If hands are not contaminated, wash to one inch above the wrists. Fifteen seconds should be the minimum time allotted for this.
8. Rinse hands well under running water. If hands have been heavily contaminated, repeat steps 6, 7, and 8.
9. Clean fingernails with a brush or an orange stick carefully once each day before beginning work and again if hands become heavily contaminated. Scrubbing heavily contaminated nails with a brush is recommended.
10. Rinse fingers well under running water.
11. Repeat washing procedure as described above after cleaning nails.
12. Turn off the water. If the handles are hand-operated, use a paper towel to turn them off to avoid contaminating hands.
13. Dry arms and hands using as many paper towels as necessary to do the job well.
14. Use lotion on hands and forearms frequently. It helps to keep the skin from cracking and thereby prevents infection.

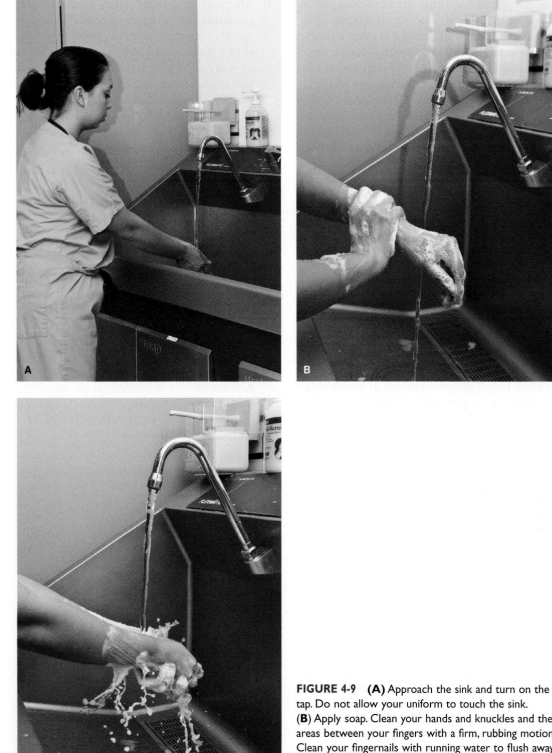

FIGURE 4-9 **(A)** Approach the sink and turn on the tap. Do not allow your uniform to touch the sink. **(B)** Apply soap. Clean your hands and knuckles and the areas between your fingers with a firm, rubbing motion. Clean your fingernails with running water to flush away dirt and microorganisms. **(C)** Clean your wrists and forearms with a firm, circular motion.

Perform the foregoing procedure at the beginning of each workday, when in contact with a patient's blood or body substances, when preparing for invasive procedures, before touching patients at greatest risk for infection, and after caring for patients with known communicable diseases. This is the case even if gloves are worn. A 15-second hand washing should precede and follow each patient contact.

Because of the high degree of non-compliance with handwashing before and after each patient contact, waterless alcohol-based hand rubs are now used effectively in place of many handwashing situations. The availablility of sinks and running water is often a problem. If this is the case, waterless alcohol-based handrubs now available are to be used. A small amount is applied to the hands, and the hands are rubbed together rapidly making sure that all surfaces of the hands, fingers, and between the fingers are covered. Rub vigorously until the solution dries. If hands have been heavily contaminated, hands must first be washed as described earlier and then the antiseptic rub used.

📢 CALL OUT!

Remove gloves after each patient care situation and then wash hands. Do not wear gloves to another area or touch other items with gloves worn for one patient!

STANDARD PRECAUTIONS (TIER 1)

In 2005 the CDC published revised guidelines for infection control for all persons working in health care settings. A two-tier system was established to be applied as prescribed for patients with particular diagnoses. The first tier is called Standard Precautions and is to be used at all times when any health care worker is caring for a patient. Tier 2 is to be used when called for (see next section). The new guidelines are attentive to the importance of body fluids, secretions, and excretions in the transmission of nosocomial infections. Radiographers must learn and abide by the rules of Standard Precautions at all times in their practice.

The threat of infection with HIV, hepatitis A, B, C, D, E, MRSA, VRE, VRSA, ESBLs, and tuberculosis was the impetus for establishing these guidelines. Use of Standard Precautions in all patient care relieves the health care worker of the unnecessary burden and the unreliable result of trying to differentiate persons with an infectious disease from those who are not. Standard Precautions are effective because they are based on the assumption that every patient has the potential for having an infectious disease. Strict adherence to these principles greatly reduces the threat of infection.

The Occupational Safety and Health Administration (OSHA) amended federal regulations concerning infection control in the workplace. OSHA states that all workplaces in which employees may be exposed to human blood or body substances shall formulate a plan to control employee exposure to pathogenic microorganisms borne by these substances. This plan was to be implemented in all affected workplaces by spring of 1992. These precautions must be followed at all times. The regulations required of all employers are as follows:

1. An infection control policy conforming to OSHA guidelines must be developed. This policy must specify when personal protective equipment (PPE) is required and how to clean spills of blood or body substances, how to transport specimens to the laboratory, and how to dispose of infectious waste.
2. All staff must be instructed in the application of these policies.
3. Hepatitis B immunizations are to be provided to staff who might be exposed to blood or body substances free of charge.
4. Follow-up care must be provided to any staff member accidentally exposed to splashes of blood or body fluids or to needle-stick injuries.
5. Personal protective equipment must be readily accessible to any staff member who needs it.
6. Impermeable, puncture-proof containers that are disposable must be provided for all used needles, syringes, and other sharps; they must be changed frequently or when full (Fig. 4-10).
7. All health care workers without exception are obliged to follow Standard Precautions and Tier 2 precautions as indicated. If an employee or the institution in which he or she is employed is remiss in this practice, legal action should be taken to enforce these rules.

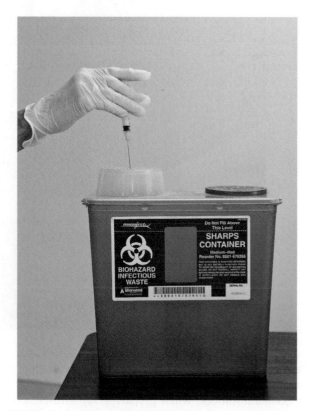

FIGURE 4-10 Place used needle uncapped into a puncture-resistant container.

8. Body substance isolation procedures define body fluids and substances as infectious (National Safety Council, 1993). Body substances and fluids that may be infectious include vaginal secretions, breast milk, cerebrospinal fluid, synovial fluid, pleural fluid, peritoneal fluid, pericardial fluid, and amniotic fluid. Urine, feces, nasal secretions, tears, saliva, sputum, and any purulent or non-purulent drainage from wounds are also considered potentially infectious.

> ### 📢 CALL OUT!
>
> If a needle-stick or sharps injury occurs, report the incident immediately and follow the procedure dictated to repair the injury according to institutional policy as quickly as possible.

Additional Infection Control Considerations

Items to be reused must be placed in designated puncture-resistant containers for transport to the area designated for cleaning and disinfecting. Mouthpieces and resuscitation bags must be kept in all diagnostic imaging examination and treatment rooms so that mouth-to-mouth contact with the patient can be avoided in the event of cardiopulmonary resuscitation (Fig. 4-11).

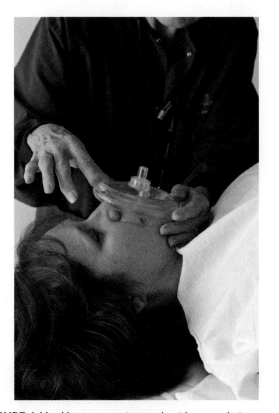

FIGURE 4-11 Use a protective mask with a mouthpiece to perform cardiopulmonary resuscitation.

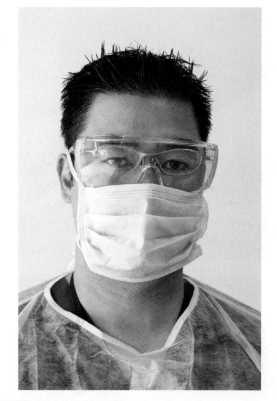

FIGURE 4-12 Wear goggles to protect your eyes.

The patient may not be familiar with the requirements dictated for infection control and may feel that the radiographer may be questioning his or her sanitation practices when he wears gloves and other protective items. Tell the patient about these required precautions, and make the patient understand that these precautions also protect him or her from infection.

Eye Protection

If the radiographer is in a patient care situation in which a spattering of blood or body fluids is possible, he must wear goggles to protect his eyes from becoming contaminated. These goggles must have side protectors. If eyeglasses are worn for vison enhancement, the goggles must fit over the glasses (Fig. 4-12). Keep hands away from eyes during the course of work so that infection is not introduced into them.

Gloves

Any time it is potentially possible that a patient's blood or body secretions may be touched, disposable, single-use gloves must be worn. These gloves should be readily available in containers in each treatment room. Since these gloves are to be used for medical aseptic purposes and not for surgically aseptic purposes, the radiographer may simply pull them on after hand washing. When they are no longer needed, remove the

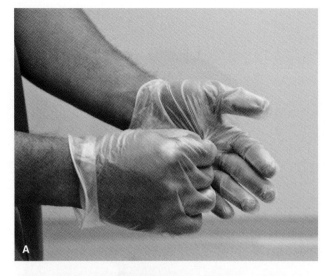

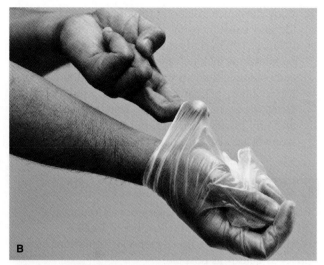

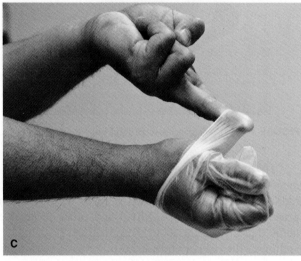

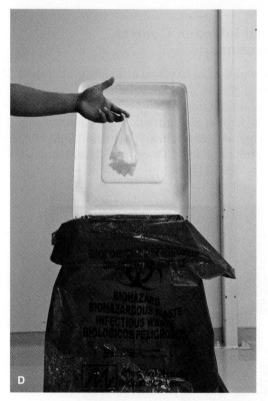

FIGURE 4-13 (**A**) Pull the first glove off by grasping it on the outside with the other gloved hand. Hold the glove that has been removed in the remaining gloved hand. (**B**) With the bare fingers, reach inside the top of the remaining soiled glove and pull it off. (**C**) Turn the glove inside out and encase the other glove inside it. (**D**) Drop the soiled gloves into a designated waste receptacle.

gloves by use of the following technique to prevent contamination of the radiographer's hands or clothing:

1. With the gloved right hand, take hold of the upper, outside portion of the left glove and pull it off, turning it inside out as you do so (Fig. 4-13A).
2. Hold the glove that you have just removed in the palm of the remaining gloved hand (Fig. 4-13B).
3. With the clean, bare index and middle fingers, reach inside the top of the soiled glove and pull it off, turning it inside out and folding the first glove

inside it as you do so. Be careful to touch only the inside of the glove (Fig. 4-13C).
4. Drop the soiled gloves into a receptacle for contaminated waste (Fig. 4-13D).
5. Wash your hands.

CALL OUT!

If exposure to blood or body fluids is possible, wear gloves, gown, mask, and eye protection!

Latex Sensitivity

Approximately 8% to 12% of health care workers have reported a latex sensitivity. Reactions range from local skin reactions to urticaria (hives) to systemic anaphylaxis, an exaggerated allergic reaction that can result in death (OSHA, 2005). The powder placed on the gloves may exaggerate this allergic response. It is the employer's responsibility to make non-latex, powder-free gloves available for any employee that has a need. A policy must be in place to deal with latex-sensitive employees and patients.

Cleaning and Proper Waste Disposal

Not all disinfectants are equally effective. Before a disinfectant is chosen for the diagnostic imaging department, it should be thoroughly studied by an infection-control consultant. Microorganisms begin to grow in disinfectant solutions left standing day after day. This is also true in liquid-soap containers. If such items are used, they should be changed and cleaned every 24 hours. A more detailed description of disinfection and sterilization methods is presented in a later chapter. The following are guidelines for the disposal of waste or the cleaning of equipment after each patient use in the diagnostic imaging department.

1. Wear a fresh uniform each day. Do not place your uniform with other clothing in your personal closet. Shoes should be cleaned and stockings should be fresh each day.
2. Pillow coverings should be changed after each use by a patient. Linens used for drapes or blankets for patients should be handled in such a way that they do not raise dust. Dispose of linens after each use by a patient.
3. Flush away the contents of bedpans and urinals promptly unless they are being saved for a diagnostic specimen.
4. Rinse bedpans and urinals and send them to the proper place (usually a central supply area) for re-sterilization if they are not to be reused by the same patient.
5. Use equipment and supplies for one patient only. After the patient leaves the area, supplies must be destroyed or re-sterilized before being used again.
6. Keep water and supplies clean and fresh. Use paper cups in the diagnostic imaging department and dispose of them after a single use.
7. Floors are heavily contaminated. If an item to be used for patient care falls to the floor, discard it or send it to the proper department to be recleaned.
8. Avoid raising dust because it carries microorganisms. When cleaning, use a cloth thoroughly moistened with a disinfectant.

9. The radiographic table or other imaging or treatment equipment should be cleaned with a disposable disinfectant towelette or sprayed with disinfectant and wiped clean and dried from top to bottom with paper towels after each patient use.
10. When cleaning an article such as an imaging table, start with the least soiled area and progress to the most soiled area. This prevents the cleaner areas from becoming more heavily contaminated. Use a good disinfectant cleaning agent and disposable paper cloths.
11. Place dampened or wet items such as dressings and bandages into waterproof bags, and close the bags tightly before discarding them to prevent workers handling these materials from coming in contact with bodily discharges. Place in contaminated waste containers.
12. Do not reuse rags or mops for cleaning until they have been properly disinfected and dried.
13. Pour liquids to be discarded directly into drains or toilets. Avoid splashing or spilling them on clothing.
14. If in doubt about the cleanliness or sterility of an item, do not use it.
15. When an article that is known to be contaminated with virulent microorganisms is to be sent to a central supply area for cleaning and re-sterilizing, place it in a sealed, impermeable bag marked "BIOHAZARD." If the outside of the bag becomes contaminated while the article is being placed in the bag, place a second bag over it (Fig. 4-14).
16. Always treat needles and syringes used in the diagnostic imaging department as if they are contaminated with virulent microbes. Do not recap needles or touch them after use. Place them immediately (needle first) in a puncture-proof container labeled for this purpose. Do not attempt to bend or break used needles because they may stick or spray you in the process.
17. Place specimens to be sent to the laboratory in solid containers with secure caps. If the specimen is from a patient with a known communicable disease, label the outside of the container as such. Avoid contaminating the outside of the container, and place the container in a clean bag. If a container becomes contaminated, clean it with a disinfectant before placing it in the bag. Specimens must be sent to the laboratory immediately after collection for examination (Fig. 4-15).
18. Medical charts that accompany patients to the diagnostic imaging department must be kept away from patient care areas to prevent contamination. Keep charts in an area where only those directly involved in patient care may read them.

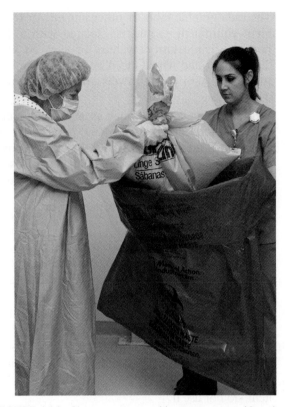

FIGURE 4-14 Place contaminated bag into a second bag that is not contaminated.

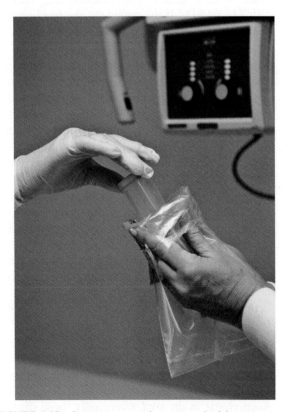

FIGURE 4-15 Specimens must be sent to the laboratory in a clean container and then encased in an outer bag.

Disinfection

Disinfection is a term used to describe the removal, by mechanical and chemical processes, of pathogenic microorganisms, but frequently not their spores, from objects or body surfaces. Usually in reference to body surfaces, the term *antisepsis* or *antiseptic* is used rather than disinfect or disinfectant. Items are disinfected when they cannot withstand the process necessary to sterilize them or when it is not practical to sterilize. This is often the case with objects leaving an isolation unit. If an object leaving an examining room or isolation unit has been contaminated, it is cleaned first by vigorous scrubbing (mechanical means) and then disinfected by wiping it with, or soaking it in, a chemical selected by the institution for this purpose.

When a patient enters the diagnostic imaging department and it is known or suspected that this patient has a contagious disease, it is the radiographer's responsibility to prevent the spread of infection. If the patient is coughing and sneezing, the patient must be provided with tissues and a place to dispose of them. Instruct the patient to cough and sneeze into the tissues and then discard them safely. The patient should be removed from a crowded waiting room to prevent infecting other persons. The radiographer must put on a gown to protect his uniform. Put on a mask and goggles, if necessary. The patient should be cared for and returned to his or her room or discharged as quickly as possible.

After the patient has been cared for and leaves the imaging department, wash your hands thoroughly and then disinfect the imaging table and anything in the room that the patient has touched. This can be accomplished with a disinfectant solution designated by the infection control department to be acceptable for this use. Then remove your gown, goggles, and gloves and scrub your hands again. The room used for imaging of patients with airborne diseases should be left vacant for a designated amount of time before bringing another patient into that room.

TRANSMISSION-BASED PRECAUTIONS (TIER 2)

Standard precautions to prevent spread of infection are used daily for all persons cared for in all health care settings. Some diseases, or the suspicion of a communicable disease, require radiographers and all health care workers to take additional precautions, as well as standard precautions to prevent infection of other health care workers, patients, other persons in the health care setting, and oneself. These precautions are presently called *transmission-based precautions* or Tier 2 precautions and are designed to place a barrier to the spread of highly infectious diseases between persons with such diseases and the persons caring for them.

It is believed that there are three specific routes or modes of disease transmission, which may differ with each disease. These routes are by airborne, by droplet, and by contact. Isolation precautions are meant to separate the patient who has a contagious illness from other hospitalized patients and from the health care workers. This separation may be accomplished in a hospital ward or in a private hospital room. The method chosen depends on how the pathogenic microorganism is transmitted and on the reliability of the patient with the disease. If the patient is very young or cannot be relied on to use necessary hygienic practices to control infection, he or she must be placed in a private room. In some institutions, Tier 2 guidelines continue to be referred to as *category-specific* guidelines. If this is the case, there may be a card posted on the patient's door with instructions informing the staff and visitors of the isolation requirements to be observed (Fig. 4-16).

If a disease can be transmitted only by direct contact, the reliable patient may remain in a ward or a room with another patient. If the disease is spread by airborne route, a private room is necessary; however, two patients who have the same disease may share a room. Some diseases may be spread by more than one route, and so more than one method of isolation is required. Following are the transmission-based precautions for the three modes of preventing transmission of infectious diseases.

Airborne Isolation

This method of transmission occurs when microbes are spread on evaporated droplets that remain suspended in air or are carried on dust particles in the air and may be inhaled by persons in that room or air space. In some instances, air currents carry microorganisms, and special air handling and ventilation are required to prevent infectious microbes from circulating. Diseases that are spread by airborne route are sudden acute respiratory syndrome (SARS), smallpox, tuberculosis, varicella "chicken pox," and rubeola. When diseases require this type of isolation, the following precautions are required.

- A private room, negative air-pressure ventilation, and an N95 respirator mask for health care workers (Fig. 4-17); a surgical mask for visitors; door closed
- Standard Precautions
- A surgical mask for a patient to be transferred within the hospital

Droplet Isolation

Transmission by droplets occurs when droplets contaminated with pathogenic microorganisms are placed in the air from a person infected with a droplet-borne infection. This happens when a patient sneezes, coughs, talks, or deposits infection from his or her eyes, nose, or mouth in other ways, and these droplets are inhaled or internalized in other ways to an uninfected person. Usually, droplets are not spread for more than 3 feet by coughing, sneezing, or talking. Diseases spread by this route are influenza, rubella, mumps, pertusis (whooping cough), most pneumonias, diptheria, pharyngitis, scarlet fever, and meningococcal meningitis. The following are requirements for precautions for disease spread by droplet transmission:

- A private room or a room with another person infected with the same disease; door may be left open
- A mask for any procedure that requires less than 3 feet in proximity to the infected patient
- Standard Precautions

Contact Isolation

There are two types of contact spread of infection, *direct contact* and *indirect contact.* Direct contact occurs when a susceptible person actually touches an infected or colonized person's body surface in an area where infectious microbes are present. *Colonization* is defined as the presence of microorganisms on the skin or body surface of an individual who has no symptoms of the disease.

Indirect contact occurs when a susceptible person touches or comes into contact with an object that has been contaminated with infectious microorganisms. These contaminated objects are called *fomites.* A fomite can be a soiled instrument, a used syringe, a food or beverage container, or contaminated hands.

Diseases transmitted by contact are drug-resistant wound infections; gastroenteritis caused by: *Clostridium difficile, Escherichia coli, Rotavirus, Shigella* and other gastrointestinal infectious diseases; hepatitis A; herpes simplex; herpes zoster; impetigo; scabies; drug-resistant gastrointestinal, respiratory, and skin diseases (i.e. MRSA, VRE, VRSA, ESBL); draining abscesses; cellulites; conjunctivitis; diphtheria cutaneous; scabies, lice; and all multidrug resistant organisms (infection or colonization). The following are precautions to prevent disease spread by contact:

- A private room or a room with another person infected with the same disease if the patient cannot be relied on to maintain adequate precautions or is too young to do so
- Gloves to be worn by health care workers before entering the patient's room and removed before leaving it
- Wearing a gown if there is a possibility of touching the patient or items in the room or if the patient is incontinent or has diarrhea, an

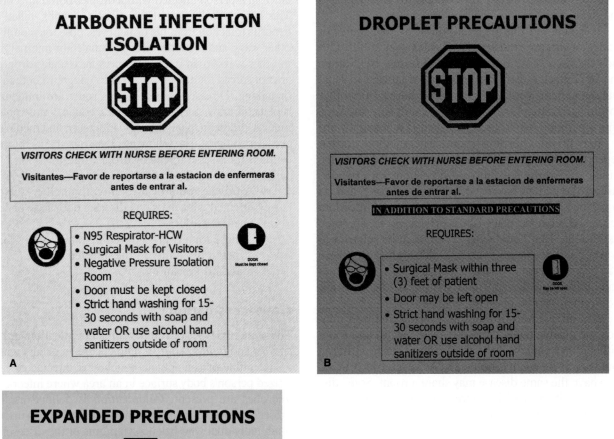

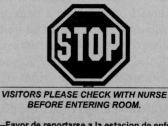

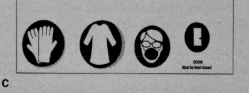

C

FIGURE 4-16 Category-specific cards.

ileostomy, a colostomy, or a draining wound that does not have a barrier dressing in place
- Careful handling of any dressing materials, linens, clothing to prevent cross contamination
- Visitors must wash hands before and after entering room

- Standard Precautions
- Precautions to minimize disease transmission if the patient is to be transported within the hospital and PPE as necessary
- Equipment used in patient's room must stay in patient's room

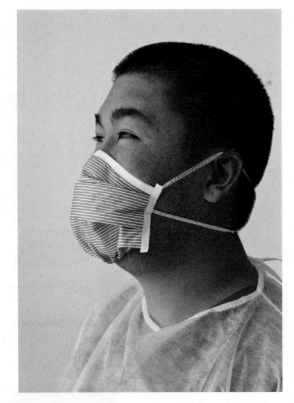

FIGURE 4-17 The N95 respirator mask for tuberculosis isolation.

Expanded Precautions

Standard Precautions are used for all patients; however, if a patient has a disease that can be transmitted by airborne contact, a private room is recommended. There are specific diseases that also require what is called negative-pressure air flow. This prevents pathogenic microorganisms from flowing out of the isolation room.

In some situations, if a patient is highly susceptible to becoming infected because of a particular treatment or condition, isolation precautions are used to protect the patient from becoming infected. These conditions include patients with neutropenia, pronounced immune compromise, transplant recipients who may be rejecting the transplanted organ, and others designated by the physician or infection control officer.

In these cases and in some cases in which diseases may be contracted by direct or airborne contact, you must adhere to a strict method of entering and leaving the isolation unit, which encompasses airborne, droplet, and contact precautions. These are known as *expanded precautions* in some institutions and *strict isolation* in others. The procedure for expanded precautions follows:

1. Wash hands using the procedure prescribed earlier in this chapter before entering and after providing care to patient

2. Cover gown and gloves are required at all times while in patient's room
3. Regular face mask may be required in select cases
4. Equipment such as stethoscopes, blood pressure cuffs, and thermometers stay in room
5. No flowers, plants, fresh fruits, or vegetables are allowed for immune-compromised patients
6. No visitors or staff with signs or symptoms of infection (colds, rashes, etc.) must go into room

To enter and leave a unit with expanded precautions, the radiographer will need the assistance of another radiographer or member of the nursing team who is caring for the patient in the unit. Remember that the patient who is in this type of isolation unit may feel alone and rejected. Such patients are forced to remain in solitude for long periods of time and are often treated by visitors and hospital personnel as if they are undesirable. It is possible to carry out expanded precautions and at the same time treat the patient as a human being with dignity and worth. Before beginning your work with the patient, spend a few moments explaining the imaging procedure. When the procedure is complete, allow a few moments for discussion, and respond in a therapeutic manner to any questions that the patient may have.

When a patient is placed in an Expanded Precautions unit in the hospital setting, a special room is set aside for this purpose. At the entrance to the room, there is a sink for hand washing, a stack of paper or cloth gowns, a container for masks and caps, and a box filled with clean, disposable gloves. Many items in the isolation unit that are used for patient care remain in the unit until the patient leaves.

Before entering the isolation room, the radiographer must have the portable imaging machine prepared with as many image receptors on hand as are needed. Make sure they are covered with protective plastic cases to keep them from becoming contaminated. Also, place an extra pair of clean gloves on the machine before placing it in the patient's room. Have an assistant available and then use the following procedure:

1. Assemble the supplies and equipment needed (Fig. 4-18A).
   Rationale: Prevents loss of time and reduces risk of breaking isolation procedure.
2. Stop in area to don protective clothing. Remove any jewelry that you are wearing and pin it into your uniform pocket so it will not be lost.
3. Wash hands as for medical aseptic practice.
   Rationale for steps 2 and 3: Prevent transmission of microorganisms.

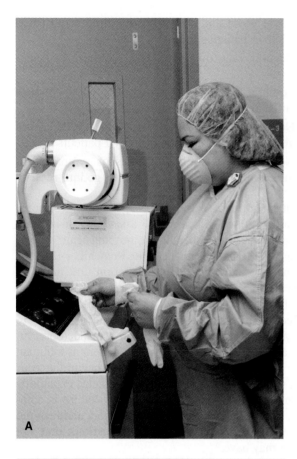

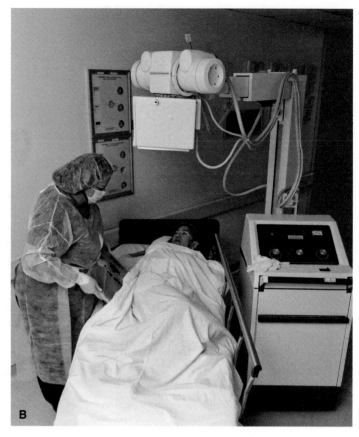

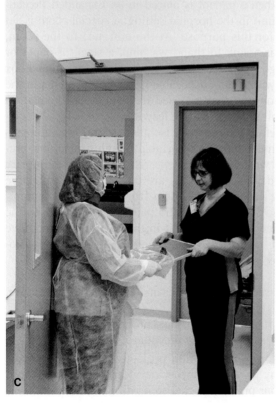

FIGURE 4-18 (**A**) Assemble the supplies and equipment needed. (**B**) Place image receptor under the patient. (**C**) Slide the image receptor from its covering, and allow the assistant to take it.

4. If your hair touches your collar, you must wear a cap.
   Rationale: Hair collects and transmits microorganisms.

5. Remove a mask from the container and put it on, making certain that it covers mouth and nose tightly. Put on a lead apron.

6. Take a gown from the stack. Hold it in front of you and let it unfold. Place arms into the sleeves and pull it on at the shoulders.

7. Tie the back of the gown, making certain that the gown covers all of your clothing.

8. Put gloves on, making certain that the cuffs of the gloves cover the cuffs of the gown.

9. Push machine into the room; introduce yourself to the patient and explain the procedure. Make necessary adjustments to the machine at this time.
   Rationale: The patient will have less anxiety if he or she understands what is to occur. It also gives the patient the opportunity to refuse the procedure. Once you have touched the patient, change gloves before touching the machine again.

10. Place the image receptor for the exposure (Fig. 4-18B).

11. Remove contaminated gloves as described earlier in this chapter, and discard them in a waste receptacle.

12. Put on clean gloves that were placed on the portable machine before entering the room.
    Rationale for steps 10, 11, and 12: Once the patient is touched, gloves are contaminated. To prevent the machine from being contaminated, change gloves before touching.

13. Make the exposure. If additional exposures are necessary, change gloves again. Place image receptor in contaminated plastic covers at the end of the patient's bed or on a bedside stand.
    Rationale: The machine is not to be touched with contaminated gloves or it will be contaminated. The image receptors that have been placed near or against the patient are contaminated and cannot be replaced in the portable machine until the plastic covers are removed.

14. When imaging exposures are completed and before gloves are contaminated by removing the last image receptor, push the machine out of the room and notify the assistant to prepare to receive the image receptors.

15. Take the covered image receptors to the door of the unit where the assistant is waiting. Slide the plastic covering back from the cassette and allow the assistant to remove it (Fig. 4-18C). Discard the contaminated image receptor covers in the waste receptacle in the patient's room.

Rationale: Prevents contamination of image receptors that must be taken to another part of the hospital for processing.

16. Return to the patient. Make the patient comfortable. Place the bed in the low (closest to the floor) position; put the side rails up and the call button within the patient's reach.
    Rationale: The patient's safety and comfort are the highest priority and must always be every health care worker's first concern.

17. Leave the patient's room, and return to the area prepared to receive your contaminated garments.

Infection Control in the Newborn and Intensive Care Nurseries

The radiographer is often called to a nursery to make portable images on infants who are ill. Prior to entering the newborn or intensive care nursery, the radiographer must carefully clean his portable machine with disinfectant wipes. He must request a diaper or cover from the nursery staff to cover image receptors.

Hands must be scrubbed for three minutes with an antibacterial soap before working with all infants. If the infant has or is suspected of having an infectious disease such as MRSA, VRSA, or ESBL, Tier 2 precautions are to be used as specified.

◀))) CALL OUT!

The radiographer must never enter a nursery if he has, or is suspected of having, an infection of any type.

Transferring the Patient with a Communicable Disease

Occasionally, it is necessary for a patient with a communicable disease to come to the diagnostic imaging department for images or treatment. The following precautions must be taken to prevent infecting anyone else and also to prevent contaminating a room or the equipment:

1. The patient must be transported by wheelchair or by gurney. If he or she has a disease that may be transmitted by droplet, airborne, or contact route, place a mask properly on the patient's face and wear a gown and mask to protect yourself.

2. Place a sheet on the gurney or wheelchair and then cover it completely with a cotton blanket. Wrap the cotton blanket around the patient and then complete the transfer (Fig. 4-20).

PROCEDURE

Removing Contaminated Garments

1. Untie waist ties of gown (Fig. 4-19A).

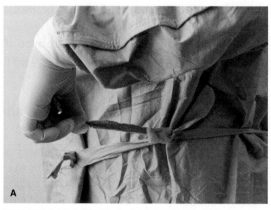

FIGURE 4-19   (A) Untie lower waist ties of gown.

2. Remove gloves according to the procedure for removing contaminated gloves, and place them in the waste receptacle (Fig. 4-19B).

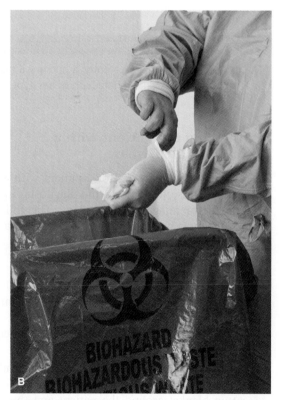

FIGURE 4-19   (B) Remove gloves as described earlier in this chapter.

3. Untie top gown ties (Fig. 4-19C).

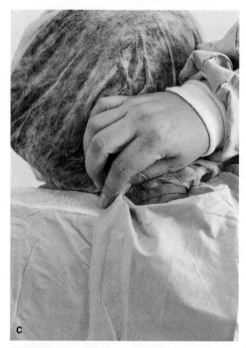

FIGURE 4-19   (C) Untie top gown ties.

4. Remove the first sleeve of the gown by placing fingers under the cuff of the sleeve and pulling it over the hand (Fig. 4-19D).

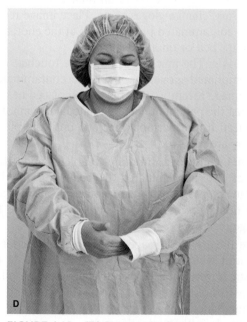

FIGURE 4-19   (D) Remove the first sleeve.

5. Remove the other sleeve with protected hand inside the gown (Fig. 4-19E).

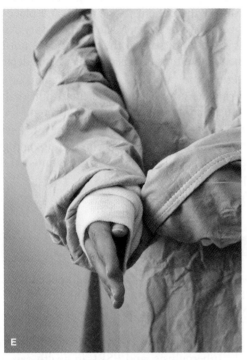

FIGURE 4-19   (E) Remove the other sleeve

6. Slip out of the gown, and hold it forward so that the inside of the gown is facing the outside (Fig. 4-19F).

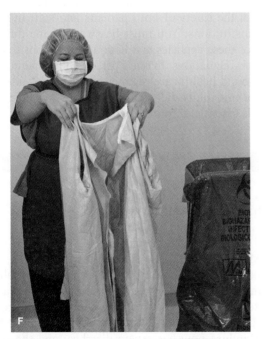

FIGURE 4-19   (F) Fold the gown forward.

7. Place the gown in the waste container (Fig. 4-19G). If gown has been contaminated with blood or infectious material, place it in a biohazard container.

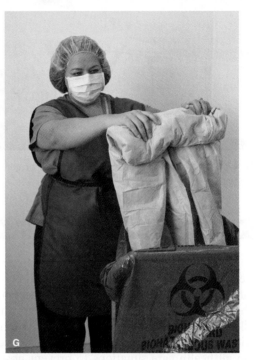

FIGURE 4-19   (G) Place gown in waste container.

8. Remove the cap and mask. Place them in the waste container, and leave the room (Fig. 4-19H).

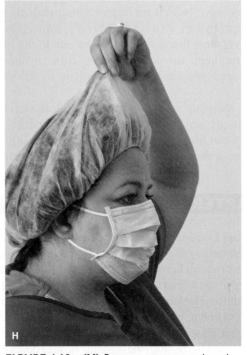

FIGURE 4-19   (H) Remove your cap and mask.

9. Wash hands as previously described in this chapter.

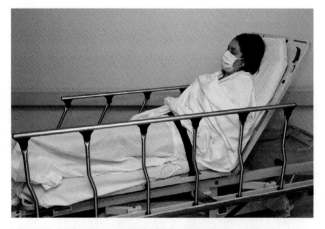

FIGURE 4-20   Place cotton blanket on wheel chair or gurney and wrap patient in blanket.

3. When the patient arrives at the destination, open the blanket without touching the inside.

4. Place a protective sheet on the radiographic table, transfer the patient to the table, and place a draw sheet over him or her. Make the necessary exposures. Arrange work so that the patient does not have to spend more time than is necessary in the department.

5. Return the patient to the wheelchair or gurney. Wrap the cotton blanket around him or her and return the patient to the hospital room.

6. Adjust the bed to the position that is lowest to the floor, put the side rails of the bed up, and give the patient the call button. Notify the unit staff that the patient has been returned.

7. Wash hands.

SUMMARY

Infection control is the obligation of all persons entering a health care facility. This includes hospital personnel, patients, and their visitors. Radiographers must learn the concepts and procedures for infection control and follow them at all times. It is the legal and ethical obligation of a radiographer to practice these procedures in all health care situations to prevent nosocomial infections and the spread of infectious diseases.

Nosocomial infections are caused by four basic types of microorganisms: bacteria, fungi, parasites, and viruses. Various forms of these microbes produce "hospital infections," which are becoming increasingly difficult to control in spite of the body's own elaborate defenses against disease. This may be due to the hospital environment, the patient's therapeutic regimen, or the lowered resistance of the patient to infectious agents.

The elements needed to transmit an infection are a reservoir, or an environment, in which pathogenic microbes can live and multiply; a portal of exit from the reservoir; a means of transmission; and a portal of entry into a new host. The radiographer must adhere strictly to infection control techniques to break the cycle of infection.

The threat of HIV and the disease that it produces, AIDS; the prevalence of HBV, MRSA, VRSA, VRE, *C. difficile*, tuberculosis, and ESBL in health care institutions; and the increasing resistance of all microorganisms to standard treatments create an increased need for the radiographer to practice strict infection control measures. This can be done by always adhering to Standard Precautions, Tier 1 and Tier 2 as required; by practicing safe hand hygiene between each patient care situation; and by correct disposal of waste.

There are federal, state, and local agencies that control the safety of both patients and staff in health care institutions. You must be aware of the duties of each of these agencies and of your obligations to abide by their regulations. In one's personal life, maintenance of a sound health care regimen that includes adequate rest, a nutritious diet, and meticulous hygienic practices is essential to preventing infections.

CHAPTER 4 TEST

1. Jonas Goodstart has been a patient at Happy Valley Community Hospital for 5 days. During his stay in the hospital, he was taken to the diagnostic imaging department several times for diagnostic imaging procedures. He was cared for each time he went to that department by a radiographer who had a severe upper respiratory infection. Two days after he returned home from the hospital, he also developed a severe upper respiratory infection. It would be appropriate to say that Mr. Goodstart had developed:

a. An iatrogenic infection
b. A nosocomial infection
c. A community-acquired infection
d. A bloodborne infection

2. Mary Mandura, an 82-year-old white female, has been hospitalized for several weeks as a result of multiple injuries suffered in an automobile accident. She has been treated with a series of broad-spectrum antibiotics to discourage infection. Ms. Mandura now has severe diarrhea, and the stool

culture has produced *Clostridium difficile*. This would be called:

a. A bloodborne infection
b. A community-acquired infection
c. A viral infection
d. A superinfection

3. Match the following:

1. The skin, the hair, the acidic condition of the stomach and intestines	a. Active production or receipt of antibodies
2. Antigen-antibody response	b. The second line of defense against infection
3. Acquired immunity	
4. The inflammatory response	c. The first line of defense against infection
5. Natural active acquired immunity	d. Antibodies acquired by having a particular disease
	e. The third line of defense against infection

4. There is currently less reason to be concerned about contracting HIV because there is improved treatment and the disease is no longer fatal.

a. True
b. False

5. Hepatitis B and hepatitis C are bloodborne viral infections. When you are caring for persons known to have either of these diseases, use the following infection control techniques:

a. Wear gloves if you may come in contact with blood or body substances.
b. Wear goggles if there is a possibility of your being splashed with blood or body substances.
c. Wear a particulate mask at all times.
d. Wear a waterproof gown or apron if there is a possibility that your clothing may be splashed by blood or body substances.
e. a and b are correct.

6. Explain the difference between Tier 1 and Tier 2 infection control precautions.

7. A person who has recently been infected with HIV may have no symptoms of disease but is able to transmit HIV to another person.

a. True
b. False

8. HIV, or the disease that it produces, is transmitted by direct or indirect contact with infected blood or body substances.

a. True
b. False

9. Match the following agencies with their particular function:

1. Food and Drug Administration	a. Conducts multicenter studies on diseases and publishes a weekly outline on the statistics of infectious diseases in the United States
2. Centers for Disease Control and Prevention	
3. World Health Organization	b. Receives data concerning infectious disease from all countries and compiles a report for every country
4. The Joint Commission	
5. The U.S. Department of Health and Human Services	c. Regulates the manufacture and sale of medications to protect health of U.S. citizens
	d. Sets requirements for hospital safety and infection control practices
	e. Controls disposal of medical waste

10. The radiographer should always dress for the workplace with infection control in mind. This means that:

a. Clothing must be washable; fingernails must be kept short; shoes must be comfortable and have closed toes; and no jewelry is worn except a wristwatch and a wedding band.
b. The radiographer must look unattractive because anything that looks good spreads infection.
c. A scrub suit must be worn at all times.
d. The rules are to be followed when JCAHO is inspecting the institution in which you work.

11. Microorganisms that need a host cell to reproduce and are virtually unresponsive to antimicrobial drugs are:

a. Bacteria
b. Fungi
c. Protozoa
d. Viruses

12. When a person is in the incubation period of the disease process, the radiographer has no control over its transmission.

a. True
b. False

13. The radiographer must use strict infection control measures that include blood and body substance precautions for:

a. Every patient who enters the diagnostic imaging department
b. Patients who have known communicable diseases
c. Only patients who have AIDS and hepatitis B
d. Patients who seem ill

14. Blood and body substance precautions include:

a. Use of clean, disposable gloves for sick persons

b. Use of clean, disposable gloves for contact of the hands with blood or body fluids, a mask and goggles if blood or body fluids may spray on your face, and a gown if the blood and body fluids may touch your clothing for any patient care that may involve contact with blood or body fluids

c. Clean, disposable gloves as necessary

d. Gown, gloves, mask, and goggles for all patient care

15. The most common means of spreading infection are:
   a. Soiled instruments
   b. Infected patients
   c. Human hands
   d. Domestic animals

16. The elements needed to produce an infection are a source, a host, and a means of transmission. An example of a source of infection might be:
   a. A radiography student who has a cold and comes to work
   b. A visitor in the hospital who has a "fever blister" on her mouth
   c. A patient who develops pneumonia
   d. a, b, and c

17. A safety precaution that must be taken when disposing of used hypodermic needles and syringes is:
   a. To place tie needles in tie waste basket as soon as possible
   b. To recap the needle and dispose of it quickly
   c. To place the syringe immediately after use with the uncapped needle attached directly into the contaminated waste receptacle provided
   d. To detach the needle from the syringe and place only the needle in the contaminated waste receptacle

18. Match the following means of transmitting infection with the correct definition:
   1. Touching objects that have been contaminated with disease-producing microbes
   2. Ingesting contaminated water, food, drugs, or blood
   3. Inhaling air contaminated with infectious microbes
   4. Contact with secretions transferred by sneezing, coughing, or talking

   a. Direct contact
   b. Indirect contact
   c. Droplet contact
   d. Vehicle contact
   e. Airborne contact

5. Touching contaminated material with hands

19. When caring for a patient whom you know to be infected with HIV and who does not have AIDS, you use standard blood and body fluid precautions and:
   a. Share the information with the technologist in the next room who has no contact with the patient
   b. Keep all information concerning the patient confidential
   c. Keep the patient's chart in a place where it cannot be read by others
   d. b and c are correct

20. The radiographer who has received a needle-stick injury is obliged to notify his supervisor at the end of the work day.
   A. True
   B. False

21. Hand hygiene is to be used in the following situations by radiographers in the workplace:
   a. Before caring for a patient
   b. After caring for a patient
   c. When preparing for invasive procedures
   d. a and c are correct
   e. a, b, and c are correct

22. If it is not possible to find a sink to wash hands, it is safe to use alcohol-based hand rubs.
   a. True
   b. False

23. The route of transmission of MRSA, VRE, VRSA, and ESBL is
   a. Droplet contact
   b. Airborne contact
   c. Direct contact
   d. Vector contact

24. When the radiographer is to enter the newborn nursery, he must do the following:
   a. Always wear a cap and mask
   b. Always scrub his hands for 3 minutes
   c. Always clean his equipment with disinfectant solution
   d. a and b are correct
   e. b and c are correct

25. The radiographer entering the room of a patient with tuberculosis must wear the following:
   a. Gloves
   b. An N95 respirator mask
   c. Gown and waterproof apron
   d. a and b are correct
   e. Only b is correct

CHAPTER 5

Surgical Asepsis and the Radiographer

STUDENT LEARNING OUTCOMES

After studying this chapter, the student will be able to:

1. Define surgical asepsis and differentiate between medical and surgical asepsis.
2. Explain the radiographer's responsibility for maintaining surgical aseptic technique when it is a required part of patient care.
3. Differentiate between **disinfection** and **sterilization.**
4. Explain the methods the radiographer must use to determine the sterility of an item or pack to be used for an invasive procedure.
5. List the rules for surgical asepsis.
6. Demonstrate the correct method of opening a sterile pack and placing a sterile object on a sterile field.
7. Demonstrate the correct method of donning a sterile gown and sterile gloves.
8. Demonstrate the skin preparation for a sterile procedure.
9. Explain the radiographer's responsibilities for the safety of the surgical team, the patient, and himself in the operating room.
10. Demonstrate the correct method of removing and reapplying a sterile dressing.

KEY TERMS

Aseptic technique: Use of methods that totally exclude microorganisms as one works

Being scrubbed: Indicates that the person is dressed in sterile gown and gloves and is engaged in a sterile procedure

Disinfectant: A chemical capable of destroying microorganisms or inhibiting their growth; same as antiseptic

Disinfection: Destruction of microorganisms and their spores by means of chemicals or physical agents

Fenestrated drape: A drape with one or more openings

Sterilization: Destruction of microbes by steam under pressure or other means, both chemical or physical

Surgical asepsis differs from medical asepsis. Medical asepsis is defined as any practice that helps reduce the number and spread of microorganisms. *Surgical asepsis* is defined as the complete removal of microorganisms and their spores from the surface of an object. The practice of surgical asepsis begins with cleaning the object in question using the principles of medical asepsis followed by a sterilization process.

Any medical procedure that involves penetration of body tissues (an invasive procedure) requires the use of surgical aseptic technique. This includes major and minor surgical procedures, administration of parenteral medications, invasive imaging procedures, catheterization of the urinary bladder, tracheostomy care, and dressing changes. Skin preparation including scrubbing and, at times, hair removal precede invasive procedures. This prevents contamination of the operative site, thereby reducing chances of infection. The radiographer may be responsible for the skin preparation in his department and must learn to perform this procedure effectively.

The radiographer will be required to perform diagnostic radiography in the operating room (also called the OR or surgical suite) where he must work without contaminating the sterile fields. Without an understanding of surgical asepsis, this would not be possible. Surgical asepsis is also routinely practiced in the special procedures areas of the imaging department. The radiographer must be able to recognize breaches in **aseptic technique** and be able to remedy the problem quickly if he is responsible. If contamination is unrecognized, infection may result. It is the duty of all health care workers who participate in procedures requiring the use of surgical asepsis to be able to maintain strict surgical aseptic technique at all times to ensure the well-being of the patient.

ENVIRONMENT AND SURGICAL ASEPSIS

To review, in Chapter 4 of this text, the methods of microbe transmission are by direct, indirect, vehicle, and airborne routes. Every possible effort is made in the surgical suite and in special procedures areas to protect the patient from infection. Barriers that limit the source of contamination are used for this purpose. All persons who enter the surgical suite or special procedure areas are expected to follow the rules established to maintain these barriers. There are theoretically three zones designated in the surgical suite to help decrease the incidents of infection. They are:

Zone 1: An unrestricted zone: persons may enter in street clothing.

Zone 2: A semi-restricted zone: only persons dressed in scrub dress with hair covered and shoes covered may enter.

Zone 3: A restricted zone: only persons wearing scrub dress, shoe covers, and masks are allowed to be present. If a surgical procedure is in progress, the doors to this area are kept closed, and only persons directly involved in the procedure may be present. Those directly involved in the operation are dressed in sterile gowns and sterile gloves. They are often referred to as **"being scrubbed."**

Surgical departments have dress and behavior protocols that are strictly enforced. The radiographer who is assigned to work in this area is expected to follow these protocols as designated by OSHA. They are as follows:

1. Shoes must be comfortable with closed heel and toe and not cloth covered. Cloth-covered shoes may allow blood, body fluids, and other liquids to permeate. Cloth-covered shoes will not protect the feet should a heavy object fall on them.

2. Personal hygiene must be meticulous. A shower should be taken shortly before beginning a work day in the operating room or special procedure area.

3. Jewelry, long or artificial fingernails, and nail polish are prohibited. Jewelry harbors microorganisms as do long, polished, or artificial nails.

4. Any body piercing jewelry must be removed as it may become loose and fall onto the sterile field.

5. All persons who expect to proceed from the unrestricted zone into the semi-restricted zone must go to the dressing area, don a scrub suit, and tuck the blouse of the suit into the pants or wear a scrub blouse that fits close to the body.

6. All hair, beards, or mustaches must be covered with a surgical cap and mask. Hair must be confined as it sheds microorganisms with movement (Fig. 5-1).

7. Shoe covers must be placed over shoes to reduce contamination and to protect shoes from coming in contact with blood and body fluids.

8. Before proceeding into Zone 3, all persons must scrub hands and arms for medical asepsis. It is believed that bare skin may shed microorganisms. In many institutions, all who are not scrubbed for the surgical procedure must wear a scrub jacket to cover bare arms.

9. Before entering a room where a surgical procedure is in progress, a mask must be donned. The masks worn in the OR must be single, high-filtration masks (Rothrock, 2007).

The mask protects the patient from droplets expelled by personnel and protects the health care worker from pathogenic organisms in the surgical environment. The mask must cover nose and mouth and must not gap. The ties should not cross because it may create venting (Fig. 5-2). Since they are regarded as highly contaminated, masks must be worn for only one procedure and then discarded by touching only the ties of the mask and dropping into the receptacle for this purpose. A mask must not be placed around the neck to be worn again (Fig. 5-3).

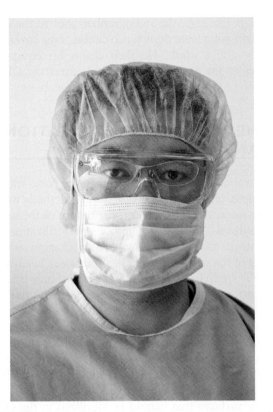

FIGURE 5-1   All hair, beards, or mustaches must be covered by surgical cap and mask.

Sterile linens and other equipment and supplies used for sterile procedures must be packaged in a particular manner to be considered safe for use. They are also stored in a particular manner that protects them from contamination. Any break in sterile technique increases the patient's susceptibility to infection. Those involved in carrying out a sterile procedure must constantly be aware of which areas and articles are sterile. If a sterile article is touched by a nonsterile one, it must be replaced by an article that is sterile. The radiographer must learn correct methods of opening sterile packs and donning sterile gown and gloves.

The use of contaminated instruments or gloves, a wet or damp sterile field, or microorganisms blown onto a surgical site are the most common causes of contamination. Ventilating ducts in the operating room must have special filters to prevent dust particles from entering the room. Airflow and humidity must be controlled to prevent static electricity. Doors must remain closed and traffic into and out of the room must be carefully controlled. When the radiographer must use radiographic equipment that is not stationary in the OR suite, he must carefully clean it with a disinfectant solution before bringing it into the operating room.

Conversation in the OR or special procedures room is kept to a minimum. The radiographer must always be aware that the surgeon is in charge while performing a surgical or invasive procedure. The

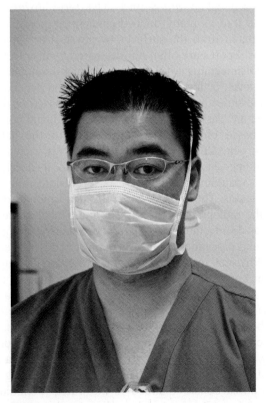

FIGURE 5-2   Mask must cover the nose and mouth and must not gap.

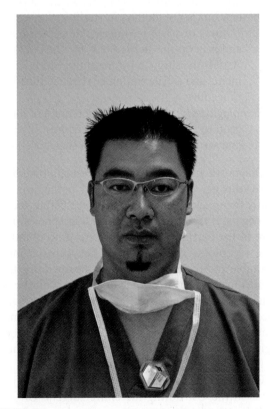

FIGURE 5-3   A mask must not be placed around the neck to be worn again.

environment is often tense as the patient's life is at risk and needless conversation is not welcome.

The radiographer or student radiographer whose work involves sterile procedures must develop a sense of responsibility and maintain the highest standards possible when practicing surgical asepsis. The patient's welfare depends on this.

THE SURGICAL TEAM

The surgical team consists of a variety of staff members who serve the patient prior to and during surgery. They are as follows:

Surgeon: the physician who plans and performs the surgical procedure and makes surgical decisions.
Surgical assistant: usually another surgeon or surgical resident. There may be several assistants if the patient's surgical needs require this.
Anesthesiologist: a physician with special education in anesthesia who makes the decisions concerning type of anesthesia required.
Nurse anesthetist: a registered nurse who has had special education in anesthesia who administers anesthesia and monitors the anesthetized patient under the supervision of the anesthesiologist.
Circulating nurse: oversees the safety of the patient and maintains the surgical environment; is attired in scrub suit, cap, mask, and shoe covers, but is not clothed in sterile attire.
Scrub nurse or scrub technician: dons sterile attire and sets up the sterile fields for the operation. Assists the surgeon by presenting sterile instruments and sterile equipment needed during the procedure.
Radiologic technologist: present at request of the surgeon to perform imaging procedures; is clothed in a scrub suit, cap, mask, and shoe covers.

Diagnostic imaging is often performed immediately before, during, and after a surgical procedure. Frequently the image receptors are in place before the surgery begins. If this is the case, the radiographer must be aware of the corridor that he must travel to obtain the image receptors. The corridor is between the instrument table and the sterile drapes on the operating table. He must take care not to come in contact with the sterile fields. Each situation varies; however, the maintenance of the sterile fields is mandatory. Many members of the surgical team work behind the scenes to prepare surgical packs; procure, clean, and repair instruments; and limit contamination of the surgical suite.

Often procedures are planned, and the radiographer is in the OR during the entire surgery. On some occasions, the need for a radiographer is not planned, and he is called to come to the OR at a moment's notice.

If this is the case, the radiographer goes to the designated dressing area, dons scrub clothes, hair cover, shoe covers, and a mask. He then cleans his equipment, washes as for medical asepsis, and enters the OR. He will then receive direction from the surgeon.

METHODS OF STERILIZATION AND DISINFECTION

Removal of microorganisms and their spores must be complete, or the article is not sterile. Methods used to attain sterilization depend on the nature of the item to be sterilized. All effective methods of sterilization have advantages and disadvantages. The packaging and sterilizing of items used for medical purposes has become a highly specialized field and is described only briefly in this text as it is not within the scope of the radiographer's practice to perform these tasks.

Whatever method of sterilization is used, there are indicators placed in the center and outside of each pack to indicate that an item is sterile. The radiographer must learn the code used in his institution and always be certain that the items are sterile prior to use. Articles or surfaces that cannot be sterilized in the OR or special procedures areas must be disinfected. Tables, floors, walls, and equipment used in areas where the patient is to have an invasive procedure are included in this category. Skin around the area to be penetrated is also disinfected. When skin is disinfected, the solutions used are called *antiseptics*. The term *disinfection* means that as many microorganisms as possible are eliminated from the surfaces by physical or chemical means. Spores are often not destroyed by disinfection.

Disinfectants are categorized as high-level, intermediate-level, or low-level. This classification depends on their disinfecting ability. Items to be sterilized or disinfected are classified as critical, semicritical, and noncritical based on the risk of infection for the patient (Rothrock, 2007). This classification is called the Spaulding Classification System named for its developer, Earle Spaulding. Table 5-1 lists the disinfectants and their status. The information in this text is not adequate for the radiographer to use if he must incorporate the use of disinfectants into his practice. Further information and precautionary measures must be researched.

Physical methods of disinfecting are boiling in water and ultraviolet irradiation. Boiling may be used as a means of disinfection if no other method is available; however, many spores are able to resist the heat of boiling (212°F or 100°C) for many hours. To increase the effectiveness of boiling, sodium carbonate may be added to the water in quantity to make a 2% solution. If an object is to be disinfected by boiling and sodium carbonate is added to the water, it should be boiled for 15 minutes. If sodium carbonate is not added, boiling time should be 30 minutes.

TABLE 5-1   Commonly Used Disinfectants

Disinfectant	Status	Use
Alcohols (70% or 90%) (intermediate-level)	bactericidal, tuberculocidal, fungicidal, and virucidal	to disinfect thermometers, medication vials, etc.
Glutaraldehyde (high-level)	broad antimicrobial range, fungicidal and virucidal	to disinfect endoscopes, thermometers, and rubber items
Chlorine Compounds (dilution of 1:50 is high-level)	concentrations of 1000 ppm inactivate bacterial spores	to disinfect countertops, floors, other surfaces
Orthophthalaldehyde (high-level)	bactericidal, virucidal, fungicidal, tuberculocidal in 12 minutes at room temperature	to clean and process endoscopes
Hydrogen Peroxide (low-level)	6% solutions effective against some bacteria, fungi, and viruses	may be used to clean work surfaces, not widely used in health care settings
Iodine and Iodophors (intermediate-level)	vegetative bactericidal, *M. tuberculosis*, most viruses and fungi, no sporicidal capability	may be used as disinfectant or antiseptic
Phenolics (intermediate- or low-level)	most formulations are tuberculocidal, bactericidal, virucidal, and fungicidal	have toxic effects, used as environmental not sporicidal disinfectants
Quaternary Ammonium Compounds	not recommended for high-, intermediate- or low-level disinfection	cleaning agents for noncritical surfaces

This is not a practical means of disinfecting for hospital use, because there is no assurance that the ultraviolet has actually come into contact with the microbes, which are constantly in a mobile state because of air currents.

METHODS OF STERILIZATION

Removal of microorganisms and their spores must be complete or the article is not sterile. Methods used to attain sterilization depend upon the nature of the item to be sterilized. Table 5-2 lists the common methods used with a brief description of each.

RULES FOR SURGICAL ASEPSIS

The basic rules for surgical aseptic technique apply whenever and wherever the sterile procedure is performed. The radiographer must commit these rules to memory and use them in his own department and elsewhere as necessary.

1. Know which areas and objects are sterile and which are not.
2. If the sterility of an object is questionable, it is *not* to be considered sterile.
3. Sterile objects and persons must be kept separate from those that are nonsterile.
4. When any item that must be sterile becomes contaminated, the contamination must be remedied immediately.
5. When tabletops are to be used as areas for creating a sterile field, they must be clean, and a sterile drape must be placed over them.
6. Personnel must be clothed in a sterile gown and sterile gloves if they are to be considered sterile.
7. Any sterile instrument or sterile area that is touched by a nonsterile object or person is considered contaminated by microorganisms.
8. A contaminated area on a sterile field must be covered by a folded sterile towel or drape of double thickness.
9. If a sterile person's gown or gloves become contaminated, they must be changed.

TABLE 5-2   Methods of Sterilization

Steam Under Pressure: Item are double-wrapped and placed in an autoclave.
Autoclaves are manufactured to sterilize by *gravity displacement and dynamic air removal.*
High-speed sterilizers or *flash sterilization* is an abbreviated gravity displacement method.

Chemical Sterilization: Referred to as *low-temperature sterilization.* A maximum temperature of 54° C to 60° C of gaseous sterilization is used. An antimicrobial and sporicidal agent must be used.

Ethylene Oxide: Used for items that cannot withstand moisture and high temperatures.
All items sterilized in this manner must be cleansed and dried since water united with ethylene oxide forms ethylene glycol, which cannot be eliminated by aeration and is toxic.

10. A sterile field must be created just prior to use.
11. Once a sterile field has been prepared, it must not be left unattended as it may become contaminated and presumed to be sterile.
12. An unsterile person does not reach across a sterile field.
13. A sterile person does not lean over an unsterile area.
14. A sterile field ends at the level of the tabletop or at the waist of the sterile person's gown.
15. Anything that drops below the tabletop or sterile person's waistline is no longer sterile and may not be brought up to the sterile tabletop. The only parts of the sterile gown considered sterile are the areas from the waist to the shoulders in front and the sleeves from 2 inches above the elbow to the cuffs.
16. The cuffs of the sterile gown are considered non-sterile because they collect moisture. Cuffs must always be covered by sterile gloves.
17. The edges of a sterile wrapper are not considered sterile and must not touch a sterile object.
18. Sterile drapes are placed by a sterile person. The sterile person places the drapes on the area closest to him first to protect his sterile gown.
19. A sterile person must remain within the sterile area. He must not lean on tables or against the wall.
20. If one sterile person must pass another, they must pass back-to-back.
21. The sterile person faces the sterile field and keeps sterile gloves above the waist in front of his chest. The sterile person must avoid touching any area of his body.
22. Any sterile material or pack that becomes damp or wet is considered unsterile.
23. Any objects that are wet with disinfectant solution and are to be placed on a sterile field must be placed on a folded sterile towel for the moisture to be absorbed.
24. A wet area on a sterile field must be covered with several thicknesses of sterile toweling or an impervious drape.

25. When pouring sterile solution, place the lid face upward and do not touch the inside of the lid or the lip of the flask. Pour off a small amount of solution before the remainder is poured into the sterile container.
26. When a sterile solution is to be poured into a container on a sterile field, the container is placed at the edge of the sterile field by the sterile person (Fig. 5-4).

CALL OUT!

If the sterility of an item is questionable, it is not to be considered sterile.

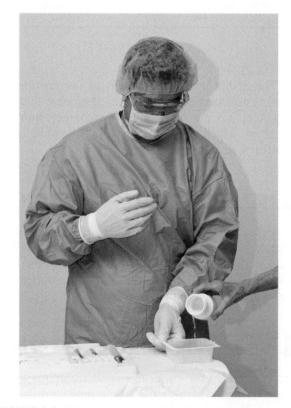

FIGURE 5-4   Place container at edge of sterile field to pour sterile liquid.

Opening Sterile Packs

The radiographer will be called upon to open commercially wrapped sterile packs and place sterile objects on sterile fields. He must be able to do this without contaminating the sterile object or the sterile field.

Commercial packs are usually wrapped in paper or plastic wrappers. They are frequently sealed in plastic to ensure prolonged sterility. Directions for opening the containers to avoid contamination are usually printed on the pack and should be read before opening. Never cut packs open or pierce them with a knife or sharp object. Do not tear packs open and do not allow the contents to slide over the edges of the pack. The usual procedure for opening a sterile pack is as follows:

1. Place the pack on a clean tabletop with the sealed end toward the radiographer.

2. Remove the outer plastic as directed and place the sealed end toward the radiographer (Fig. 5-5A).

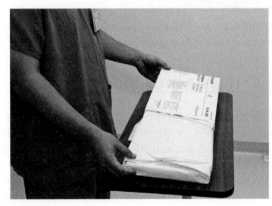

FIGURE 5-5   (A) Place sealed end of sterile pack toward radiographer.

3. Open corner 1 back and away from the pack (Fig. 5-5B).

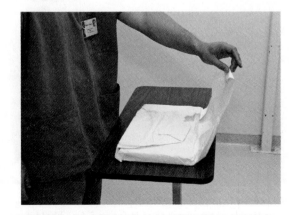

FIGURE 5-5   (B) Open first corner back and away.

4. Next, open corners 2 and 3 (Fig. 5-5C).

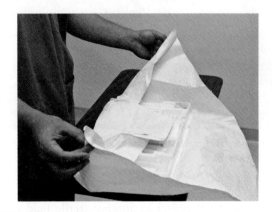

FIGURE 5-5   (C) Open corners 2 and 3.

5. Then open corner 4 and drop it toward the radiographer (Fig. 5-5D).

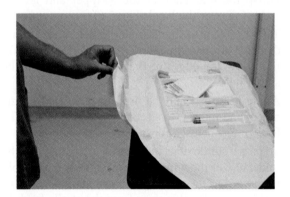

FIGURE 5-5   (D) Open corner and drop it toward radiographer.

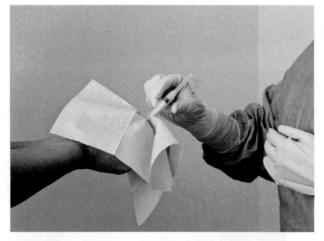

FIGURE 5-6   Grasp the underside of the wrapper and let edges fall over hand.

To move a sterile object to another sterile field or to pass a sterile object to a sterile person, the procedure is as follows:

1.   Open the package as directed in Figure 5-5A-D.
2.   Grasp the underside of the wrapper and let the edges fall over the hand (Fig. 5-6).
3.   Take the item to the next sterile field and, from a distance, drop or flip it onto the field (Fig. 5-7). Do not allow the edges of the wrapper to touch the sterile field.
4.   A sterile forcep may be used to pick up a sterile object and move it to a second field (Fig. 5-8). The forcep may be used for one transfer only.
5.   To pass a sterile object to a sterile person, grasp the underside of the wrapper as in Figure 5-6 and hold it forward to the sterile person so that he may take it (Fig. 5-9). Do this away from the sterile field.

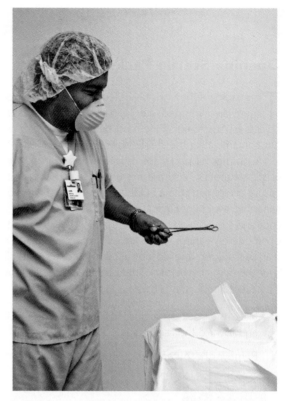

FIGURE 5-8   A sterile forceps may be used to pick up a sterile object and move it to a second sterile field.

▮ THE SURGICAL SCRUB

Although the radiographer is not often the "sterile person" in the OR or the special procedures rooms, he must be able to perform the surgical scrub if the situation calls for it. Before entering the surgical suite, the radiographer must change into a scrub suit, cover hair with a cap, cover shoes, and place a mask over mouth and nose. Remove all jewelry. If ear studs are worn,

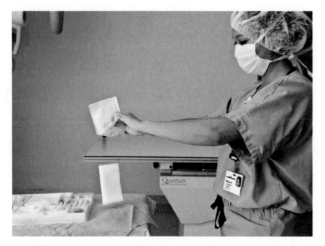

FIGURE 5-7   Take the item to sterile field and drop it on sterile field from a distance.

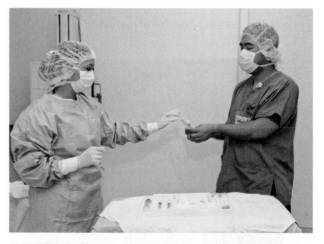

FIGURE 5-9   To pass a sterile object to a sterile person, grasp the underside of the wrapper as in Figure 5-6 and hold it forward to sterile person away from sterile field.

they must be covered by the cap. If the radiographer is not to scrub, he must perform hand washing for 3 minutes using an antiseptic soap.

The surgical scrub varies from institution to institution, but the purpose is always the same—that is, to remove as many microorganisms as possible from the skin of the hands and lower arms by mechanical and chemical means and running water before a sterile procedure is begun. If the radiographer is known to have an allergy to latex, he must inform the person preparing sterile gloves, so that a pair that is latex free can be in place. The procedure in this text is adequate for most cases. It is as follows:

1. Any person, including the radiographer, who will be present and unable to protect himself from radiation must don a lead apron prior to beginning the scrub. Arms should be bare to at least 4 inches above the elbow.

2. Approach the sink. Adjust the water temperature and pressure. Most surgical scrub areas have either foot or knee pedals to regulate water flow.

3. Obtain a scrub brush. Brushes must be single-use and disposable. Many have an antimicrobial agent permeated through them. The hands and forearms are wet to approximately 2 inches above the elbow. Hands must be held up to allow the water to drain downward toward the elbow from cleanest to dirtiest area. Apply the antimicrobial agent (Fig. 5-10).

4. Scrub hands and arms using a firm, rotary motion. Fingers, hands, and arms should be considered to have four sides, all of which must be thoroughly cleansed. Follow an anatomical pattern, beginning with the thumb and proceeding to each finger. Next, do the dorsal surface of the hand, the palm, and up the wrist, ending 2 inches above the elbow. Wash all four sides of the arm. The surgical scrub always begins with the hands because they are in direct contact with the sterile field (Fig. 5-11A-C). Rinse the soap from hands and arms and repeat the procedure.

5. When the scrub is completed, drop the brush into the sink or a receptacle prepared to receive used brushes. Do not touch the sink or the receptacle. Hold hands up above the waist and higher than the elbows during the surgical scrub.

6. Proceed to the area where a sterile towel, sterile gown, and sterile gloves have been prepared.

7. Pick up the towel, which is folded on top of the sterile gown, by one corner and let it drop and unfold in front of you at waist level. Do not let the towel touch the scrub suit (Fig. 5-12).

8. Dry one hand and one arm with each end of the towel. Do not go over areas already dried (Fig. 5-13).

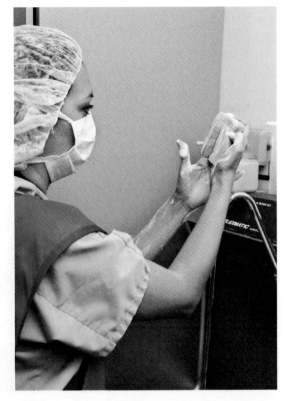

FIGURE 5-10 Approach sink, wet arms from hands and arms to 2 inches above elbows, and apply antimicrobial agent.

9. When hands and arms are dry, drop the towel to the floor or into a receptacle for this purpose. Do not let hands drop below the waist.

STERILE GOWNING AND GLOVING

If the radiographer must open his own sterile gown and towel pack, he must do this before he begins the surgical scrub. The gown is made either of a synthetic nonwoven material or of cloth. To put it on, follow these simple steps:

1. Grasp the gown and remove it from the table.

2. Step away from the table. The gown is folded inside out.

3. Hold the gown away from the body and allow it to unfold lengthwise without touching the floor (Fig. 5-14).

4. Open the gown and hold it by the shoulder seams. Place both arms into the armholes of the gown and wait for assistance (Fig. 5-15).

An assistant or the circulating nurse will place their hands inside the gown over your shoulders and pull the

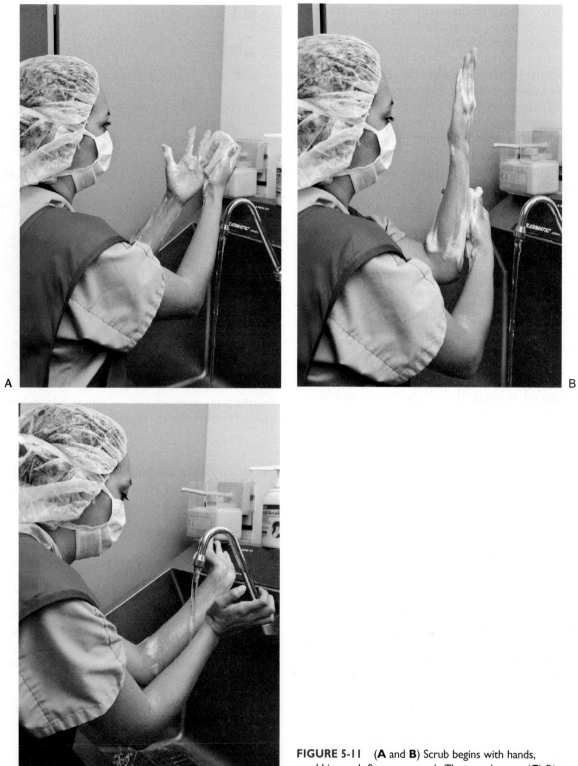

A

B

C

FIGURE 5-11 (**A** and **B**) Scrub begins with hands, scrubbing each finger separately. Then scrub arms. (**C**) Rinse from hands to arms.

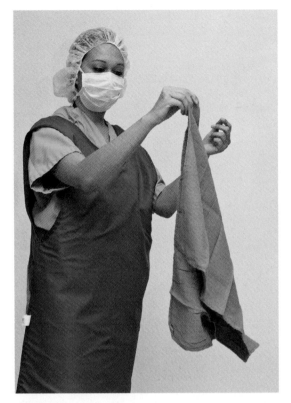

FIGURE 5-12 Pick up towel by one corner and let it drop in from of the radiographer at waist level.

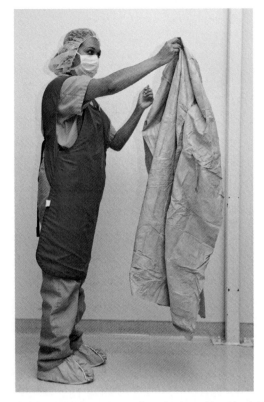

FIGURE 5-14 Hold gown away from body and let it unfold.

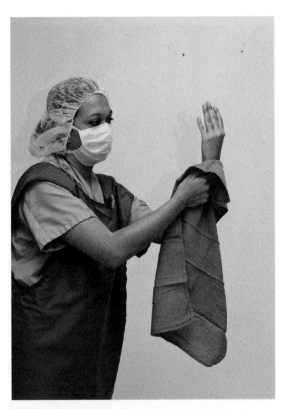

FIGURE 5-13 Dry one hand and one arm with each corner of the towel.

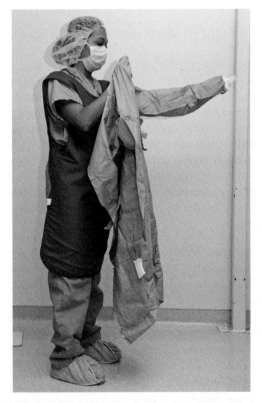

FIGURE 5-15 Open gown and hold it at shoulder seams and place arms in sleeves.

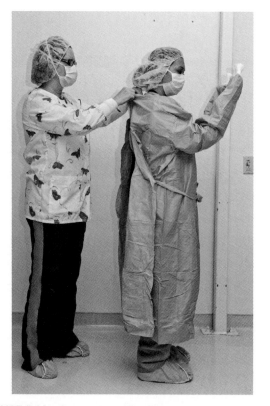

FIGURE 5-16   An assistant will pull gown over shoulders until hands are exposed.

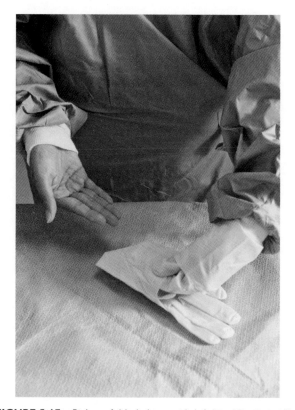

FIGURE 5-17   Pick up folded glove with left hand leaving cuff folded.

gown over the shoulders until your hands are exposed (Fig. 5-16).

The radiographer is then ready to don sterile gloves. There are two methods of gloving, open and closed. For the radiographer's purposes, open gloving is most practical and will be discussed. Setting up for a sterile procedure, catheterization of the urinary bladder, and several other procedures require the radiographer to don sterile gloves, but not a sterile gown. If this is the case, the radiographer must wash his hands according to the rules of medical asepsis and then don the gloves by the open method. The procedure is as follows:

1. Open the wrapper as directed for opening sterile packs. Sterile gloves are always packaged folded down at the cuff and powdered so they may be put on more easily.
2. Glove the dominant hand first. Assuming that the right hand is the dominant hand, pick up the right glove with the left hand at the folded cuff and slide the right hand into the glove, leaving the cuff folded down (Fig. 5-17).
3. When the glove is over the hand, leave it and pick up the left glove with the gloved right hand under the fold (Fig. 5-18).

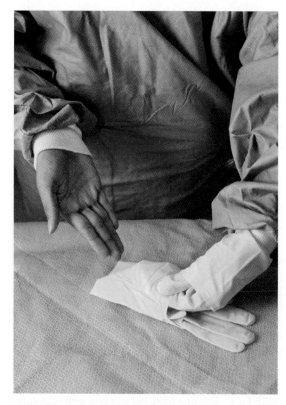

FIGURE 5-18   When the glove the is over the hand, leave it and pick up the left glove with gloved right hand under fold.

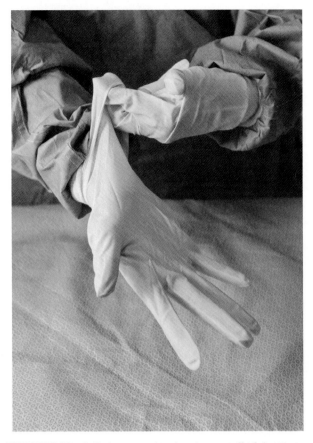

FIGURE 5-19   Pull glove over hand and over cuff of the gown.

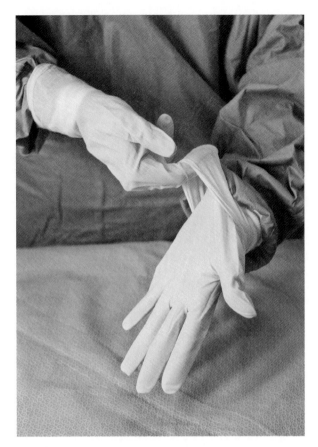

FIGURE 5-20   Place fingers of gloved left hand under cuff of right glove and pull it over cuff of gown.

4. Pull the glove over your hand and over the cuff of the gown (if you are wearing a sterile gown) in one motion (Fig. 5-19).

Next, place the fingers of the gloved left hand under the cuff of the right glove and pull it over the cuff of the gown (Fig. 5-20). The gloves may then be adjusted if necessary to disinfect thermometers, medication vials, etc.

RADIOGRAPHY IN THE OPERATING ROOM AND SPECIAL PROCEDURE AREA

The radiographer is responsible for protecting himself and all persons in the OR and special procedure areas from radiation. He is also expected to be knowledgeable concerning the areas that are sterile. He must protect sterile areas and the patient from contamination in the process of his duties.

The most common types of imaging equipment used in the OR are fixed ceiling or table mounted portables and image intensifiers or C-arms for fluoroscopy. The radiographer is responsible for making certain that any radiographic equipment used during a sterile procedure is clean and dust-free before use. Following are some guidelines for working in the OR or special procedure areas:

1. Overhead units must be cleaned with a disinfectant solution, and portable radiographic machines and image receptors to be used must be cleaned with a disinfectant solution.

2. Sterile technique must be maintained for all items and persons involved in the invasive procedure.

3. If possible, place image receptors and take scout films before draping the patient for the procedure.

4. If the image receptors must be placed after the procedure is begun, the radiographer may pass the image receptor to the scrub nurse who receives the image receptor in a sterile plastic bag and places it at the radiographer's direction.

5. If the radiographer places the image receptor himself, the surgical team must make room for

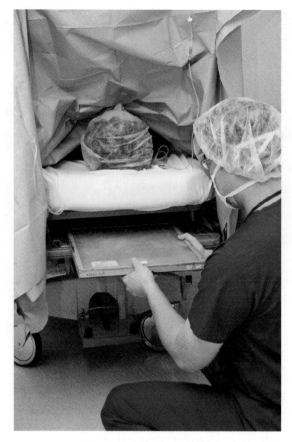

FIGURE 5-21   Raise sterile drapes and place image receptor.

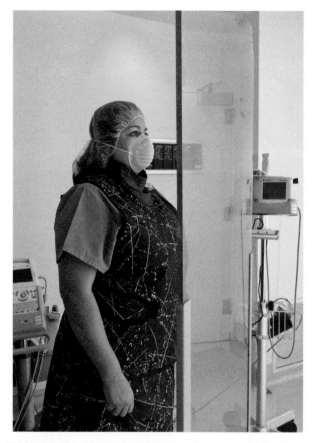

FIGURE 5-22   All members of team who are not involved must step behind protective leaded screen.

him. He may place the image receptor by raising the sterile drapes touching only the inside of the drape, or the circulating nurse may lift the drapes and assist in placing the cassette into the image receptor holder (Fig. 5-21).

6. If multiple images are to be taken, all personnel who are not scrubbed must leave the OR if at all possible. The scrubbed members of the team must wear protective radiation apparel. They may also step behind protective lead-lined screens (Fig. 5-22).

7. When hands are directly exposed to radiation, leaded sterile gloves as well as all other protective equipment must be worn.

8. Pregnant female personnel should not be present in the OR when radiographic imaging is in progress.

9. The radiographer must wear his radiation detection badge on the outside of the lead apron and under the sterile gown during imaging procedures. The badge must be checked at prescribed intervals.

10. During imaging, all unnecessary instruments must be removed from the operative field and a sterile drape must be placed over the open incision.

CALL OUT!

The radiographer must wear his radiation detection badge outside of the lead apron while working in the operating room.

DRAPING FOR A STERILE PROCEDURE

Following the skin prep for a sterile procedure, sterile drapes may be applied. These are used to provide a barrier to infection and also to create a sterile field on which to place sterile instruments. Usually single use, single thickness, impermeable drapes are used; however, some cloth drapes may be chosen. Whatever the material on hand, the process is the same. A **fenestrated drape** is often used, and, if so, the drape should be applied in such a way that the opening leaves only the operative site exposed.

Sterile drapes must be handled as little as possible. They must not be flipped or fanned. If sterile towels are used, place them so that they are within the limits of the area prepared. They are folded so that they overlap

PROCEDURE

Skin Preparation for Sterile Procedures

The radiographer may be called upon to prepare a patient's skin for an invasive procedure in the special procedures area. This is referred to as "*skin prep.*" The purpose of the skin prep is to remove as many microorganisms as possible by mechanical and chemical means to reduce the chances of infection. The antimicrobial agents used for this purpose may vary; however, it must prevent tissue irritation and the rebound growth of microbes. If hair removal from the site is indicated, it will be completed by the radiology nurse. If ordered, it is done as close to the procedure as possible to prevent growth of microorganisms. If no hair removal is required, or is complete, the skin prep follows. For special imaging procedures, a commercial skin prep pack is used. Items the radiographer must have on hand are:

1. Sterile gloves if they are not included in the commercial pack.

2. The sterile prep tray that includes a sterile drape, two small basins, and a set of large sponges with handles to distance the operator's hand from the site. The sponges are permeated with antiseptic soap.

3. A flask of sterile water and a flask of antiseptic solution as recommended by the physician.

4. A sterile towel.

The radiographer proceeds as follows:

1. Approach the patient, explain the procedure, and ascertain allergies to antiseptic to be used. Open the sterile pack as directed earlier in this chapter.

2. Pour sterile water into one small basin and antiseptic solution into the other as directed earlier in this chapter.

3. Don sterile gloves.

4. Inspect the area of skin to be prepped for lesions or unusual appearance. If there is no problem, you may proceed.

5. Pick up one sponge permeated with antiseptic soap and dampen it in the sterile water. Then begin scrubbing in the center of the area to be prepared. The physician will explain how large an area must be prepped; usually an area approximately 6 to 10 inches in diameter is prepped. Work outward in a circular motion using a firm stroke as friction is as important in the removal of microorganisms as the antiseptic soap (Fig. 5-23A).

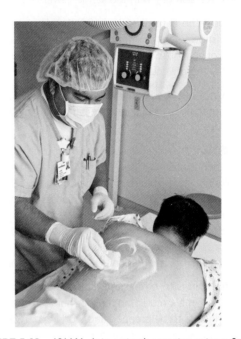

FIGURE 5-23 (**A**) Work in a circular motion using a firm stroke from center outward.

6. Do not go back over the skin that has already been scrubbed with this sponge. When the edges of the area being scrubbed are reached, drop the sponge off the sterile field and repeat the procedure with a second sponge (Fig. 5-23B).

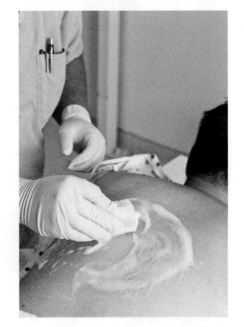

FIGURE 5-23 (**B**) Drop soiled sponge off field and repeat.

(continued)

7. Following the scrub, rinse the skin well with sterile water or wipe away the lather without rinsing if that is the institution's procedure.

8. Blot the skin dry with the sterile towel.

9. Inspect the patient's skin during the skin prep. If the skin shows signs of irritation, stop the procedure and thoroughly rinse off the soap with sterile water and notify the physician.

10. Do not allow solution to drain off the area being prepped or to pool under the patient during the procedure as this may burn the skin.

11. Following the initial scrub, the skin around the area to be penetrated is often painted with an antiseptic solution. This destroys some of the remaining microbes and acts as a deterrent to further microbial growth for a brief period of time. Agents commonly used for skin prep are chlorhexidine and hexachlorophene. Alcohol is not used on mucous membranes or on open wounds as it may cause harm.

12. If the skin is to be painted after the scrub, it is performed in a circular motion beginning in the center of the area to be prepped and working outward (Fig. 5-23C). Allow the skin to dry.

13. If there are no long-handled sponges available, 4 by 4 sterile sponges may be folded and grasped with a sterile ring forceps and dipped into a container of antiseptic solution.

CALL OUT!

Sterile technique is maintained during the skin prep for sterile procedures!

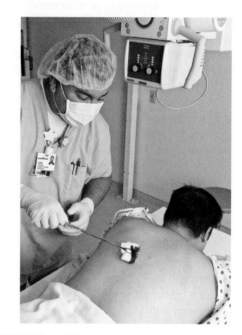

FIGURE 5-23   (C) Paint skin in circular motion beginning at center and working outward.

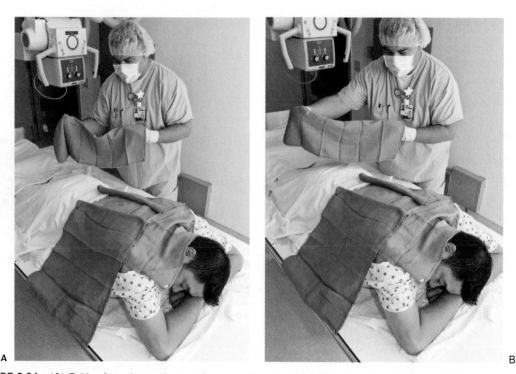

A   B

FIGURE 5-24   (A) Folds of sterile towels must face operative site. **(B)** Pick up first drape holding drape to protect sterile gloves.

and the folds face the operative site. If the radiographer is to place the sterile drapes, the procedure is as follows:

1. Place the pack of sterile drapes on the table on which they are to be opened.
2. Open a pack of sterile gloves.
3. Open the packs as directed earlier in this chapter and don the sterile gloves.

4. Pick up the first drape holding the drape in such a manner that your sterile gloves are protected (Fig. 5-24A). Do not allow the drape to fall below waist level or touch the uniform.
5. Drop the drape in place and do not move it again as the underside is now contaminated (Fig. 5-24B).
6. Add additional drapes as required. If a drape is contaminated during the draping process, it must be replaced.

PROCEDURE

Removing and Re-applying Dressings

If a dressing is to be removed or re-applied, there must be an order from the physician in charge of the patient. If an order has been obtained and a dressing is to be removed for a procedure, the radiographer must be able to remove it without contaminating the wound or himself in the process.

All dressings must be treated as if they are contaminated, because drainage from wounds may harbor pathogenic microorganisms. Before removing a dressing, the radiographer will obtain a plastic bag for infectious waste, a bag closure, clean gloves, and a drape sheet. The procedure is as follows:

1. Wash hands as for medical aseptic procedure.

2. Explain the procedure to the patient and place him or her in a comfortable position.

3. Provide privacy for the patient by closing the door. Keep all of his body covered except the area where the dressing is in place.

4. Loosen the tape holding the patient's dressing in place and then don the clean gloves. It is difficult to manage tape while wearing gloves. Remove the tape with care; if it adheres to the skin and the patient complains of pain, use a commercial tape remover. Pull the tape off toward the wound while supporting the skin with the non-dominant hand.

5. Don the gloves and remove the dressing carefully (Fig. 5-25A). Be cautious when removing the dressing because it may adhere to the wound or there may be a drain in place. If the dressing does adhere to the wound, stop the procedure and call for assistance from the physician or the nurse. Do not forcefully remove a dressing. To do so may damage tissues around the wound or dislodge a drain.

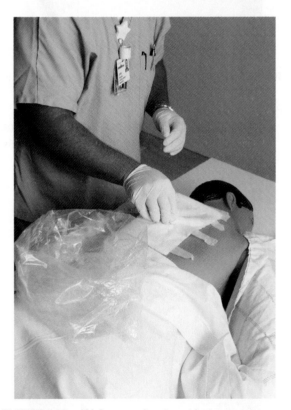

FIGURE 5-25   (A) Remove dressing with care.

6. Assess the dressing for drainage or blood when removed. Inform the physician if a large amount of either is observed.

7. Place the soiled dressing into the bag prepared for it (Fig. 5-25B). Remove the gloves as previously instructed.

(continued)

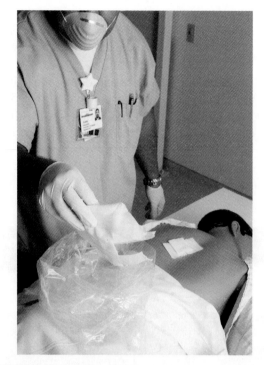

FIGURE 5-25 (B) Place soiled dressing in bag prepared for it.

8. Place your hands under the cuff of the refuse bag and unfold it upward; close the bag with a closure and place it into a receptacle for contaminated waste (Fig. 5-25C). Wash hands.

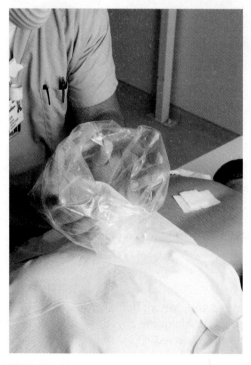

FIGURE 5-25 (C) Place hands under cuff of refuse bag and unfold it upward.

When the radiographer receives an order to reapply a dressing, sterile technique must be used. The procedure is as follows:

1. Assemble the necessary equipment and wash hands. Equipment needed is:

   - A sterile towel or small sterile drape
   - Sterile dressings of the appropriate size and type
   - A sterile container for normal saline if cleansing is necessary
   - A sterile forcep
   - Tape
   - A refuse bag and closure
   - Sterile gloves

2. Approach the patient and explain the procedure.

3. If the soiled dressing has not been removed, remove it in the manner described above.

4. Open the sterile towel or drape to double thickness and use it as a sterile field on which to place the sterile dressings.

5. Open the dressings and drop them onto the sterile field without contaminating them (Fig. 5-26).

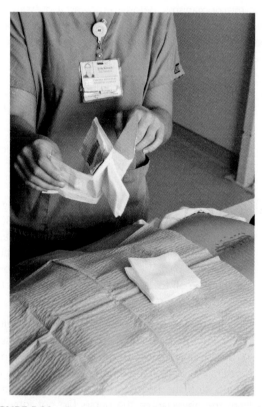

FIGURE 5-26 Open dressings and drop them onto sterile field.

(continued)

6. Prepare the tape by having it cut or torn into lengths needed to keep the new dressing in place. Place tape in a convenient place away from the sterile field.

7. If plan includes cleansing the skin around the wound, pour normal saline into the container prepared for it.

8. Don sterile gloves.

9. Cleanse the skin around the wound with sterile normal saline if necessary. In the following manner: fold gauze sponges and grip them with a sterile forcep; moisten several of the gauze sponges with normal saline and gently cleanse the skin, beginning in the area closest to the wound and moving outward (Fig. 5-27); drop soiled sponges into waste receptacle being careful not to contaminate gloves. Repeat the process if necessary. Do not wash the wound and do not apply medication or antiseptics.

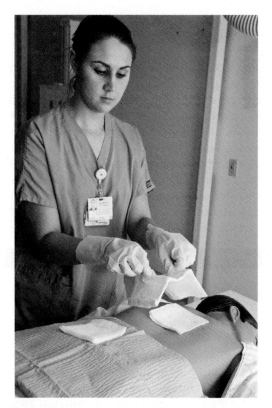

FIGURE 5-28   Apply new sterile dressing.

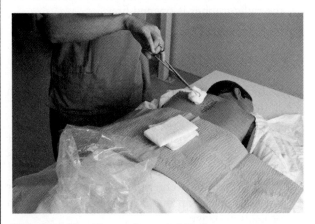

FIGURE 5-27   Cleanse skin with folded gauze sponges.

10. Allow skin to dry. Then apply new sterile dressing (Fig. 5-28). If there is drainage from the wound, apply additional dressing to absorb the drainage.

11. Remove gloves and drop them into the refuse bag.

12. Apply tape to the dressing by applying pressure evenly on both sides of the tape away from the direction of the wound. Do not apply excessive pressure as it may traumatize the skin. Cover the patient and make him comfortable. Dispose of waste correctly.

SUMMARY

Surgical asepsis is defined as the complete removal of microorganisms and their spores. The radiographer must participate in imaging procedures that require the use of surgical asepsis, both in the surgical suite and in his own department. Any health care worker who participates in invasive procedures must practice meticulous surgical asepsis to prevent contamination that may result in infecting the patient. The most common means of spreading microbes in the OR and during special procedures are by using contaminated instruments and gloves, by allowing a sterile field to become damp, and by failing to control air currents across sterile fields. All of these situations are avoidable.

There are several methods of rendering an article sterile, that is, completely removing microorganisms and their spores. These methods are steam under pressure, chemical sterilization, and gas sterilization.

The radiographer must learn the rules of surgical asepsis because all invasive medical procedures require its use. He must learn to differentiate sterile objects from non-sterile objects and to open sterile packs correctly to prevent contamination. When there is a question about the sterility of an item, it is always considered to be nonsterile.

The radiographer must learn to conduct himself in the surgical suite in a manner that prevents contamination. The surgical team is comprised of the surgeon, the surgical assistant, the anesthesiologist, the nurse anesthetist, the circulating nurse, the scrub nurse or operating room technologist, and the staff who prepares and maintains the surgical suite.

A surgical scrub is performed in the OR before a sterile gown and gloves are donned for a surgical procedure. The radiographer is not usually the sterile person in the OR because he will be there to make radiographic images and for operation of the fluoroscope. He is also expected to assist with special procedures in his own department. This may require the use of aseptic technique and, in some instances, the surgical scrub.

Preparation of the skin for surgical penetration involves removing as many microorganisms as possible from the operative site to reduce the possibility of infection. Mechanical and chemical methods are used to prepare the skin, followed by application of sterile drapes around the operative site.

The radiographer may be required to remove or reapply a dressing. He must perform these procedures using aseptic technique. Any dressing that is removed must be assumed to harbor pathogenic microorganisms. Soiled dressings must not be touched with bare hands. The soiled dressings must be wrapped in a waterproof bag and disposed of correctly to prevent contamination.

When dressings are removed or reapplied, the patient must be protected from infection and injury. The radiographer must also protect himself and others in his department. Use of aseptic technique and proper methods of waste disposal will accomplish these goals.

CHAPTER 5 TEST

1. Differentiate between medical and surgical asepsis.
2. Match the need for medical or surgical asepsis to the following procedures:
   a. Measuring vital signs
   b. Administering an intravenous contrast agent
   c. Taking a flat plate image of the abdomen
   d. Re-applying a dressing
   e. Catheterization of the urinary bladder

   1. Surgical asepsis
   2. Surgical asepsis
   3. Surgical asepsis
   4. Medical asepsis
   5. Medical asepsis

3. When entering a surgical suite and preparing to enter Zone 2, the radiographer must:
   a. Change into a scrub suit
   b. Change his shoes
   c. Change into a scrub suit, don shoe covers, and cover his/her hair
   d. Perform a surgical scrub
   e. Wear a mask
4. List the three most common causes of contamination of a surgical site.
5. Maintenance of the sterile field is the duty of only the circulating nurse.
   a. True
   b. False
6. Disinfectants are categorized depending on their ability to disinfect. Alcohol is considered an intermediate-level disinfectant. This means that it:
   a. May be used to disinfect surgical instruments
   b. May be used to disinfect work surfaces
   c. May be used to disinfect thermometers and medication vials
   d. Is toxic and may not be used
7. If there is a question about the sterility of an item, the radiographer must:
   a. Use it as if it were sterile
   b. Call the radiologist and ask him about the item
   c. Consider it unsterile and replace it

8. When opening a sterile wrapper, the fold closest to the radiographer is opened first.
   a. True
   b. False
9. The purpose of the surgical scrub is:
   a. To sterilize the skin of the person scrubbing
   b. To remove as many microbes as possible from the skin
   c. To cleanse the skin of the person scrubbing
10. List three responsibilities of the radiographer in the operating room or special procedures room.
11. When preparing to enter the OR, the radiographer must don a lead apron. He may wear his radiation protection badge:
    a. Inside the lead apron
    b. Outside the lead apron
    c. He does not need to wear a radiation protection badge in the OR
12. Any dressing removed in the imaging department must be considered:
    a. Sterile
    b. Contaminated
    c. Surgically aseptic
    d. Medically aseptic
13. When sterile drapes are placed by the sterile person. The drape is placed:
    a. In the area farthest away from the sterile person first
    b. In the area nearest the sterile person first
    c. Over the operative site first
14. If the radiographer is allergic to latex, he must:
    a. Decline to participate in any procedure that requires him to wear sterile gloves
    b. Request gloves that are not of latex material
15. Sterile technique must be used during a dressing change only if the dressing is not contaminated.
    a. True
    b. False

Vital Signs and Oxygen Administration

STUDENT LEARNING OUTCOMES

After studying this chapter, the student will be able to:

1. Define vital signs and explain when assessment should be done.
2. List the rates of temperature, pulse, respiration, and blood pressure that are considered to be within normal limits for a child and an adult, male and female.
3. Identify sites and methods available for measuring body temperature and correctly read a clinical thermometer.
4. Identify the most common types of oxygen administration equipment and explain their potential hazards.
5. Describe the equipment that must be available and functional in all radiographic imaging departments to monitor blood pressure and to administer oxygen.
6. List the precautions that must be taken when oxygen is being administered.
7. Accurately monitor pulse rate, respiration, and blood pressure.

KEY TERMS

Bradycardia: A slow heart rate of less than 60 beats per minute

Chronic Obstructive Pulmonary Disease (COPD): Disease of the lungs in which inspiratory and expiratory lung capacity is diminished

Cyanosis: A condition in which the blood does not supply enough oxygen to the body, causing a bluish tone to the lips and fingertips

Diastolic: The blood pressure reading that occurs during the relaxation of the ventricles

Dyspnea: Difficult breathing resulting from insufficient air-flow to the lungs

Korotkoff sounds: Extraneous sounds heard during the taking of a blood pressure and may be a tapping, knocking, or swishing sound

Sphygmomanometer: A blood pressure cuff

Systolic: The blood pressure reading taken during the contraction of the ventricles while the blood is in the arteries

Tachycardia: A fast heart rate of more than 100 beat per minute

Tympanic: Bell-like; resonance pertaining to tympanum

Volatile: Easily vaporized or evaporated; unstable or explosive in nature

MEASURING VITAL SIGNS

Taking a patient's vital signs (also called cardinal signs) is an important part of a physical assessment and includes measurement of body temperature, pulse, respiration, and blood pressure. The radiographer must know how to measure each vital sign to be prepared in case an emergency situation in which these skills are needed is ever encountered. It is also important to learn what the patient's vital signs are under normal circumstances because everyone has some variation from what is considered normal for their particular age group. After the baseline vital signs for a patient have been established, it will be easy to determine if the patient's vital signs are deviating from that baseline. Changes in vital signs can be an indication of a problem or a potential problem. A patient's baseline vital signs cannot be established with one reading of pulse, respiration, or blood pressure because of the many variables that can make one reading unreliable. Vital signs must be measured if the patient comes to the diagnostic imaging department for an extensive procedure or examination without a chart and no registered nurse is available.

Oxygen is an essential physiologic need for survival. It comes from the environment to the lungs and then is transported to the bloodstream and body tissues. The human brain cannot function for longer than 4 to 5 minutes without an adequate oxygen supply.

It is occasionally necessary to administer oxygen in the diagnostic imaging department. The radiographer is expected to assist in its administration. Also, a patient receiving oxygen therapy in the hospital room may be unable to leave the room to go to the diagnostic imaging department for necessary procedures. In this instance, the mobile units will be required to make the radiographic exposure at the bedside. Because oxygen is a potentially toxic and **volatile** substance, the radiographer needs to understand the precautions that are to be taken when assisting with oxygen administration or when using radiographic equipment while oxygen is in use.

It is the responsibility of the radiographer to make certain that there is a functioning sphygmomanometer, a stethoscope, and the equipment necessary to administer oxygen in each diagnostic imaging room at the beginning of each shift. Emergencies requiring these items arise, and there is no time to look for this equipment.

A physician's order is not required for vital signs to be measured. Unless a registered nurse is present to do so, vital signs should be taken by the radiographer when a patient is brought into the diagnostic imaging department for any invasive diagnostic procedure or treatment, before and after the patient receives medication, any time the patient's general condition suddenly changes, or if the patient reports nonspecific symptoms of physical distress such as simply not feeling well or feeling "different."

BODY TEMPERATURE

Body temperature is the physiologic balance between heat produced in body tissues and heat lost to the environment. It must remain stable if the body's cellular and enzymatic activities are to function efficiently. Changes in the body's physiology occur when the body temperature fluctuates even 2 to 3 degrees. Body temperature is controlled by a small structure in the basal region of the diencephalon of the brain called the *hypothalamus*, sometimes referred to as the body's thermostat.

Chemical processes that result from metabolic activity produce body heat. When the body's metabolism increases, more heat is produced. When it decreases, less heat is produced. Both normal and abnormal conditions in the body can produce changes in body temperature. The environment, time of day, age, weight, hormone levels, emotions, physical exercise, digestion of food, disease, and injury are some factors that influence body temperature. The body's cellular functions and cardiopulmonary demands change in proportion to temperature variations outside of normal limits.

A patient whose body temperature is elevated above normal limits is said to have a fever, or *pyrexia*. Fever indicates a disturbance in the heat-regulating centers of the body, usually as a result of a disease process. As body temperature increases, the body's demand for oxygen increases.

The normal body temperature remains almost constant; however, a variation of 0.5 to 1 degree above or below the average is within normal limits. The normal body temperature of infants and children up to 13 years of age varies somewhat from these readings. Average body temperature in well children from ages 3 months to 3 years is from 99°F (37.2°C) to 99.7°F (37.7°C); from 5 years to 13 years, the normal temperature is from 97.8°F (36.7°C) to 98.6°F (37°C).

Symptoms of a fever are increased pulse and respiratory rate, general discomfort or aching, flushed dry skin that feels hot to the touch, chills (occasionally), and loss of appetite. Fevers that are allowed to remain very high for a prolonged period of time can cause irreparable damage to the central nervous system (CNS).

A person with a body temperature below normal limits is said to have hypothermia, which may be indicative of a pathological process. Hypothermia may also be induced medically to reduce a patient's need for oxygen. It is rare for a person to survive with a body temperature between 105.8°F (41°C) and 111.2°F (44°C) or below 93.2°F (34°C).

Measuring Body Temperature

There are four areas of the body in which temperature is usually measured: the oral site, the tympanic site, the rectal site, and the axillary site.

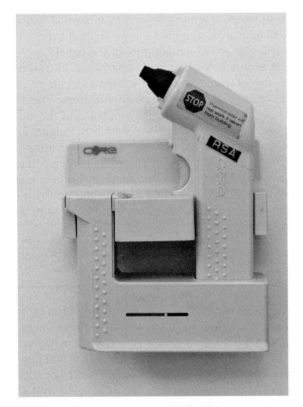

FIGURE 6-1   Tympanic membrane thermometer.

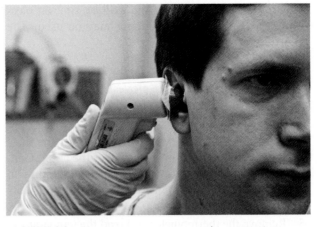

FIGURE 6-2   Measuring temperature with a tympanic thermometer. The probe is placed inside the external auditory canal.

The Tympanic Membrane Thermometer

The **tympanic** membrane thermometer (also called an *aural thermometer*) is a small, hand-held device that measures the temperature of the blood vessels in the tympanic membrane of the ear (Fig. 6-1). This provides a reading close to the core body temperature if correctly placed. The patient may be sitting upright or in a supine position. The procedure for use is:

1. Place a clean sheath on the probe that is to be inserted into the external auditory canal.
2. Place the probe into the external auditory canal and hold it firmly in place (Fig. 6-2) until the temperature registers automatically on the meter held in the non-dominant hand.
3. Remove the probe and read the indicator.
4. Remove the probe's cover and dispose of it correctly. Remove any gloves and wash hands.
5. Record the reading. Immediately report any abnormal temperature to the radiologist in charge of the procedure.

The Electronic Thermometer for Oral Temperature

The procedure for the electronic thermometer is the same as for the tympanic membrane thermometer, except that the probe is placed under the patient's tongue and held in place until the instrument signals that it has registered a temperature.

Taking an Axillary Temperature

Use of the axillary site is the safest method of measuring body temperature because it is noninvasive. It is particularly useful when measuring an infant's temperature. Unfortunately, the time and precision of placement needed to obtain an accurate reading make this method somewhat unreliable. When it is necessary to

Oral temperature is taken by mouth under the tongue; the average oral temperature reading is 98.6°F (37°C). The axillary temperature is taken in the axilla or armpit. The average axillary temperature is 97.6°F to 98°F (36.4°C to 36.7°C). Rectal temperature is taken at the anal opening to the rectum. The average rectal temperature is 99.6°F (37.5°C).

The site selected for measuring body temperature must be chosen with care depending on the patient's age, state of mind, and ability to cooperate in the procedure. Because the reading will vary depending on where it is measured, be sure to specify the site used when reporting the reading. Temperature readings are reported in most health care facilities as follows:

- A rectal temperature of 99.6°F is written 99.6 R.
- An oral temperature of 98.6°F is written 98.6 O.
- An axillary temperature of 97.6°F is written 97.6 Ax.
- A tympanic temperature of 97.6°F is written 97.6 T.

Whatever method of measuring body temperature is chosen, the radiographer must assemble the necessary equipment and abide by medically aseptic technique (such as washing the hands and wearing gloves if there is a possibility of coming in contact with blood or other body fluids).

measure temperature using the axillary site, an electronic or disposable thermometer may be used. The procedure is as follows:

1. Obtain the instrument to be used.
2. After putting on clean gloves, dry the patient's armpit with a paper towel or dry washcloth.
3. Place the thermometer into the center of the armpit.
4. Place the patient's arm down tightly over the thermometer with the arm crossed over the chest. Gently hold the arm of a child or a restless adult in place until the thermometer has registered, usually about 1 minute.
5. Remove the thermometer and read the temperature.
6. Record the reading and dispose of the thermometer as appropriate.

Taking a Rectal Temperature

The rectal site is considered to provide the most reliable measurement of body temperature because factors that can alter the results are minimized. It is also in close proximity to the pelvic viscera or "core" temperature of the body. Body temperature should not be measured rectally if the patient is restless or has rectal pathology such as tumors or hemorrhoids.

To take a rectal temperature, use a thermometer with a blunt tip. Never use an oral thermometer to take a rectal temperature. Probe covers are often colored red for rectal temperature. The procedure is as follows:

1. Obtain the correct thermometer.
2. Put on clean gloves.
3. Assure the patient's privacy and place him or her in the Sim's position.
4. Expose only as much of the patient as necessary for clear viewing of the rectal area.
5. Lubricate the thermometer tip (or probe cover if one is used) with lubricating gel.
6. Separate the patient's buttocks with the heel of one hand so that rectum is clearly visible.
7. Gently insert the tip of the thermometer into the rectum about 1 to 1.5 inches and hold it in place for 2 to 3 minutes. Do not leave a patient with a rectal thermometer in place. It must be held in place for an accurate reading.
8. Remove the thermometer, read it, and dispose of it as appropriate.
9. After removing the gloves in the correct manner and performing a minimum 30-second hand wash, record the temperature.

Other Instruments Used to Measure Body Temperature

Temperature-sensitive patches are available that can be placed on the abdomen or forehead of infants or children to measure temperature. If an abnormal temperature is indicated, a more accurate method can be used to verify the actual temperature of the patient.

If a patient's behavior is unreliable, an unbreakable, disposable, single-use thermometer can be used. Wear gloves as in previous descriptions. The thermometer is removed from its wrapper, and the indicator end is placed under the patient's tongue for 1 minute. The beads change color, indicating the patient's temperature. After recording the temperature, discard the thermometer. The accuracy of these instruments is uncertain but will provide the radiographer with an estimate of what a temperature might be in an unstable situation.

PULSE

As the heart beats, blood is pumped in a pulsating fashion into the arteries. This results in a throb, or pulsation, of the artery. At areas of the body in which arteries are superficial, the pulse can be felt by holding the artery beneath the skin against a solid surface such as bone. The pulse can be detected most easily in the following areas of the body:

- *Apical pulse*: over the apex of the heart (heard with a stethoscope) (Fig. 6-3A)
- *Radial pulse*: over the radial artery at the wrists at the base of the thumb (Fig. 6-3B)
- *Carotid pulse*: over the carotid artery at the front of the neck (Fig. 6-3C)
- *Femoral pulse*: over the femoral artery in the groin (Fig. 6-3D)
- *Popliteal pulse*: at the posterior surface of the knee (Fig. 6-3E)
- *Temporal pulse*: over the temporal artery in front of the ear (Fig. 6-3F)
- *Dorsalis pedis pulse* (*pedal*): at the top of the feet in line with the groove between the extensor tendons of the great and second toe (may be congenitally absent) (Fig. 6-3G)
- *Posterior tibial pulse*: on the inner side of the ankles (Fig. 6-3H)
- *Brachial pulse*: in the groove between the biceps and triceps muscles above the elbow at the antecubital fossa (Fig. 6-3I)

Usually, the pulse rate is rapid if the blood pressure is low and slower if the blood pressure is high. The patient who is losing blood has an unusually rapid pulse rate and a very low blood pressure. The normal average pulse rate in an adult man or woman in a resting state is between 60 and 90 beats/min. The normal average pulse rate for an infant is 120 beats/min. A child from 4 to 10 years of age has a normal average pulse rate of 90 to 100 beats/min.

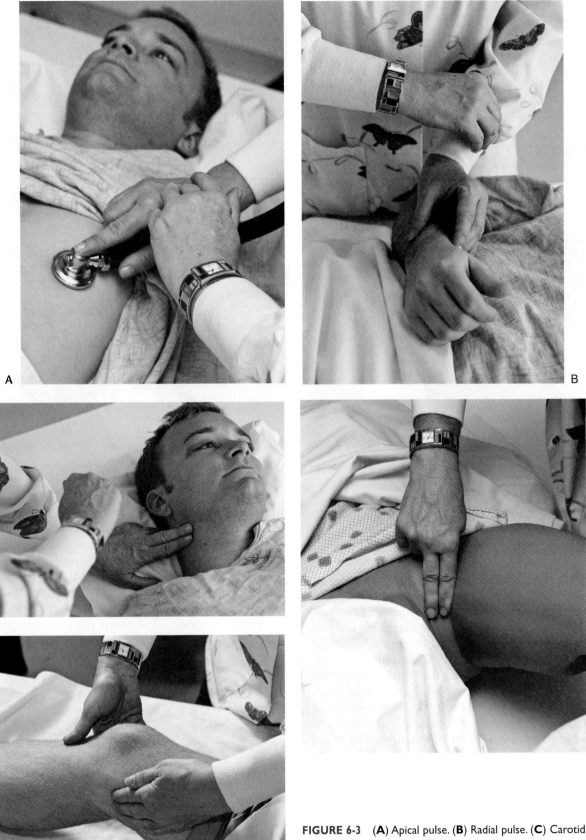

FIGURE 6-3 (**A**) Apical pulse. (**B**) Radial pulse. (**C**) Carotid pulse. (**D**) Femoral pulse. (**E**) Popliteal pulse.

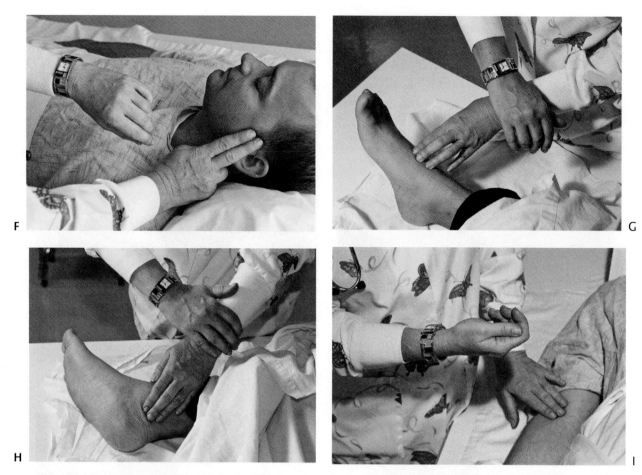

FIGURE 6-3 (continued) (**F**) Temporal pulse. (**G**) Dorsalis pedis pulse (pedal). (**H**) Posterior tibial pulse. (**I**) Brachial pulse.

Assessment of the Pulse

The pulse rate is a rapid and relatively efficient means of assessing cardiovascular function. **Tachycardia** is an abnormally rapid heart rate (over 100 beats/min), and **bradycardia** is an abnormally slow heart rate (below 60 beats/min). If a registered nurse is not present to take the pulse rate, be prepared to make this assessment before beginning any invasive diagnostic imaging procedure in order to establish a baseline reading and to reassess it frequently until the procedure is complete and the patient leaves the department. The radial pulse is usually the most accessible and can be taken most conveniently on an adult patient. It should be counted for 1 full minute. If there is any irregularity of the radial pulse rate, take the apical pulse. The apical pulse is also monitored if the patient's radial pulse is inaccessible.

For infants and children, the apical pulse is the most accurate for cardiovascular assessment. The femoral, popliteal, and pedal pulses are assessed bilaterally if peripheral blood flow is to be assessed.

When assessing pulse rate, report the strength and regularity of the beat as well as the number of beats per minute. The normal rhythm of the pulse beat is regular,

with equal time intervals between beats. The pressure of the fingers should not obliterate the pulse. When this does happen, report the pulse as weak or thready. If the beat is irregular, unusually rapid, unusually slow, or unusually weak, immediately report this to the physician in charge of the patient. Changes in pulse rate during a procedure must also be reported.

Equipment needed to assess the pulse includes a watch with a second hand and a pad and pencil to record the findings. For monitoring the apical pulse, a stethoscope that has been cleaned will be needed. To assess the radial, femoral, carotid, popliteal, pedal, and temporal pulses, observe the following guidelines:

1. After completing the necessary hand washing, place the index finger and middle finger flat over the artery chosen for assessment. Do not press too hard or the artery will be compressed and no beat will be felt. Do not use the thumb when counting the pulse rate as it too has a pulse that may be mistaken for the patient's pulse.

2. When the throbbing of the artery is felt, count the throbs for 1 minute.

CALL OUT!

Be careful not to press too hard with the finger or the pulse will be compressed and not felt.

CALL OUT!

Do not use the thumb to count the pulse because it has its own pulse.

The pedal, popliteal, and femoral pulses are often monitored during special diagnostic imaging procedures to ascertain that the patient's circulatory status in the lower extremities is satisfactory. When this is done, the pulses are not always counted. Instead, they are palpated and assessed as present and strong, weak, regular, or irregular. Mark the areas where the pedal and popliteal pulses are palpated so that they may be checked as necessary.

Apical Pulse

To assess the apical pulse, a stethoscope and alcohol wipes are needed. The procedure is as follows:

1. Clean the earpieces and the bladder of the stethoscope with alcohol wipes, and then wash hands.
2. Place the patient in a semi-Fowler's or supine position.
3. Drape the patient so the lower chest area is exposed.
4. Place the bladder of the stethoscope at the fifth intercostal space 5 cm from the left sternal margin (the nipple of the breast can be used as a landmark for 5 cm).
5. If the beat cannot be heard, move the stethoscope slightly in every direction until it can be heard.
6. Count the beats for 1 minute and assess for regular rate and rhythm.
7. Remove the stethoscope and cover the patient. Clean the earpieces and bladder again with alcohol.
8. After completing a 30-second hand wash, record the pulse rate and report any irregularities.

When recording pulse rate, use the abbreviation P for pulse and AP for apical pulse. For example, P 80 equals a pulse rate of 80 beats/min. AP 88 equals an apical pulse rate of 88 beats/min. Record any abnormalities and immediately report these to the patient's physician.

RESPIRATION

The function of the respiratory system is to exchange oxygen and carbon dioxide between the external environment and the blood circulating in the body. Oxygen

is taken into the lungs during inspiration. It passes through the bronchi, into the bronchioles, and then into the alveoli, which are the gas-exchange units of the lungs. Oxygen is transported to the body tissues by the arterial blood. Deoxygenated blood is returned to the right side of the heart through the venous system. It is then pumped into the right and left pulmonary arteries and reoxygenated by passing through the capillary network on the alveolar surfaces. The blood is then returned to the left side of the heart though the pulmonary veins for recirculation. During this process, carbon dioxide is also deposited in the alveoli and exhaled from the lungs during expiration.

The average rate of respiration (one inspiration and one expiration) for an adult man or woman is 15 to 20 breaths/min, and for an infant it is 30 to 60 breaths/min. Respiration of fewer than 10 breaths/min for an adult may result in **cyanosis**, apprehension, restlessness, and a change in level of consciousness because the supply of oxygen is inadequate to meet the needs of the body.

Normal respirations are quiet, effortless, and uniform. Medication, illness, exercise, or age may increase or decrease respirations, depending on the body's metabolic need for oxygen. When a patient is using more than the normal effort to breathe, he or she is described as dyspneic or as having **dyspnea**.

Assessment of Respiration

As with other vital signs, it is important to establish a baseline respiratory rate because changes in respiration are often an early sign of a threatened physiologic state. Remember, however, that the rate of respiration increases with physical exercise or emotion. Respiration is also quicker in newborns and infants. When assessing respiration, observe the rate, depth, quality, and pattern. The assessment procedure is as follows:

1. *Keep the patient in a seated or supine position.* The patient should be in a quiet state and be unaware that the breathing pattern is being observed. The most convenient time to count respirations is immediately after the pulse count. This gives the appearance of continuing to count the pulse rate and helps to keep the patient unaware of the respiratory movement. Patients that become aware that respiration is being assessed may consciously or unconsciously alter the pattern.
2. *Observe the chest wall for symmetry of movement.* There should be an even rise and fall of the chest with no involvement of muscles other than the diaphragm. In the adult patient, abdominal, intercostal, or neck muscle involvement in breathing is a sign of respiratory distress and should be noted. Other signs of respiratory distress in an adult

patient include the need to assume a sitting position or the need to lean forward and place the arms over the back of a chair or on the knees in order to breathe easily.

3. *Observe skin color.* Cyanosis, or bluish discoloration, is easily observed around the mouth, in the gums, in nail beds, or in the earlobes. Cyanosis may be a sign of respiratory distress.

4. *Count the number of times the patient's chest rises and falls for 1 full minute.* An easy way to count respirations is to cross the patient's arm across the chest and count the rise and fall of the arm.

When recording respiration, use the abbreviation R. R 20 equals 20 rises and falls of the chest wall. Any abnormalities or deviations from the baseline should be reported to the physician in charge of the patient and recorded, for example, *R 28, shallow and labored.*

CALL OUT!

Patients who are aware of respiration assessment may alter their normal pattern of breathing.

BLOOD PRESSURE

In general terms, pressure is defined as the product of flow times resistance. Blood pressure is the amount of blood flow ejected from the left ventricle of the heart during systole and the amount of resistance the blood meets due to systemic vascular resistance. Maintenance of blood pressure depends on peripheral resistance, pumping action of the heart, blood volume, blood viscosity, and the elasticity of the vessel walls.

If the volume of blood decreases because of hemorrhage or dehydration, the blood pressure falls because of a diminished amount of fluid in the arteries. Fluid or blood replacement reverses the problem.

The number of red blood cells in the blood plasma determines the viscosity of the blood. With an increased number, the blood thickens or becomes more viscous and subsequently increases the blood pressure.

The arteries are normally elastic in nature; however, age or build-up of atherosclerotic plaque reduces flexibility of the arteries and increases blood pressure.

The peripheral blood vessels distribute blood ejected into the circulatory system to the various body organs. When the peripheral blood vessels are in normal physiologic state, they are partially contracted. If this normal physiologic state is changed because of changes in environmental factors such as heat or cold, medication, disease, or other obstructive conditions, peripheral blood vessel resistance may increase. This increase causes an increase in blood pressure. Or, the peripheral blood vessel resistance may decline, thus causing a decrease in blood pressure.

Blood pressure normally varies with age, gender, physical development, body position, time of day, and health status. As a person ages, the blood pressure usually increases as the body systems that control blood pressure deteriorate.

Physiologic factors that may increase blood pressure are increased cardiac output, increased peripheral vascular resistance, increased blood volume, increased blood viscosity, and decreased arterial elasticity. Physiologic factors that decrease blood pressure are decreased cardiac output, decreased peripheral vascular resistance, decreased blood volumes, decreased blood viscosity, and increased arterial elasticity.

Blood pressure is usually lower in the morning after a night of sleep than later in the day after activity. Blood pressure increases after a large intake of food. Emotions and strenuous activity usually cause systolic blood pressure to increase.

Men usually have higher blood pressure than women. Infants generally have higher blood pressure than adults, and adolescents have the lowest overall blood pressure. Because the range of blood pressure varies in these age groups, measurements for infants and children should be taken in series.

The instrument used to measure blood pressure is called a **sphygmomanometer**. Two numbers, read in millimeters of mercury (mm Hg), are recorded when reporting blood pressure: systolic pressure and diastolic pressure. The **systolic** reading is the highest point reached during contraction of the left ventricle of the heart as it pumps blood into the aorta. The **diastolic** pressure is the lowest point to which the pressure drops during relaxation of the ventricles and indicates the minimal pressure exerted against the arterial walls continuously.

In men and women, the normal ranges are 90 to 120 mm Hg for systolic pressure and 50 to 70 mm Hg for diastolic pressure. Adolescent patients' blood pressure ranges from 85 to 130 mm Hg systolic and 45 to 85 mm Hg diastolic.

Pulse pressure is the difference between the systolic and diastolic blood pressure and is an indicator of the stroke volume of the heart (the amount of blood ejected by the left ventricle during contraction). Pulse pressure decreases when a patient is in a state of hypovolemic shock.

The patient's baseline blood pressure reading must be taken so that the blood pressure can be evaluated effectively if necessary. A patient is considered to be hypertensive if the systolic blood pressure is consistently greater than 140 mm Hg and if the diastolic blood pressure is consistently greater than 90 mm Hg. A patient is considered hypotensive if the systolic blood pressure is less than 90 mm Hg.

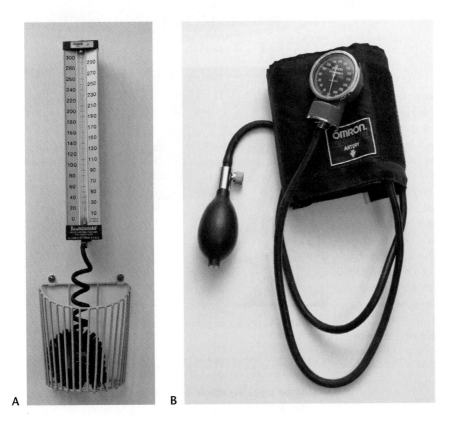

A   B

FIGURE 6-4   (**A**) A mercury manometer
and (**B**) an Aneroid manometer.

Equipment Needed to Measure Blood Pressure

There are two types of sphygmomanometers, a mercury manometer and aneroid manometer (Fig. 6-4A and B). Each has a cloth cuff, which comes in a variety of sizes. Within the cuff is an inflatable bladder, which should be nearly long enough to encircle the arm. Each also has a pressure manometer, a thumbscrew valve to maintain or release the pressure, a pressure bulb to inflate the bladder, and rubber tubings that lead to the gauge and to the pressure bulb. The bulb and the tubing must be free of leaks.

The mercury manometer is the more accurate of the two, but it is less convenient to use. The aneroid manometer needle should point to zero before the bladder of the cuff is inflated. Its calibration should be checked for accuracy and recalibrated by means of a perfectly accurate mercury manometer at least once each year.

The blood pressure cuffs should be selected according to patient size. A cuff that is too large or too small for the patient's arm will give an incorrect reading.

A good-quality stethoscope (Fig. 6-5) has a bladder and a bell, strong plastic or rubber tubing 12 to 19 inches (30 to 40 cm) in length that leads to firm but flexible binaural tubes (the metal tubings leading to the earpieces), and earpieces that fit snugly and securely into the ears. The bladder or the bell of the stethoscope can be used for assessing blood pressure. The bell

transmits low sound and should be held lightly against the skin; the bladder transmits high-pitched sound and is held firmly against the skin.

An automated vital sign monitor is used during special diagnostic imaging procedures when it is necessary to know the patient's circulatory status at all times. The pulse, blood pressure, and mean arterial pressure are measured with this instrument. (Many types of Doppler and electronic blood pressure monitoring devices are used in clinical practice. Their methods of operation vary and are not discussed in this chapter.

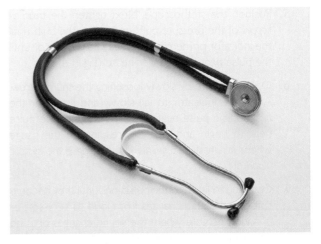

FIGURE 6-5   Stethoscope.

Measuring Blood Pressure

Have the patient sit in a chair with his or her arm supported or recline in a supine position. Although a pressure can be taken while the patient is standing, it is not recommended. Most often, the patient will be recumbent when it becomes necessary for the radiographer to perform a blood pressure reading.

The room should be as quiet as possible to facilitate hearing the pulsations. Make sure that no clothing is between the blood pressure cuff and the skin. The brachial artery of the left arm should be used as it is a direct line from the patient's heart and gives the truest indication of the blood pressure. The bladder and bell of the stethoscope and the earpieces should be cleansed with alcohol sponges before and after each use to prevent passing infection indirectly from one person to another.

The procedure for taking blood pressure is as follows:

1. Roll up the patient's sleeve, if necessary. The brachial artery must be free of clothing.

2. Place the deflated sphygmomanometer cuff evenly around the patient's upper arm above the elbow; secure it so that it will not work loose. Make sure that the cuff is facing the correct direction and that the arrow indicating the artery is placed appropriately.

3. Place the bladder or bell of the stethoscope over the brachial artery. This artery is located at the center of the anterior elbow and may be identified by feeling its pulsations. Place the instrument flat against the brachial artery. Do not allow the stethoscope or the tubing to touch the patient's clothing because it will create sounds that may confuse the reading.

4. Place the gauge of the sphygmomanometer on a flat surface or attach it to the top edge of the cuff so that it can be easily read.

5. Position the stethoscope. Next tighten the thumbscrew of the pressure bulb, and pump the bulb until the indicator or mercury reaches 180 mm Hg or until the pulse beat is no longer heard (Fig. 6-6).

6. Open the valve by slowly loosening the thumbscrew. Allow the indicator to fall slowly and listen for the first audible pulse beat. Listen carefully for the pulse beat to begin and take the reading on the gauge where it is first heard. *This first reading is the systolic blood pressure.*

7. Continue to listen to the pulsations until they become soft or the sound changes from loud to very soft or is inaudible. Note where the sound changes or is no longer heard. *This is the diastolic reading.*

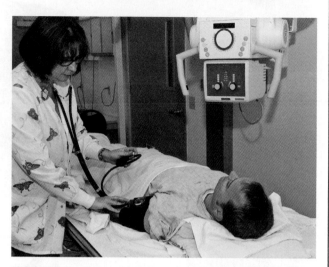

FIGURE 6-6 Measuring blood pressure.

CALL OUT!

Blood pressure should be taken on the left arm above the brachial artery.

CALL OUT!

Clothing must be removed from the area prior to placing the cuff of the sphygmomanometer on the arm.

When the diastolic pressure is heard, there may be a change in intensity of the sound before the sound is completely muffled. Note the point at which the softer sound is heard, and then note the point at which the pulsations are completely absent. This reading is a more accurate indication of intra-arterial diastolic pressure. Record both readings, but record the softer sound first. There are times when extraneous sounds such as tapping, knocking, or swishing may be heard. These are known as **Korotkoff sounds** and they must be recorded as well.

If the systolic reading is 120 and the diastolic reading is 80, the blood pressure is recorded as BP 120/80 and is read "one twenty over eighty." If the diastolic reading is soft at 80 and then completely muffled at 60, it should be written 120/80/60 (the 60 reading being the Korotkoff sound).

Blood pressure measurement for infants and small children is a more complex procedure and requires a smaller sphygmomanometer cuff and less pressure exerted upon inflation. A physician or nurse educated in this skill should perform this. Usually, a nurse is on hand to monitor when invasive diagnostic imaging procedures are to be done for patients in this age group.

OXYGEN THERAPY

An adequate oxygen supply is essential to life. Because oxygen cannot be stored in the body, the supply from the external environment must be constant. When a human being's oxygen supply is suddenly interrupted or interfered with in any manner, it is an emergency that must be dealt with immediately to prevent a life-threatening situation. This type of emergency may occur in the diagnostic imaging department; therefore, the radiographer performing the procedure may be the first person to observe such a problem. It is that person's responsibility to ensure that the equipment needed to administer oxygen is available at all times and in functioning condition in the work area. It is also that person's responsibility to assist with oxygen administration in emergency situations. Therefore, understanding the methods of oxygen administration that may be encountered in the care of the patient is critical.

The lungs supply oxygen and remove carbon dioxide from the body. Oxygen and carbon dioxide are carried to and from the various body systems in the blood. Only small amounts of oxygen are carried in solution in the blood. The major supply of oxygen is carried in chemical combination with hemoglobin. The oxygen capacity of the blood is expressed in percentage of the volume. The amount of oxygen in either air or blood is called the oxygen tension (partial pressure) and is written PO_2. Carbon dioxide is described similarly as PCO_2.

Carbon dioxide diffuses into the plasma of systemic capillary blood, but the major part enters the red blood cells. Carbon dioxide also is carried in combination with hemoglobin, which assists with its removal from the body. When there is an excessive build-up of carbon dioxide in the bloodstream, the pH (acidity or alkalinity) of the blood changes, often with dire physiologic effects. Prevention of excessive acidity of the blood is achieved through the presence of a bicarbonate (HCO_3) buffer in the bloodstream.

The effectiveness of pulmonary function (the lungs' ability to exchange oxygen and carbon dioxide efficiently) is most accurately measured by laboratory testing of arterial blood for the concentrations of oxygen, carbon dioxide, bicarbonate, acidity, and the saturation of hemoglobin with oxygen (SaO_2). Laboratory values (called *arterial blood gases* or *ABG*) considered within normal limits are:

pH: 7.35 to 7.45
$PaCO_2$: 32 to 45 mm Hg
PaO_2: 80 to 100 mm Hg
HCO_3: 20 to 26 mEq/L
SaO_2: 97%

When pulmonary function is disturbed, the level of oxygen in the arterial blood becomes inadequate to meet the patient's physiologic needs. This condition is referred to as *hypoxemia*. Carbon dioxide may be retained in the arterial blood, which results in a condition called *hypercapnia*. When the PaO_2 is below 60 mm Hg or the hemoglobin saturation is less than 90%, it can be assumed that adequate oxygenation of the blood is not taking place. Physical symptoms of this problem, discussed in the next chapter, will be a good indicator that hypoxemia is occurring.

CALL OUT!

Hypoxemia may happen with little warning. There may not be time for lab analysis of the ABG.

Pulse Oximetry

A pulse oximeter is frequently used to monitor the oxygen saturation of hemoglobin (SaO_2). This is a fast, noninvasive method of monitoring the patient for sudden changes in oxygen saturation, such as when a patient has just been removed from a ventilator. A sensor is attached to a fingertip or an earlobe (Fig. 6-7). A photodetector attached to the sensor is able to distinguish between oxygenated and deoxygenated hemoglobin of the blood pulsing through the tissue at the location of the sensor. Normal SaO_2 values are 95% to

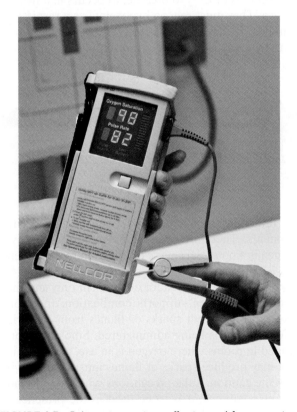

FIGURE 6-7 Pulse oximetry is an effective tool for measuring subtle changes in oxygen saturation.

100%. Values of less than 85% indicate that the tissues are not receiving adequate oxygen. The pulse oximeter is used in all areas of acute health care as well as in the special procedures areas of radiographic imaging.

Hazards of Oxygen Administration

Oxygen is considered to be a medication and, like all other forms of medical therapy, must be prescribed by a physician. Excessive amounts of oxygen may produce toxic effects on the lungs and central nervous system or may depress ventilation.

Varying degrees of oxygen toxicity may result from inhalation of high concentrations of oxygen for more than a brief period of time. Mild oxygen toxicity may produce reversible tracheobronchitis. Severe oxygen toxicity may cause irreversible parenchymal lung injury. Because of the potential for adverse effects from excessive amounts of oxygen, oxygen should be administered as prescribed and in the lowest possible amount to achieve adequate oxygenation.

Special care is necessary when oxygen is administered to patients who have **chronic obstructive pulmonary disease (COPD).** Excessive oxygen in the blood of the patient who has COPD may depress the respiratory drive, and the patient may stop breathing. This occurs because patients with a chronic lung disease have chemoreceptors that no longer respond to the stimulus of CO_2 to breathe, as occurs in a healthy person. They must rely on hypoxemia as a respiratory stimulus. If they receive an excessive amount of oxygen, hypoxia is no longer present and respiration ceases.

> ⚠ **WARNING!**
>
> High flow rates of oxygen are toxic to patients who have COPD because their respiration is controlled by higher levels of carbon dioxide in the blood.

Infection and bacteria thrive in oxygenated environments. Therefore, the equipment used to deliver oxygen is a potential source of infection to the patient. Be certain that the tubing, cannulas, and masks for oxygen delivery are used for one patient only and then discarded. Oxygen supports combustion; therefore, take care to prevent sparks or flames from occurring where oxygen is being administered. Smoking is prohibited in rooms where oxygen is in use, and anything that may produce sparks or flames must be used with extreme caution. Take precautions when mobile radiographic equipment is to be used in the presence of pure oxygen to be certain that it will not produce sparks.

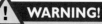

> ⚠ **WARNING!**
>
> Oxygen is combustible, so great care must be taken to prevent sparks from occurring while radiographing a patient with the mobile unit.

Oxygen Delivery Systems

Oxygen is administered by artificial means when the patient is unable to obtain adequate amounts from the atmosphere to supply the needs of the body. If the patient requires supplementary oxygen, it is delivered to the respiratory tract under pressure. When the flow rate is high, the oxygen is humidified to prevent excessive drying of the mucous membranes. Passing the oxygen through distilled water can do this, because oxygen is only slightly soluble in water. The procedure for moisturizing oxygen varies somewhat from one institution to another, but often, the receptacle for distilled water is attached at the wall outlet, and the oxygen passes through the water and then into the delivery system.

In most hospitals, oxygen is piped into patient rooms, post-anesthesia areas, emergency suites, and the diagnostic imaging department. Wall outlets make it readily available. Oxygen supplied in this fashion comes through pipes from a central source at 60 to 80 pounds of pressure per square inch. A flow meter is attached to each wall outlet to regulate flow.

If oxygen is not piped in through wall outlets, it is available compressed and dispensed in tanks of varying sizes (Fig. 6-8). A large, full tank contains 2,000 pounds of pressure per square inch. These tanks have two regulator valves—one valve indicates how much oxygen is in the tank, and the other valve measures the rate of oxygen flow through the delivery tubing. If this type of system is used, take care not to allow the tank to fall or the regulator to become cracked. If this were to happen, the buildup of pressure within the tank may cause the regulator to act as a dangerous projectile.

Twenty-one percent of the air we breathe normally is composed of oxygen, often abbreviated as FiO_2. This percentage of oxygen may need to be increased if a patient is in respiratory distress and unable to inspire enough room air to fulfill his body's oxygen needs.

There are many types of oxygen delivery systems that transport oxygen from wall outlets or tanks. The more complex systems deliver a controlled amount of premixed room air and oxygen. The simpler systems deliver a prescribed amount of oxygen mixed with room air, but the concentration varies as the patient's rate of respiration varies because they are not closed systems. The physician determines the amount of oxygen that the patient needs and the type of delivery device needed. The flow rate of oxygen is measured in

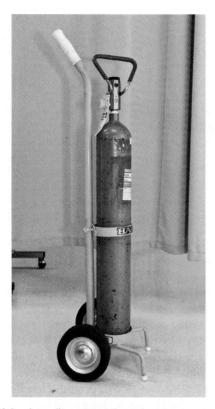

FIGURE 6-8   A small oxygen tank used to transport patients from hospital room to the diagnostic imaging department.

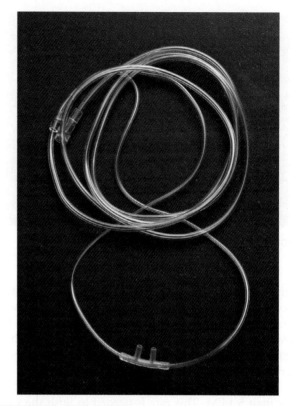

FIGURE 6-9   Nasal cannula.

liters per minute (LPM). The systems that the radiographer will see most often deliver low to moderate concentrations of oxygen.

Nasal Cannula

The nasal cannula is a disposable plastic device with two hollow prongs that deliver oxygen into the nostrils (Fig. 6-9). The other end of the cannula is attached to the oxygen supply, which may or may not pass through a humidifier, and it has a flow meter attached. The cannula is held in place by an elastic strap that fits over the patient's ears and behind the head. This device is the most commonly seen delivery system in the diagnostic imaging department. Patients on long-term oxygen delivery have a nasal cannula because of the comfort and convenience of the cannula.

The concentration of oxygen delivered by nasal cannula varies from 21% to 60%, according to the amount of room air inspired by the patient. Oxygen delivery by nasal cannula is indicated for patients whose breathing range and depth are normal and even. With this method, 1 to 4 LPM of oxygen is usually prescribed for adults. For children, the rate is much lower (1/4 to 1/2 LPM). Rates at higher levels dry the nasal mucosa because of the position of the tubes against the skin of the nostrils.

The oxygen should be turned on and flowing at the desired rate before placing any low-flow device on a patient. This prevents a sudden burst of oxygen into the patient's nostrils when the regulator is first turned on. The nasal prongs must be kept in place in both nostrils.

Nasal Catheter

A nasal catheter is another means of low-flow delivery of oxygen. While this method of oxygen delivery is not routinely used, it warrants description in the event that the radiographer may come in contact with it. In this system, a French-tipped catheter is inserted into one nostril until it reaches the oral pharynx. This type of catheter is used to deliver a moderate to high concentration of oxygen. As with the nasal cannula, the other end of the French-tipped catheter is attached to the oxygen supply with a flow meter attached. The prescribed flow rate for this method of delivery is usually 1 to 5 LPM. Oxygen delivered by this method does have associated hazards. For example, oxygen may be misdirected into the stomach, causing gastric distention; or the mucous membranes may become dry, causing a sore throat.

Face Mask

A simple face mask is used to deliver oxygen for short periods of time (Fig. 6-10). It, too, is attached to an oxygen supply and a flow meter. The mask is placed over the nose and mouth and attached over the ears and behind the head with an elastic band (Fig. 6-11). A mask is uncomfortable for long periods because the

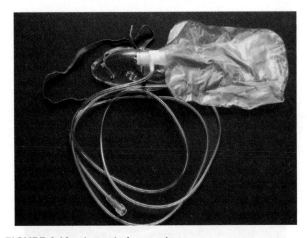

FIGURE 6-10   A simple face mask.

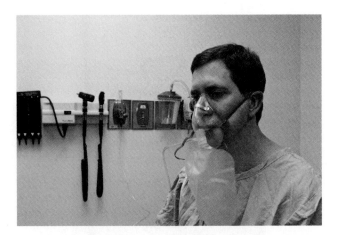

FIGURE 6-11   The face mask is secured over the head with an elastic strap.

patient is unable to eat, drink, or talk with it in place. Moreover, the percentage of oxygen is so variable with the face mask that it is not the method of choice for long periods. Because the mask does not fit tightly against the face, the concentration of oxygen delivered varies from 30% to 50%.

When the face mask is used, it should be run at no less than 5 LPM. This rate is needed to flush the CO_2 from the mask. Other face masks are usually used to administer more precise concentrations of oxygen. Several types of face mask delivery systems are available at present, and the physician will prescribe the one best suited to the patient's needs.

The different types of mask include a *nonrebreathing mask*, which, if correctly used, may supply 100% oxygen. This high-flow system has a reservoir bag attached. The bag fills with oxygen to provide a constant supply of oxygen. A valve prevents the exhaled gases from entering the reservoir bag and prevents rebreathing of exhaled gases. A *partial rebreathing mask*, which delivers 60% to 90% oxygen, operates similarly to the nonrebreather mask. The rebreather mask does not have a valve between the mask and the bag; therefore, exhaled air flows into the reservoir bag and allows the patient to breathe a mixture of oxygen and carbon dioxide. Two other types of face mask delivery systems include a *Venturi mask*, which limits oxygen to 24% to 50% by mixing room air and the oxygen in specific percentages; and an *aerosol mask,* which provides 60% to 80% oxygen mixed with particles of water.

Other Oxygen Delivery Systems

Persons who must have continuous oxygen therapy for long periods of time may have a *transtracheal delivery system*. This system has a catheter that is inserted into the trachea and tubing that is connected to a portable tank.

Patients in acute respiratory failure are often placed on *mechanical ventilators* (also known as respirators), which control or partially control inspiration and expiration and FiO_2. The radiographer usually encounters these patients in the critical care units of the hospital while performing mobile radiography. These patients are generally unable to breathe on their own accord. The rate of oxygen flow is determined by many factors and is regulated by the equipment. Because the ventilator tubing is generally over the patient during the performance of the procedure, adequate help must be obtained prior to moving the patient and placing the image receptor. The nurse in charge of the patient in the critical care unit who is on high-flow oxygen therapy or a mechanical ventilator must be consulted so that the patient's care is not jeopardized.

Oxygen Tent

Oxygen tents are used when there is a need for humidity and a higher concentration of oxygen than is present in the natural environment of the patient. This method of delivery is rarely used for adults, but one may be encountered in a pediatric unit. If this is the case, the oxygen may be turned off for a brief period while the required exposures are made with the mobile equipment. The hazard of fire is especially great with an oxygen tent. Smoking is not permitted, nor is the use of any equipment that might generate sparks.

Home Oxygen Delivery Systems

There are agencies that hire radiographers to take radiographs in the home of a patient who is unable to be transported to a health care facility. These patients are often using oxygen, and the oxygen may be delivered as compressed gas, as a liquid, or by means of an oxygen concentrator.

Compressed oxygen comes in tanks, which are usually smaller than the tanks used in the hospital; however, the principles of delivery are similar. Pure oxygen may be delivered by this method.

Liquid oxygen is a liquefied gas that concentrates oxygen into a lightweight container the size of a thermos bottle. It is conveniently portable and lasts longer than other forms of oxygen; therefore, people who must take oxygen with them when they leave home use it. This is an expensive method, chiefly because the oxygen evaporates quickly.

The oxygen concentrator is economical and is an excellent source of oxygen. Oxygen is concentrated by means of an electric machine that removes the nitrogen, water vapor, and hydrocarbons from room air. Oxygen is delivered at 90% by this means.

Oxygen Delivery Equipment for the Imaging Department

The following is a list of equipment that must be on hand for oxygen administration in the diagnostic imaging department:

1. An oxygen source, either a piped-in source or a tank. If the source of oxygen is a tank, the tank must be checked daily to make certain that it is filled. Tanks should be stored on their side and not in the upright position if standard carriers are not available. This is to avoid accidental falling of the tank, which may cause an explosion.

2. A sterile nasal cannula or simple face mask that is packaged and has not been used. These are disposable items.

3. Connecting tubing and an adapter to fit into a wall unit or tank.

4. A humidifier, if indicated. Humidifiers are not always used for short-term oxygen administration.

5. A flow meter.

6. A "no smoking" sign.

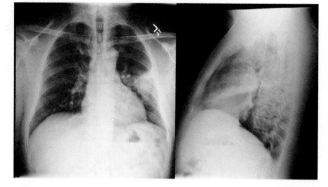

FIGURE 6-12 PA and lateral chest images showing pneumonia.

RADIOGRAPHIC EXAMINATIONS OF THE CHEST

Normal lung tissue is radiolucent; therefore, pathological conditions that produce opacities may be detected by radiographic imaging techniques (Fig. 6-12). Posterior/anterior and lateral radiographic images are frequently ordered to diagnose pulmonary pathology and to determine placement of endotracheal tubes and hemodynamic devices. These radiographic images are frequently taken at the patient's bedside because he or she is too ill to be moved. If this is the case, the patient may have difficulty complying with directions for positioning and breathing. Critical thinking and problem-solving skills will need to be employed in order to obtain a diagnostically acceptable image.

Before taking the image, the oxygen delivery system, the oxygen monitoring equipment, and the placement of associated tubing must be assessed to prevent repeating the exposure. Transporting patients or moving patients from a wheelchair or stretcher to the table or to the upright position can pull on oxygen tubes and cause pain to the patient.

SUMMARY

Body temperature is a physiologic balance between heat produced in body tissues and heat lost to the environment. Fever indicates a disturbance in the heat-regulating centers of the body. It can be detected by an elevation in body temperature, which can be measured by oral, tympanic, rectal, and axillary methods. The site and device selected to measure body temperature depend on the patient's age, as well as the mental and physical status. The reading varies depending on the site used for measurement. The body temperature of a normal adult man or woman is:

- 97.6°F (36.7°C) axillary
- 98.6°F (37°C) oral
- 99.6°F (38°C) rectal

These readings vary somewhat in infants and children. Time of day, age, exercise, environmental temperature, and pathology also alter body temperature.

The pulse is a reflection of the heartbeat, which sends blood to the arteries and causes them to throb. The areas where pulse can be measured best are at the radial artery (radial pulse), the temporal artery (tem-

TABLE 6-1	**Equipment Needed to Assess Patients' Vital Signs**				
	Thermo-meter	**Watch w/ Second Hand**	**Alcohol Wipes**	**Sphygmo-manometer**	**Stetho-scope**
Temperature	X		To clean thermometer		
Pulse		X			
Respiration		X			
Blood Pressure			To clean ear pieces & bladder	X	X

poral pulse), the carotid artery (carotid pulse), the femoral artery (femoral pulse), the apex of the heart (apical pulse), the dorsalis pedis artery (pedal pulse), and the posterior tibial artery (popliteal pulse). The apical pulse is measured by listening to it through a stethoscope. The average adult man or woman has a pulse rate of 60 to 90 beats/min. This rate varies in infants and children. The rate changes with age, exercise, time, and physiologic disturbances.

The exchange of oxygen and carbon dioxide between the atmosphere and the circulating blood is accomplished by respiration, which involves the inspiration of air containing oxygen and the expiration of air containing carbon dioxide. The rate of respiration for a normal adult male or female is from 15 to 20 breaths/min. This varies in infants and small children. Exercise, medication, age, or disease may change the respiratory rate.

Pressure is exerted by the blood on the walls of the blood vessels during the expulsion of blood from the heart and during the resting phase of the heart. It is measured with a sphygmomanometer and a stethoscope or with an electron device. The most practical place to measure blood pressure is at the brachial artery of the left arm, located at the center of the anterior elbow.

To record blood pressure, two or three readings are noted. The systolic reading is the highest point of pressure reached during a heart contraction. The diastolic reading is the lowest point to which the pressure drops during the relaxation of the ventricles and indicates the minimal pressure exerted against the arterial walls continuously. The diastolic reading is heard first as a softening and then as a disappearance of sound, in which case both readings are recorded. Blood pressure readings are influenced by age, exercise, medication, disease, and time of day.

To determine critical changes in a patient's vital signs, a radiographer must know what the patient's usual or baseline vital sign readings are. If these are not available, established norms must be relied upon to detect critical changes in the patient's vital signs.

Life cannot continue without oxygen; yet, oxygen cannot be stored in the human body. When a patient has a disease that prevents the body from taking in enough oxygen, the necessary oxygen must be supplied to the patient by artificial means. Oxygen may be administered in the diagnostic imaging department in emergency situations, or when a patient who is on oxygen is brought to the department, and it is frequently administered on hospital wards. Pure oxygen is a hazardous substance to be used only when prescribed by a physician. It supports combustion, so all health care workers need to take precautions when it is in use. No flames or machinery that might produce sparks may be used when oxygen therapy is in progress. Oxygen may also be toxic to lung tissues and may produce other harmful physiologic effects if not used cautiously. Radiographic exposures should not be made without adequate care being taken when oxygen is in use.

There are many types of oxygen delivery systems, including nasal cannulas, catheters, face masks, nonrebreather masks, partial rebreather masks, rebreather masks, Venturi masks, aerosol masks, and oxygen tents and ventilators.

The rebreather masks deliver a controlled amount of oxygen mixed with room air. Patients who need continuous oxygen for long periods of time may have a transtracheal delivery system, whereas patients in acute respiratory failure may receive oxygen by means of mechanical ventilators.

The most commonly seen type of delivery system is the nasal cannula; the most infrequently seen system is the nasal catheter. Oxygen tents are generally reserved for pediatric patients. The face mask is used for short-term administration of oxygen because it is uncomfortable for the patient to wear. Nasal cannulas are used for long-term administration because they allow the patient to speak and eat with little difficulty.

The radiographer may be responsible for assisting with oxygen administration or for monitoring vital signs in emergency situations in the diagnostic imaging department. Proficiency in the use of the equipment and the skills needed to be of assistance is essential and not to be taken lightly.

Table 6-1 shows the equipment needed to assess each of the patient's vital signs.

CHAPTER 6 TEST

1. Which of the following are essential parts of the initial assessment of a patient who is in the diagnostic imaging department for an invasive procedure? Circle all that apply.
   a. Taking a blood pressure
   b. Taking a pulse
   c. Listening for rales in the lungs
   d. Taking a respiration rate
   e. Doing blood gas assessment
   f. Finding out the oxygen saturation level
   g. Taking a temperature
2. Why is the initial assessment defined in Question #1 so important to perform?
3. Systolic blood pressure can be defined as:
   a. The lowest point to which the blood pressure drops during relaxation of the ventricles
   b. The highest point reached during contraction of the left ventricle
   c. The difference between the systolic and diastolic blood pressure
   d. The pressure in the pulmonary vein
4. What range of breaths/min is the normal adult respiratory rate?
   a. 8 to 10
   b. 15 to 20
   c. 20 to 30
   d. 80 to 90
5. An adult patient is considered to be hypertensive or to have hypertension if the systolic blood pressure and diastolic blood pressure are consistently greater than:
   a. 100 systolic and 60 diastolic
   b. 120 systolic and 80 diastolic
   c. 130 systolic and 86 diastolic
   d. 140 systolic and 90 diastolic
6. Oxygen can be toxic to patients if it is incorrectly used. State 2 reasons why this is so.
7. A patient may be considered to have tachycardia if the pulse rate is higher than:
   a. 60 beats/min
   b. 80 beats/min
   c. 90 beats/min
   d. 100 beats/min
8. Which of the following items must be in the diagnostic imaging department and in working order? Circle all that apply.
   a. Catheterization sets
   b. Suture removal sets
   c. Oxygen delivery system
   d. Blood pressure monitoring equipment
9. What is the normal oral body temperature of an adult?
10. Match the following:
    a. Sphygmomanometer
    b. Clinical thermometer
    c. Stethoscope
    d. Brachial artery
    e. Radial artery
       i. Point where the blood pressure is most often measured
       ii. Measures apical pulse
       iii. Measures blood pressure
       iv. Measures body temperature
       v. Point where the pulse is most often measured
11. Name the two most commonly used oxygen delivery systems.
12. List the hazards of oxygen administration.
13. Explain why the pulse rate goes up when the blood pressure drops.
14. Ms. Gwen Knics has entered the radiography room for an intravenous urograph. After the injection of contrast, she begins to experience tightness of the chest and difficulty breathing. From the list below, identify the best response with a "B" and the worst response with a "W."
    a. Immediately call a code blue.
    b. Take the vital signs again to establish that she really is having trouble.
    c. Assure her that she will be just fine.
    d. Call for the radiography nurse.
    e. Start the flow of oxygen at 2 LPM with a face mask.

Basic Electrocardio-gram Monitoring

STUDENT LEARNING OUTCOMES

After studying this chapter, the student will be able to:

1. Briefly explain the cardiac conduction system.
2. Correctly apply the three lead cardiac monitoring electrodes.
3. Identify electrocardiogram waveform components.
4. Recognize ominous cardiac arrhythmias.
5. Explain the role of a radiographer in responding to ominous arrhythmias.

KEY TERMS

Angina: A severe, often constricting pain or sensation of pressure, usually referring to angina pectoris

Cardiogram: The tracing that depicts the heart's electrical activity

Depolarization: Process by which cardiac muscle cells change from a more negatively charged to a more positively charged intracellular state

Dysrhythmia: A disorder of the formation or conduction of the electrical impulses in the heart that alters the heart rate or rhythm or both

Hemodynamic: Factor affecting the force and flow of circulating blood

Myocardial infarction: Death of heart tissue resulting from lack of oxygenated blood flow

Myocardial ischemia: Insufficient oxygenation of the tissues of the heart muscle

Normal sinus rhythm: The pacing impulse begins in the sinus node and travels normally down the electrical conduction pathways

Oscilloscope: The screen on which ECG patterns appear

Repolarization: Cardiac muscle cells return to a more negatively charged intracellular condition (their resting state)

Thrombi: Collections of platelets, fibrin, and clotting factors that attach to the interior wall of a vein and may result in occlusion of a vessel

In the mid-1880s, it was discovered that the heart's electrical activity could be measured externally by placing an electrode on a person's skin. In 1901, Dr. Willem Einthoven improved on this initial discovery and devised a means of measuring the heart's electrical activity with a timed record. He named these measured waves or rhythmic movements the P, QRS, and T waves, and named the tracing of these movements *electrokardiogram.* In many circles, it is still known as an EKG. In the English language, we spell **cardiogram**, with a *c* and call this measurement the electrical activity of the heart an ECG. It will be known in this text as an ECG; however, EKG and ECG are the same.

The radiographer will participate in many diagnostic procedures that require continuous cardiac monitoring. In some institutions, he may be expected to prepare the patient for cardiac monitoring. In others, he may simply observe the patient who is being monitored and recognize ominous ECG patterns as they appear on the screen of an **oscilloscope**.

An ECG records the electrical activity of the heart, thereby providing a record of the heart's electrical activity and information concerning the heart's function and structure. As the heart is monitored, a tracing of its electrical activity is made on electrically sensitive paper or on the screen of an oscilloscope. This tracing is used to detect abnormal transmission of cardiac impulses from the heart through the surrounding tissues to the skin surface. When the impulses reach the skin, electrodes that have been placed in standardized anatomic positions transmit them to the ECG machine, and the impulses are then recorded in graphic form (Fig. 7-1).

ECG readings that seem abnormal are not necessarily indicative of heart disease. Conversely, a normal ECG pattern is not always an indication that the heart is healthy. The ECG cannot detect all pathological cardiac conditions.

There are several types of ECG testing. They require that electrodes be placed in varying numbers on the exterior body. A radiographer who must learn this subject in detail must plan to enroll in a special class for this purpose, which includes clinical practice in learning to read ECG rhythm strips. Continuous monitoring with the patient connected to a cardiac oscilloscope is the type of ECG to which the radiographer will most often be exposed. Blood pressure, respiratory rate, and oxygen saturation are also continuously monitored and displayed on the oscilloscope. If the patient's heart rate, rhythm, or other vital signs deviate from the normal rate or rhythm, an alarm sounds to alert the team caring for the patient. In this manner, life-threatening problems are detected instantly. A printout of the ECG pattern is made at specified times for the patient's record to compare the current pattern with previous patterns on each patient. The radiographer must be able to manually assess the patient's vital signs and the patient's visi-

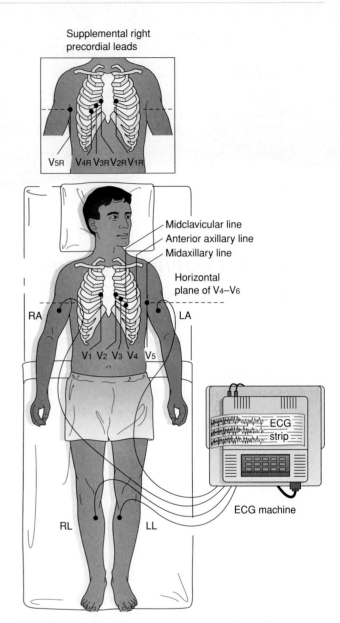

FIGURE 7-1   Recognize ominous signs on the oscilloscope.

ble signs of distress in emergency situations as he may be the first to detect a problem.

A REVIEW OF CARDIAC ANATOMY

The heart is a fist-sized muscular organ that is located in the left side of the body between the lungs and the mediastinum. It is a double pump. Its purpose is to pump deoxygenated blood through the heart to the lungs for reoxygenation and then to pump reoxygenated blood back through the heart into the aorta and ultimately to all body tissues. The student will recall that the heart has four chambers: the right and left atria and the right and left ventricles. The apex of

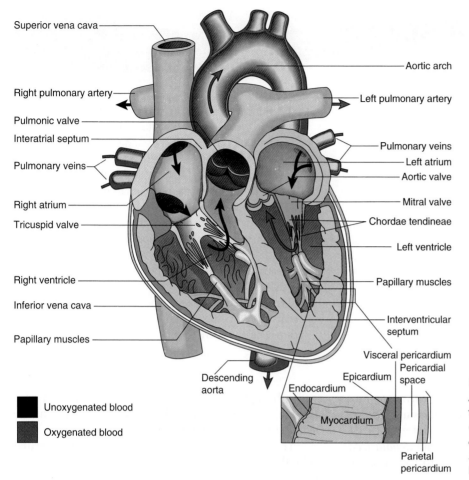

Superior vena cava

Aortic arch

Right pulmonary artery

Left pulmonary artery

Pulmonic valve

Pulmonary veins

Interatrial septum

Left atrium

Pulmonary veins

Aortic valve

Right atrium

Mitral valve

Tricuspid valve

Chordae tendineae

Left ventricle

Right ventricle

Papillary muscles

Inferior vena cava

Interventricular septum

Papillary muscles

Visceral pericardium

Descending aorta

Epicardium

Pericardial space

Endocardium

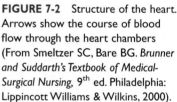

Myocardium

Parietal pericardium

Unoxygenated blood

Oxygenated blood

FIGURE 7-2   Structure of the heart. Arrows show the course of blood flow through the heart chambers (From Smeltzer SC, Bare BG. *Brunner and Suddarth's Textbook of Medical-Surgical Nursing*, 9th ed. Philadelphia: Lippincott Williams & Wilkins, 2000).

the heart is at the lowest aspect of the organ, and the base of the heart is the upper aspect. The right and left ventricles of the heart are separated by the interventricular septum. The chambers of the heart are protected from re-entry of blood that has been pumped from one chamber of the heart to another by a series of valves. The walls of the atria and ventricles are composed of three layers: the epicardium (the thin outer layer), the myocardium (the middle muscular layer), and the endocardium (the thin inner layer). The muscular layer of the atria is thinner than that of the ventricles. The blood flow through the heart is as follows:

1. Deoxygenated blood flows into the right atrium from the inferior and superior vena cava and veins draining into the heart.
2. It is then pumped through the tricuspid valve into the right ventricle.
3. The contraction of the right ventricle sends deoxygenated blood through the pulmonic (semilunar) valve into the lungs for reoxygenation through the pulmonary artery.
4. The oxygenated blood then flows through the pulmonary veins into the left atrium.

5. The contraction of the left atrium pumps the blood from the left atrium through the mitral (bicuspid) valve into the left ventricle.
6. The left ventricle then contracts, and oxygenated blood is pumped into the aorta and then to all parts of the body.

The myocardium (the heart muscle) is supplied with oxygenated blood via the right and left coronary arteries and their branches. The branches of the left coronary artery supply the interventricular septum, the walls and surfaces of the atria and ventricles, and the sinoatrial (SA) and atrioventricular (AV) nodes. The right coronary artery supplies the remainder of the myocardial blood supply (Fig. 7-2).

THE CARDIAC CONDUCTION SYSTEM

The ECG reports the electrical activity of the heart, particularly the contraction of the myocardium. It also supplies information concerning the heart's rate and rhythm. Electrical stimulation results in contraction of

Normal Cardiac Cycle

1. From the SA node, the wave of depolarization is carried through to the right atrium to the left atrium and results in nearly simultaneous contraction of the right and left atria.
2. The atrial conduction system has three internodal tracts in the right atrium (anterior, middle, and posterior) and one conduction tract in the left atrium called *Bachmann's bundle,* which depolarizes the left atrium.
3. Depolarization is then conducted to the AV node. The AV node is located in the right atrial wall near the tricuspid valve and coordinates the incoming electrical impulses from the atria.
4. After a brief delay during which the atria contracts and completes filling the ventricles, the impulse is conducted to the bundle of His.
5. The bundle of His is a group of cells that travels through the ventricular septum. It divides into the right and left bundle branches and conducts impulses to the right and left ventricles.
6. The left bundle branch bifurcates into the left anterior and left posterior bundle branches to reach the terminal point in the conduction system, the Purkinje fibers.
7. At this point, the myocardial cells are stimulated and result in ventricular contraction. This cell-to-cell passage of impulse is the *conductivity.* When the impulse spreads to all areas of the heart, the action potential is called *excitability.*
8. This leads to the shortening of the myocardial cells and *contractility.* The heart rate is determined by the myocardial cells with the most rapid firing rate (Fig. 7-3).

the heart. The cells of the heart muscle *(myocytes)* are influenced by sodium, calcium, and potassium ions. At rest, myocytes are *polarized,* and the interior of the cells is negatively charged. When they are *depolarized,* the interior of the myocytes become positive. When an electrical impulse is initiated, potassium rushes out of the myocytes and sodium rushes in. Calcium also enters the cells at this stage, but at a slower rate, and acts as a regulator of cardiac contraction. This initiates **depolarization** and converts the electrical charge of the cell into a positive charge. Depolarization acts as a wave throughout the myocardium and results in contraction of the heart. **Repolarization** takes place as the cells return to a resting state.

The conduction system of the heart has myocardial cells that have the properties of automaticity, conductivity, excitability, and contractility. The SA node, located in the upper posterior wall of the right atrium, is the dominant pacemaker of the heart. At rest under normal conditions, the SA node initiates 60 to 100 impulses per minute. It is responsible for the rate and rhythm of the cardiac cycle or the automaticity.

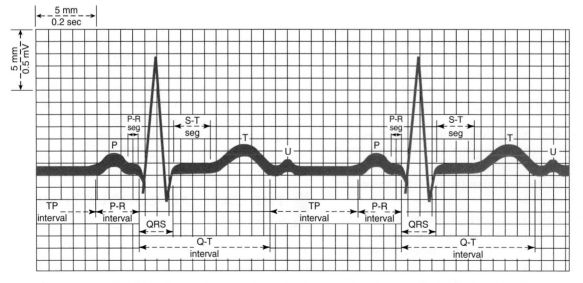

FIGURE 7-3 ECG graph (From Smelzer S, Bare B, Hinkle J, Cheever K. *Brunner and Suddarth's Textbook of Medical-Surgical Nursing,* 11th ed. Philadelphia: Lippincott Williams & Wilkins, 2008).

Display 7-1 describes the automaticity of the cardiac cycle when functioning in a normal fashion.

ELECTROPHYSIOLOGY OF THE CARDIAC CYCLE

The depolarization-repolarization cycle goes through five phases, which can be seen as it registers on the ECG monitor. When the electrical activity of the heart is normal, it is referred to as being in **normal sinus rhythm**. The P wave records the contraction of the atria (atrial depolarization). The QRS complex records contraction of the ventricles. The ST segment follows (the cell membrane is neutral in electrical charge). A U wave may follow the T wave and is associated with repolarization of the Purkinje fibers. (Fig. 7-4).

LEAD PLACEMENT

There are several methods of placing electrodes to monitor the electrical activity of the heart. The radiographer will rarely be called on to place the electrodes for a 12-lead ECG. The lead placement does not change the heart's electrical activity, but it does change the angle from which the activity is recorded. When a depolarization wave moves toward a positive electrode, the deflection on the ECG will be upward.

The two leads most often used for continuous monitoring are placed on the subclavicular and the midclavicular line (Fig. 7-5). If a third electrode (a ground electrode) is used, it may be positioned anywhere on the upper anterior chest.

The preparation of a patient for cardiac monitoring is as follows:

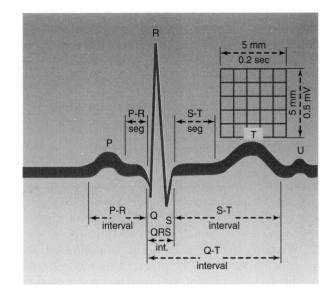

FIGURE 7-4 ECG graph and commonly measured complex components. Each small box represents 0.04 second on the horizontal axis and 1 mm or 0.1 millivolt on the vertical axis. The PR interval is measured from the beginning of the QRS complex; the QRS complex is measured from the beginning of the Q wave to the end of the S wave; the QT interval is measured from the beginning of the Q wave to the end of the T wave (From Smeltzer SC, Bare BG. *Brunner and Suddarth's Textbook of Medical-Surgical Nursing,* 9th ed. Philadelphia: Lippincott Williams & Wilkins, 2000).

1. Approach the patient, explain the procedure, and provide privacy.
2. Inform the patient that the monitor does not detect chest pain or dyspnea, and, if these symptoms occur, the patient must immediately inform the person who is caring for him. Also inform the patient that he will feel no electricity although he is wired as if he might.

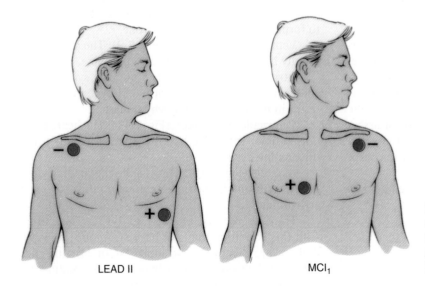

LEAD II   MCI₁

FIGURE 7-5 Placement of 2 leads for continuous monitoring (From Smeltzer SC, Bare BG. *Brunner and Suddarth's Textbook of Medical-Surgical Nursing,* 9th ed. Philadelphia: Lippincott Williams & Wilkins, 2000).

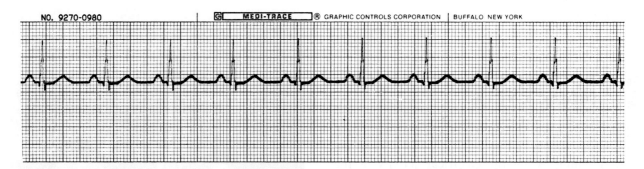

NO. 9270-0980   MEDI-TRACE   ® GRAPHIC CONTROLS CORPORATION   BUFFALO NEW YORK

FIGURE 7-6   Normal sinus rhythm (From Smeltzer SC, Bare BG. *Brunner and Suddarth's Textbook of Medical-Surgical Nursing,* 9th ed. Philadelphia: Lippincott Williams & Wilkins, 2000).

3. Wherever the electrodes are to be positioned, the patient's skin must be prepared by removing the dirt and oils present with soap and water or alcohol. Hair in those areas is sometimes removed by physician's order to reduce skin resistance.

4. Place the electrodes on flat areas of the skin. The electrodes used for continuous monitoring usually come pre-lubricated in a prepared package. If the electrodes are not pre-lubricated, an electroconductive paste is applied to each electrode before placement. The electrodes are adhesive and will remain in place if positioned on a flat surface.

5. Once the electrodes are in place, an alarm is set on the ECG machine for 30% above and 30% below the patient's baseline heart rate. Then the monitor and the electrocardiograph are activated. A deviation from the settings activates the alarm.

RADIOGRAPHER'S RESPONSIBILITIES DURING ECG MONITORING

The radiographer is expected to recognize **normal sinus rhythms** (Fig. 7-6). Cardiac **dysrhythmias** affect the heart's ability to pump an adequate supply of blood throughout the body. The ECG is used to detect cardiac dysrhythmias, conduction disorders, **myocardial ischemia**, injury, and **infarction**. A deviation from normal sinus rhythm may indicate a life-threatening emergency. The radiographer may be the first to see the change in the ECG. If this is the case, he must assess the patient's observable and reported symptoms and report them immediately to the team member in charge of the patient's care.

Signs and symptoms that may be observed and reported are:

- Anxiety
- Chest pain
- Altered level of consciousness
- Increased heart and respiratory rate

- Lightheadedness
- Cool, pale, moist skin
- Shortness of breath
- Nausea and vomiting

A radiographer's response should be:

- Use a calm, reassuring attitude toward the patient.
- Assess vital signs.
- Elevate patient's head.
- Prepare for oxygen to be administered.
- Prepare for intravenous drug administration.
- Prepare to call a code.

POTENTIALLY OMINOUS ECG DYSRHYTHMIAS

ECG rhythms that the radiographer must recognize as potential emergencies are pictured as follows:

Sinus bradycardia (Fig. 7-7): Ventricular and atrial rates are less than 60 and may result in significant **hemodynamic** changes; i.e., decreased level of consciousness, **angina**, hypotension.

Atrial fibrillation (Fig. 7-8): Atria and ventricles contracting rapidly and in an uneven pattern; may lead to formation of **thrombi** and stroke.

Ventricular tachycardia (Fig. 7-9): The patient may rapidly become unresponsive and pulseless.

Atrial flutter (Fig. 7-10): May have symptoms of chest pain, shortness of breath, and hypotension; may result in life-threatening dysrhythmias.

Ventricular fibrillation (Fig. 7-11): The heart rate is not audible; the pulse is not palpable. This is a life-threatening event.

Asystole (Fig. 7-12): This is a life-threatening emergency. Without immediate treatment, this is a fatal arrhythmia.

Third-degree AV block (Fig. 7-13): The patient with this condition may not have symptoms; however, if there are symptoms of shortness of breath, chest pain, lightheadedness, and hypotension, treatment is necessary to prevent myocardial infarction.

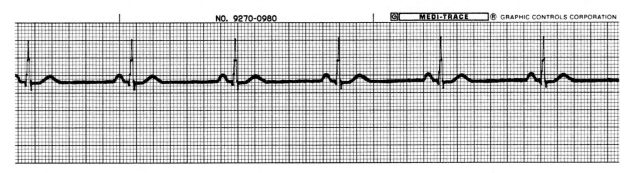

FIGURE 7-7 Sinus bradycardia (From Smeltzer SC, Bare BG. *Brunner and Suddarth's Textbook of Medical-Surgical Nursing*, 10th ed. Philadelphia: Lippincott Williams & Wilkins, 2004).

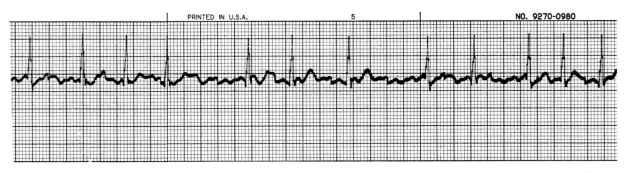

FIGURE 7-8 Atrial fibrillation (From Smeltzer SC, Bare BG. *Brunner and Suddarth's Textbook of Medical-Surgical Nursing*, 10th ed. Philadelphia: Lippincott Williams & Wilkins, 2004).

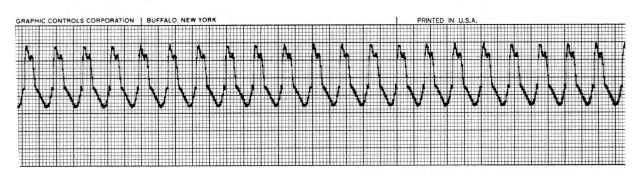

FIGURE 7-9 Ventricular tachycardia (From Smeltzer SC, Bare BG. *Brunner and Suddarth's Textbook of Medical-Surgical Nursing*, 10th ed. Philadelphia: Lippincott Williams & Wilkins, 2004).

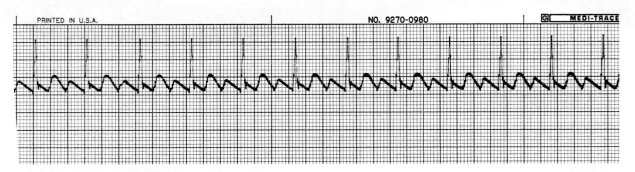

FIGURE 7-10 Atrial flutter (From Smeltzer SC, Bare BG. *Brunner and Suddarth's Textbook of Medical-Surgical Nursing*, 10th ed. Philadelphia: Lippincott Williams & Wilkins, 2004).

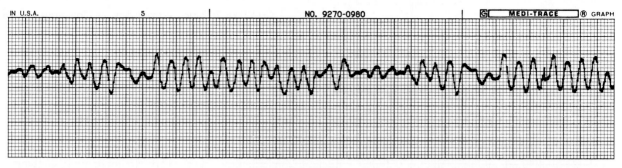

FIGURE 7-11 Ventricular fibrillation (From Smeltzer SC, Bare BG. *Brunner and Suddarth's Textbook of Medical-Surgical Nursing,* 10th ed. Philadelphia: Lippincott Williams & Wilkins, 2004).

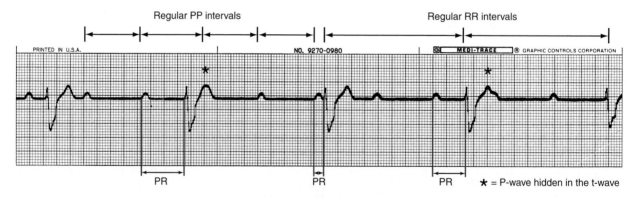

FIGURE 7-12 Asystole (From Smeltzer SC, Bare BG. *Brunner and Suddarth's Textbook of Medical-Surgical Nursing,* 10th ed. Philadelphia: Lippincott Williams & Wilkins, 2004).

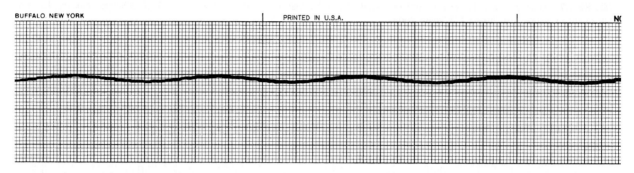

FIGURE 7-13 Third-degree AV block (From Smeltzer SC, Bare BG. *Brunner and Suddarth's Textbook of Medical-Surgical Nursing,* 10th ed. Philadelphia: Lippincott Williams & Wilkins, 2004).

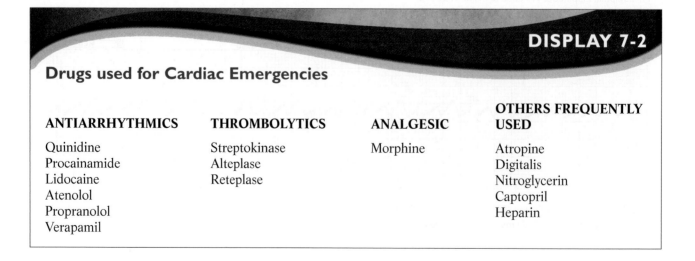

DISPLAY 7-2

Drugs used for Cardiac Emergencies

ANTIARRHYTHMICS	THROMBOLYTICS	ANALGESIC	OTHERS FREQUENTLY USED
Quinidine	Streptokinase	Morphine	Atropine
Procainamide	Alteplase		Digitalis
Lidocaine	Reteplase		Nitroglycerin
Atenolol			Captopril
Propranolol			Heparin
Verapamil			

DRUGS FREQUENTLY USED FOR CARDIAC EMERGENCIES

The radiographer will not administer the drugs called for during a cardiac emergency; however, he will find it helpful to be familiar with those most frequently used. Display 7-2 lists them and their physiologic purpose.

ECG ARTIFACTS

The radiographer must recognize artifacts when they appear on the ECG. Often seen as ominous or bizarre signs, they are simply errors in electrode connections or patient movement. Before calling a CODE, assess the patient's condition. If the patient is alert and without signs or symptoms of distress, reassess the electrode placement and connections. Be certain that an artifact is not the cause of an ominous-appearing ECG as the electrocardiograph will record any muscle movement.

SUMMARY

The radiographer will participate in and care for many patients whose cardiac status is being continuously monitored. He may be present when there is a change in the patient's condition accompanied by cardiac changes visible on the monitor (oscilloscope). He must be able to recognize ominous changes in the patient and alert the team member in charge of the patient's care. He must also be able to recognize the visible and verbal signs and symptoms that a patient in cardiac distress may display and respond to the patient's needs rapidly.

Interpreting an ECG is a complex process and is not within the scope of a radiographer's practice; however, he must be able to recognize normal sinus rhythm and ominous ECG patterns as they appear on the screen of an oscilloscope. He must be able to assess the patient, notify the team members in charge of the patient, and prepare for emergency action. The ability to correctly place chest leads on the patient to be monitored is also helpful.

Artifacts are often present as the patient moves or a lead becomes detached. The radiographer must be aware of artifacts and be able to recognize them as such.

CHAPTER 7 TEST

1. The radiographer is informed that the patient to whom he is assigned is having an EKG. The radiographer is aware that an EKG and an ECG are one and the same.
   a. True
   b. False
2. If the electrocardiogram reading is normal, the radiographer can assume that the patient does not have heart disease.
   a. True
   b. False
3. At rest, under normal conditions, the SA node initiates 60 to 100 impulses per minute.
   a. True
   b. False
4. When measuring the heart's ability to function in an adequate manner, the radiographer must also consider the following:
   a. The blood pressure
   b. The respirations
   c. The mental status of the patient
   d. The peripheral pulses
   e. All of the above

5. If the ECG rate indicates that the heart rate is 48 beats per minute, the radiographer can assume that the patient is having a problem called:
   a. Arrhythmia
   b. Tachycardia
   c. Bradycardia
   d. Flutter
   e. Fibrillation
6. Each normal ECG wave form consists of _____, _____, and _____ waves.
7. The ECG reports the following:
   a. Any pathology of the heart
   b. The heart's rate and rhythm
   c. The electrical activity of the heart
   d. a and b
   e. b and c
8. The radiographer's responsibilities in analyzing an ECG strip are:
   a. To diagnose the problem and notify the team caring for the patient
   b. To observe and report ominous changes in the ECG, assess the patient's signs and symp-

toms of distress, and prepare for emergency care
c. To observe and report ominous changes in the ECG
d. To observe changes in the ECG rhythm and notify the team caring for the patient
9. Signs and symptoms, other than changes in the ECG pattern, that indicate that the patient is in distress while he is being monitored on the oscilloscope might be:
a. Respiratory distress
b. Increased anxiety
c. Complaints of chest pain
d. a and b
e. All of the above
10. The ECG rhythm that the radiographer is expected to recognize is:
a. Atrial fibrillation
b. Sinus arrhythmia
c. Sinus tachycardia
d. Normal sinus rhythm

CHAPTER 8

Medical Emergencies

STUDENT LEARNING OUTCOMES

After studying this chapter, the student will be able to:

1. Assess the basic levels of neurological and cognitive functioning.

2. List the three classifications of shock, and describe the shock continuum.

3. Define distributive shock; list and define the three types of distributive shock.

4. Explain the role of the radiographer in recognizing and responding to the patient's immediate medical needs in the various categories of shock.

5. List the clinical manifestations of pulmonary embolus, and describe what the radiographer's response should be.

6. Differentiate among hypoglycemia, ketoacidosis, and hyperosmolar nonketotic syndrome, and explain the actions to take in response to these symptoms.

7. List the clinical manifestations of a cerebral vascular accident and explain the actions to take in response to these symptoms.

8. List the clinical manifestations of cardiac and respiratory failure and explain the actions to take in response to these symptoms.

9. Explain the symptoms of mechanical airway obstruction and the emergency intervention necessary if this is suspected.

10. Describe the action to take if a patient were to faint or have a seizure while under the radiographer's care.

11. Describe the best way to assist an agitated or confused patient and the intoxicated patient.

KEY TERMS

Anaphylaxis: The result of an exaggerated hypersensitivity reaction; an allergic reaction

Bradycardia: An abnormal circulatory condition in which the heart beats in a regular pattern but at a rate of less than 60 beats per minute

Bronchospasm: Contraction of smooth muscles in the walls of the bronchi and bronchioles causing narrowing of the lumen

Diaphoresis: Profuse sweating, heavy perspiration

Periorbital: Relating to the periosteum of the orbit, usually of the eye

Psychosis: A state in which a person's mental capacity to recognize reality, communicate, and relate to others is impaired

Syncope: Fainting

Tachycardia: An abnormal condition in which the myocardium contracts at a rate greater than 100 beats per minute

Many patients come to the radiographic imaging department in poor physical condition. This may be due to illness, injury, or a lengthy preparation for a diagnostic examination. When a person is in a weakened physical condition, physiologic reactions may not be as expected. Many abnormal physiologic reactions occur quickly and without warning and may be life threatening if not recognized and treated immediately. The non-trauma-related medical emergencies that are most likely to occur while the patient is undergoing radiographic imaging are shock, anaphylaxis (a type of shock), pulmonary embolus, reactions related to diabetes mellitus, cerebral vascular accident, cardiac and respiratory failure, syncope, and seizures. As the radiographer may be the first member of the health care team to observe these reactions, he or she must be able to recognize the symptoms and initiate the correct treatment.

The radiographer must be able to assess the behaviors that determine a patient's level of neurological and cognitive functioning on admission for a radiographic procedure. If this initial assessment is performed, the radiographer will be able to recognize changes in the patient's mental status if they occur while in the imaging department.

In most cases, the first action that should be taken in a life-threatening emergency is to call the hospital emergency team, the physician conducting the procedure, and a co-worker for assistance. Every radiographer must learn the correct procedure for calling the hospital emergency team in the institution in which he or she works. In many health care institutions, this procedure is dubbed "calling a code" or CODE BLUE. Memorize the emergency team number, and be prepared to explain the exact location of the emergency and the problem that has occurred.

All radiographic imaging departments have an emergency cart that contains the medications and equipment that are needed when a patient's condition suddenly becomes critical. This is often called the "crash cart." Know where to obtain this cart quickly and know who is responsible for maintaining the cart and having all its equipment and supplies in working order. Be familiar with the oxygen administration equipment so that assistance can be provided quickly.

Although radiographers are not the health care workers who are responsible for a patient's pain management during most of his or her medical care, the radiographer must be sensitive to complaints of pain and discomfort while the patient is in the imaging department.

ASSESSMENT OF LEVELS OF NEUROLOGIC AND COGNITIVE FUNCTIONING

The radiographer must be able to quickly assess the patient's neurologic functioning. This is important so that if the patient's condition deteriorates, you can quickly recognize this based on changes in the initial assessment data. Neurologic assessment can be highly technical and complex and is not within the scope of a radiographer's practice. However, a rapid neurologic assessment tool that is used frequently in health care institutions is the Glasgow Coma Scale. This scale addresses the three areas of neurologic functioning and quickly gives an overview of the patient's level of responsiveness. It is simple, reliable, and convenient to use.

Three areas can be readily observed—eyes opening, motor response, and verbal response (Display 8-1). A patient can be rated a maximum of 15 points for neurologic functioning. If the patient's score begins to

DISPLAY 8-1

Glasgow Coma Scale

Eyes Open

Spontaneously	14
To voice	3
To painful stimuli	2
No response	1

Motor Response

Obeys commands	6
Localized pain	5
Withdraws from painful stimuli	4
Abnormal flexion	3
Extension	2
No response	1

Verbal Response

Oriented	5
Confused speech	4
Inappropriate words	3
Incomprehensible sounds	2
None	1
Total points possible	15

drop after the initial assessment, notify the physician in charge of the patient immediately.

Another indicator that a patient's condition is deteriorating is a change in the level of consciousness (LOC). These changes can be subtle but must not be ignored. The LOC can be assessed quickly as follows:

1. Ask the patient to state his or her name, date, address, and the reason for coming to the radiographic imaging department. *If the patient gives these responses readily and correctly, then it can be assumed that the patient is responding to verbal stimuli and that he or she is oriented to person, place, time, and situation. Note any undue need to repeat questions and any slow response, difficulty with choice of words, or unusual irritability.*

2. Note the patient's ability to follow directions during instruction regarding positioning for the examination. Also note any movement that causes pain or other difficulty in movement, as well as any alterations in behavior or lack of response. Report these to the physician in charge of caring for the patient. *These measures provide a baseline against which changes in the patient's mental and neurologic status can be assessed.*

3. Assess the patient's vital signs at this time if current readings are not on the chart. Baseline readings are a must to have in order to note any changes that may occur. An increasing systolic blood pressure or widening of the pulse pressure may indicate increasing intracranial pressure. Slowing of the pulse may also indicate increasing intracranial pressure. As compression of the brain increases, the vital signs change. Respirations increase, blood pressure decreases, and the pulse rate decreases further. A rapid rise in body temperature or a decrease in body temperature is also an ominous sign.

If the patient has no complaints on initial assessment, note this. If the patient begins to complain of a headache, becomes restless or unusually quiet, or develops slurred speech or a change in the level of orientation as a procedure progresses, report this to the physician immediately, stop the procedure, stay with the patient, and summon assistance. This includes ordering the emergency cart to be brought to the patient. Then, prepare the patient for oxygen and intravenous fluid administration.

⚠ **WARNING!**

Changes in a patient's neurologic status or LOC must never be ignored! Stop your work and notify the physician of these changes.

SHOCK

Shock is the body's pathological reaction to illness, trauma, or severe physiologic or emotional stress. It may be caused by body fluid loss, cardiac failure, decreased tone of the blood vessels, or obstruction of blood flow to the vital body organs. Shock is a life-threatening condition that may occur rapidly and without warning. It may be reversible if it is not allowed to progress. The radiographer may be the first health care worker to observe the initial symptoms of shock; therefore, it is important to recognize them and begin the interventions that will halt its progress.

The Shock Continuum

The vital organs of the body depend on oxygen and other nutrients supplied by the blood for their survival. When this supply is diminished, adverse effects on normal physiologic functions occur. The shock syndrome may progress as a continuum in the patient's struggle to survive and return to a normal physiologic state.

At the onset of the shock continuum, the changes in physiologic function are in the cells of the body and are not clinically detectable except for a possible increase in heart rate. As the condition progresses, blood is shunted away from the lungs, skin, kidneys, and gastrointestinal tract to accommodate the brain's and the heart's critical need for oxygen. At this stage, called the *compensatory* stage, a host of symptoms are noticeable:

1. Skin is cold and clammy.
2. Urine output decreases.
3. Respirations increase.
4. Bowel sounds are hypoactive.
5. Blood pressure is normal.
6. Anxiety level increases; patient may begin to be uncooperative.

If shock is allowed to progress beyond the compensatory stage, the mean arterial pressure (the average pressure at which the blood moves through the vasculature of the body; abbreviated MAP) falls. All body systems are inadequately perfused, including the heart, which begins to pump inadequately.

The peripheral circulation reacts to the chemical mediators released by the body in this state, and fluid leaks from the capillaries, further decreasing the amount of fluid in circulation. The patient has acute renal failure, and the liver, gastrointestinal, and hematologic systems begin to fail. This stage in the shock continuum is called the *progressive* stage. Progressive stage symptoms are as follows:

1. Blood pressure falls.
2. Respirations are rapid and shallow.

3. Severe pulmonary edema results from leakage of fluid from the pulmonary capillaries. This is referred to as acute respiration distress syndrome or shock lung.
4. **Tachycardia** results and may be as rapid as 150 beats per minute.
5. The patient complains of chest pain.
6. Mental status changes beginning with subtle behavior alterations such as confusion with progression to lethargy and loss of consciousness.
7. Renal, hepatic, gastrointestinal, and hematologic problems occur.

If shock progresses beyond this point, it is called the *irreversible* stage. The organ systems of the body suffer irreparable damage, and recovery is unlikely.

Irreversible stage involves the following:

1. Blood pressure remains low.
2. Renal and liver failure result.
3. There is a release of necrotic tissue toxins and an overwhelming lactic acidosis.

There are different classifications of shock. These include hypovolemic, cardiogenic, and distributive or vasogenic shock. The following sections provide descriptions, clinical manifestations, and the radiographer's response to each of these.

Hypovolemic Shock

Body fluids are contained within the cells of the body and are in the extracellular compartments. The extracellular fluid is further distributed to the blood vessels (intravascular) and into the surrounding body tissues (interstitial). Approximately three or four times more body fluid is within the interstitial spaces than is within the vasculature of the body. When the amount of intravascular fluid decreases by 15% to 25% or by a loss of 750 to 1,300 milliliters, hypovolemic shock occurs. This decrease in volume may be due to internal or external hemorrhage; loss of plasma from burns; or fluid loss from prolonged vomiting, diarrhea, or medications.

Clinical Manifestations The signs and symptoms of hypovolemic shock may be placed into classes as follows:

Class I: A blood loss of 15%
* Blood pressure is within normal limits.
* Heart rate is less than 100 beats per minute.
* Respiration ranges from 14 to 20 per minute.

Class II: A blood loss of 15% to 30%
* Blood pressure is within normal limits.
* Heart rate is greater than 100 beats per minute.
* Respiration ranges from 20 to 30 per minute.

Class III: A blood loss of 30% to 40%
* Blood pressure begins to decrease to below normal limits.
* Heart rate is greater than 120 beats per minute.
* Respiration increases to 30 to 40 per minute.

Class IV: A blood loss of 40% or more
* Systolic blood pressure decreases from 90 to 60 mm Hg.
* Heart rate is now in tachycardia with a weak and thready pulse.
* Respiration is greater than 40 per minute.

The patient may become excessively thirsty as a result of the fluid loss from hypovolemic shock. The extremities are cold; the skin is cold and clammy with cyanosis starting at the lips and nails. If the patient is dark-skinned, observe for cyanosis by pressing lightly on the fingernails or earlobes. If the patient is cyanotic, the color will not return to the compressed area in the usual 1-second interval. A bluish discoloration of the tongue and soft palate of the mouth is also indicative of cyanosis. If this condition is allowed to continue, cardiac and respiratory failure follows.

Radiographer's Response

1. Stop the ongoing radiographic procedure; place the patient supine with legs elevated 30 degrees (if there is no head or spinal cord injury). Do not place the patient in Trendelenburg position.
2. Notify the physician in charge and call for emergency assistance from the radiology nurse.
3. Make certain the patient is able to breathe without obstruction caused by position or blood or mucus in the airway.
4. If there is an open wound with blood loss, don gloves and apply pressure directly to the wound with several thicknesses of dry, sterile dressing.
5. Bring the emergency cart to the patient's room.
6. Prepare to assist with oxygen, intravenous fluids, and medications.
7. Keep the patient warm and dry, but do not overheat the patient as this will increase the need for oxygen.
8. Assess vital signs every 5 minutes until the emergency team assumes this role.
9. Do not leave the patient unattended. Inform him or her as appropriate of what is happening to alleviate anxiety.
10. Do not offer fluids to the patient, even if requested. Explain that he or she may need examination or treatment that requires an empty stomach.

Cardiogenic Shock

Cardiogenic shock is caused by a failure of the heart to pump an adequate amount of blood to the vital organs. The onset of cardiogenic shock may occur over a period of time, or it may be sudden. The patient who has been hospitalized for myocardial infarction, cardiac tamponade, dysrhythmias, or other cardiac pathology is most vulnerable.

Clinical Manifestations

- Complaint of chest pain that may radiate to jaws and arms
- Dizziness and respiratory distress
- Cyanosis
- Restlessness and anxiety
- Rapid change in level of consciousness
- Pulse may be irregular and slow; may have tachycardia and tachypnea
- Difficult-to-find carotid pulse indicates decreased stroke volume of the heart
- Decreasing blood pressure
- Decreasing urinary output
- Cool, clammy skin

Radiographer's Response

1. Summon the emergency team and have the emergency cart placed at the patient's side.
2. Notify the physician in charge of the patient
3. Place the patient in semi-Fowler's position or in another position that will facilitate respiration.
4. Prepare to assist with oxygen, intravenous fluid, and medication administration. Chest pain must be controlled.
5. Do not leave the patient alone; offer an explanation of treatment as appropriate; alleviate the patient's anxiety.
6. Assess pulse, respiration, and blood pressure every 5 minutes until the emergency team arrives.
7. Do not offer fluids.
8. Be prepared to administer cardiopulmonary resuscitation (CPR), if indicated.

Distributive Shock

Distributive shock occurs when a pooling of blood in the peripheral blood vessels results in decreased venous return of blood to the heart, decreased blood pressure, and decreased tissue perfusion. This may be the result of loss of sympathetic tone. Distributive shock is characterized by the blood vessels' inability to constrict and their resultant inability to assist in the return of the blood to the heart. It may also occur when chemicals released by the cells cause vasodilation and capillary permeability, which in turn prompts

a large portion of the blood volume to pool peripherally. There are three types of distributive shock: neurogenic, septic, and anaphylactic. Each is discussed in the following text.

Neurogenic Shock

Neurogenic shock results from loss of sympathetic tone causing vasodilation of peripheral vessels. Spinal cord injury, severe pain, neurologic damage, the depressant action of medication, lack of glucose (as in insulin reaction or shock), or the adverse effects of anesthesia can all cause neurogenic shock.

Clinical Manifestations

- Hypotension
- **Bradycardia**
- Warm, dry skin
- Initial alertness if not unconscious because of head injury
- Cool extremities and diminishing peripheral pulses

Radiographer's Response

1. Summon emergency assistance.
2. Notify the physician in charge of the patient.
3. Keep the patient in supine position; legs may be elevated with physician's orders.
4. Have the emergency cart brought to the patient's side.
5. If spinal cord injury is possible, do not move the patient.
6. Stay with the patient and offer support.
7. Monitor pulse, respirations, and blood pressure every 5 minutes.
8. Prepare to assist with oxygen, intravenous fluids, and medications.

Septic Shock

Septic shock is the least likely to be observed by the radiographer in the imaging department. However radiographers must be able to recognize septic shock. Patients in the intensive care unit or emergency room who are in septic shock may need to have a portable radiograph taken. In spite of the wide availability and use of antibiotics in recent years, the incidence of septic shock has risen and has a 40% to 50% mortality rate for its victims.

Gram-negative bacteria are the most common causative organisms in septic shock; however, gram-positive bacteria and viruses can be the cause. When invaded by bacteria, the body begins its immune response by releasing chemicals that increase capillary permeability and vasodilatation, leading to the shock syndrome. The clinical manifestations of septic shock are divided into two phases.

Clinical Manifestations

First Phase:

- Hot, dry, and flushed skin
- Increase in heart rate and respiratory rate
- Fever, but possibly not in the elderly patient
- Nausea, vomiting, and diarrhea
- Normal to excessive urine output
- Possible confusion, most commonly in the elderly patient

Second Phase:

- Cool, pale skin
- Normal or subnormal temperature
- Drop in blood pressure
- Rapid heart rate and respiratory rate
- Oliguria or anuria
- Seizures and organ failure if syndrome is not reversed

Radiographer's Response The radiographer is rarely the person who initiates action if septic shock is present. However, if a patient in septic shock is in the imaging department, he or she must not become chilled as shivering increases the body's oxygen consumption.

Anaphylactic Shock

Because some imaging procedures use contrast agents that contain iodine, to which some people are allergic, this is the most frequently seen type of shock in radiographic imaging. The radiographer must be able to recognize it at its onset to prevent life-threatening consequences.

Anaphylactic shock (**anaphylaxis**) is the result of an exaggerated hypersensitivity reaction (allergic reaction) to re-exposure to an antigen that was previously encountered by the body's immune system. When this occurs, histamine and bradykinin are released, causing widespread vasodilatation, which results in peripheral pooling of blood. This response is accompanied by contraction of nonvascular smooth muscles, particularly the smooth muscles of the respiratory tract. This combined reaction produces shock, respiratory failure, and death within minutes after exposure to the allergen. Usually, the more abrupt the onset of anaphylaxis, the more severe the reaction will be.

The most common causes of anaphylaxis are medications, iodinated contrast agents, and insect venoms. The path of entry may be through the skin, respiratory tract, or gastrointestinal tract, or through injection.

The radiographer performing the procedure in which contrast media is injected is responsible for the patient. A meticulous history of previous allergic responses that the patient may have had to any medication or food, including previous incidents when receiving contrast agents in imaging, must be obtained. If any of these responses are reported, the radiologist must be informed prior to injection of any contrast media.

When iodinated contrast agents are being used for diagnostic procedures, observe the patient continuously for signs of allergic reaction. If early symptoms of anaphylactic shock are observed, quick action must be taken to halt the progression of symptoms.

Clinical Manifestations The signs of anaphylactic shock may be classified as mild, moderate, or severe as follows:

Mild Systemic Reaction:

- Nasal congestion, **periorbital** swelling, itching, sneezing, and tearing of eyes
- Peripheral tingling or itching at the site of injection
- Feeling of fullness or tightness of the chest, mouth, or throat
- Feeling of anxiety or nervousness

Moderate Systemic Reaction:

- All of the above symptoms, plus:
- Flushing, feeling of warmth, itching, and urticaria
- **Bronchospasm** and edema of the airways or larynx
- Dyspnea, cough, and wheezing

Severe Systemic Reaction:

- All symptoms listed above with an abrupt onset
- Decreasing blood pressure; weak, thready pulse either rapid or shallow
- Rapid progression to bronchospasm, laryngeal edema, severe dyspnea, cyanosis
- Dysphasia, abdominal cramping, vomiting, and diarrhea
- Seizures, respiratory and cardiac arrest

Radiographer's Response

1. Do not leave the patient. Stop any infusion or injection of contrast immediately and notify the radiologist if any of the symptoms occur.
2. If the patient complains of respiratory distress or has any of the symptoms listed in the severe reaction section, call the emergency team.
3. Place the patient in semi-Fowler position or in a sitting position to facilitate respiration.
4. Monitor pulse, respiration, and blood pressure every 5 minutes or until the emergency team arrives to assume responsibility.
5. Prepare to assist with oxygen, intravenous fluid, and medication administration. Have large-gauge venous catheters available.
6. Prepare to administer CPR as required.

The medications usually given for anaphylactic shock are epinephrine, diphenhydramine, hydrocortisone, and aminophylline.

DISPLAY 8-2

Information Requested before Administration of Contrast Agents

Name

Age

Date

Have you had the study you are having today at any other time?

If the answer is yes, did you have any allergic or unusual reaction?

Are you allergic to any food, medications or any other substance? If you are, please specify.

Recent laboratory tests performed and results

Blood urea nitrogen (BUN) and createnine

Have you had any protein in your urine? If so, to what degree?

Do you have heart disease?

Hypertension?

Diabetes mellitus?

Sickle cell anemia?

Asthma?

Have you had any procedures such as a cryptogram that involved use of contrast agents? If so, please explain.

Many radiographic imaging departments have a standardized procedure form that must be completed before the administration of contrast agents. This form may request the information shown in Display 8-2.

After the examination, the physician completes a report indicating the type of contrast agent used and any unusual responses. If the patient has an anaphylactic reaction, the nature of the reaction should be written on the patient's radiographic history. The person performing the injection and examination must also make documentation of the reaction in the patient's chart.

A copy of this report is kept in the patient's diagnostic imaging department file, and the radiography supervisor also keeps a copy. If these precautions in documentation are taken, the history of the patient's previous problem will be on record, and the correct decisions can be made subsequently.

Patients who have received contrast agents as part of the diagnostic imaging procedure should remain in the department for 30 minutes for observation if they are not patients in the hospital. If they are having no problems after 30 minutes, they may be allowed to return home, accompanied by another person. They should be clearly instructed in the signs and symptoms of an anaphylactic reaction and told to return to the hospital emergency department immediately if any of these symptoms appear. A patient who has had even a mild allergic reaction during a diagnostic procedure that involves the use of a contrast agent should be instructed to report this if he or she is ever to receive iodinated contrast media in the future. If the reaction was severe, the patient may

need to wear an alert bracelet to prevent further exposure to antigens of this sort.

Obstructive Shock

Obstructive shock results from pathological conditions that interfere with the normal pumping action of the heart; however, the heart itself may be free of pathologic conditions. The cause of obstructive shock may be pulmonary embolism, pulmonary hypertension, arterial stenosis, constrictive pericarditis, or tumors that interfere with blood flow through the heart. Because pulmonary embolism is the only condition mentioned here that might have an impact on the radiographer in the care of patients, it is the only condition discussed in this chapter.

PULMONARY EMBOLUS

A pulmonary embolus is an occlusion of one or more pulmonary arteries by a thrombus or thrombi. The thrombus originates in the venous circulation or in the right side of the heart and is carried through the vessels to the lungs, where it blocks one or more pulmonary arteries. This is a common medical emergency, which results in more than 50,000 deaths each year. The onset is sudden and requires immediate action to prevent severe consequences.

Pulmonary embolus is associated with trauma, orthopedic and abdominal surgical procedures, pregnancy, congestive heart failure, prolonged immobility, and hypercoagulable states. Emboli may also be the result of air, fat, amniotic fluid, or sepsis. The severity of symptoms depends on the size or number of emboli that disturb the pulmonary circulation. The end result is arterial hypoxemia, which may be a life-threatening emergency.

When working with postoperative patients and patients who have suffered traumatic events affecting

⚠ WARNING!

A meticulous history is mandatory when a patient is to receive a contrast agent!

the long bones of the body, the radiographer must be aware of the complication of pulmonary embolism and be prepared to initiate emergency action if it occurs.

Clinical Manifestations
- Rapid, weak pulse
- Hyperventilation
- Dyspnea and tachypnea
- Tachycardia
- Apprehension
- Cough and hemoptysis
- **Diaphoresis**
- **Syncope**
- Hypotension
- Cyanosis
- Rapidly changing levels of consciousness
- Coma; sudden death may result

Radiographer's Response
1. Stop the procedure immediately, and call for emergency assistance.
2. Notify the physician, and bring the emergency cart to the patient's side.
3. Monitor vital signs.
4. Do not leave the patient alone; reassure the patient.
5. Prepare to assist with oxygen administration and administration of intravenous medication and fluid.

◼ DIABETIC EMERGENCIES

Diabetes mellitus is now recognized as a group of metabolic diseases resulting from a chronic disorder of carbohydrate metabolism. It is caused by either insufficient production of insulin or inadequate utilization of insulin by the cells of the body. The result is an abnormal amount of glucose in the blood (hyperglycemia). The underlying cause of this disease process is a disturbance in the production, action, or utilization of insulin. Insulin is a hormone normally secreted by the islets of Langerhans located in the pancreas. In diabetes mellitus, the cells either stop responding to insulin or the pancreas ceases to produce insulin. In either case, the result is hyperglycemia, which leads to a series of metabolic complications. These complications may be diabetic ketoacidosis or hyperglycemic hyperosmolar nonketotic syndrome complications. These disease processes adversely affect the structure and function of blood vessels and other organs of the body.

There are four major types of diabetes mellitus. The causes are not identical, and the course of the disease process and the treatment vary according to the type presenting. They are as follows:

1. *Type 1 diabetes mellitus.* Usually occurs in persons younger than 30 years of age and has an abrupt onset. An autoimmune process destroys the insulin-producing pancreatic beta cells, and the affected person must receive insulin by injection to control blood glucose levels in the body and prevent ketoacidosis.

2. *Type 2 diabetes mellitus.* Usually occurs in persons older than 40 years of age and has a gradual onset. It results either from an impaired sensitivity to insulin or from a decreased production of insulin. This disease may be controlled by weight loss, dietary control, and exercise. However, if these measures do not control the problem, the person affected must take oral hypoglycemic agents to prevent hyperglycemia. Diabetic ketoacidosis does not occur in type 2 diabetes because there is enough insulin present in the body to prevent the breakdown of fat. However, a syndrome called hyperosmolar nonketotic syndrome may result and present an acute problem.

3. *Diabetes mellitus associated with or produced by other medical conditions or syndromes.*

4. *Gestational diabetes.* A diabetic condition that occurs in the later months of pregnancy. Hormones secreted by the placenta that prevent the action of insulin cause it. This condition is usually treated with diet, but insulin may be prescribed to maintain blood glucose levels.

There are other conditions or physiologic problems that result in impairment of glucose tolerance that are not discussed in this text because they do not usually result in the need for emergency care. Persons with diabetes mellitus are extremely susceptible to infections and therefore require extra skin care and infection control precautions.

Acute Complications of Diabetes Mellitus

There are three complications of diabetes mellitus that may occur when caring for a patient: hypoglycemia, diabetic ketoacidosis, and hyperosmolar nonketotic syndrome (also called hyperosmolar nonketotic coma). The descriptions and radiographer's responses follow:

- *Hypoglycemia* occurs when persons who have diabetes mellitus have an excess amount of insulin or oral hypoglycemic drug in their bloodstream, an increased metabolism of glucose, or an inadequate food intake with which to utilize the insulin. This may occur when the patient has not had anything to eat or drink prior to coming to the department for his or her procedure. The onset of symptoms is rapid, and immediate action is necessary to prevent coma.
- *Diabetic ketoacidosis* occurs when insufficient insulin causes the liver to produce more glucose, resulting in hyperglycemia. The kidneys attempt to compensate by excreting glucose with water

and electrolytes. There is excessive urination (polyuria) with an outcome of dehydration and electrolyte imbalance in the body.

- *Hyperglycemic hyperosmolar nonketotic syndrome* (coma) may be a complication of mild type 2 diabetes mellitus, or it may occur in the elderly person with no known history of diabetes mellitus.

Clinical Manifestations   The following occur in all cases:

- Tachycardia
- Headache
- Blurred or double vision
- Extreme thirst
- Sweet odor to the breath may occur in diabetic ketoacidosis

Radiographer's Response
1. Stop the procedure and notify the radiologist in charge of the procedure.
2. Do not leave the patient unattended.
3. Monitor the vital signs and prepare to administer intravenous fluids, medication, and oxygen as they may be needed and requested by an emergency team.

CEREBRAL VASCULAR ACCIDENT (STROKE)

Cerebral vascular accidents (CVAs) are caused by occlusion of the blood supply to the brain, rupture of the blood supply to the brain, or rupture of a cerebral artery, resulting in hemorrhage directly into the brain tissue or into the spaces surrounding the brain (Fig. 8-1).

Strokes vary in severity from mild transient ischemic attacks to severe, life-threatening situations. CVAs occur most frequently with little or no warning and may possibly occur in the radiographic imaging department during a stressful procedure.

Strokes are now being termed "brain attacks." A stroke is now recognized as an event that is as great a medical crisis as a heart attack. It is extremely important that the stroke victim receive immediate emergency evaluation, because being started on fibrinolytic therapy reduces the neurologic damage from an ischemic stroke. The warning signs and symptoms of this medical crisis must be recognized in order to be prepared to initiate emergency care.

Clinical Manifestations
- Possible severe headache
- Numbness
- Muscle weakness or flaccidity of face or extremities, usually one-sided

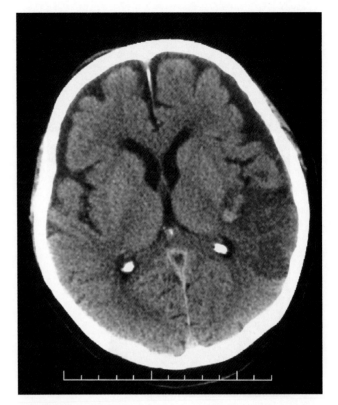

FIGURE 8-1   CT of the brain showing bleeding on the right side, which resulted in a stroke.

- Eye deviation, usually one-sided; possible loss of vision
- Confusion
- Dizziness or stupor
- Difficult speech (dysphasia) or no speech (aphasia)
- Ataxia
- May complain of stiff neck
- Nausea or vomiting may occur
- Loss of consciousness

CARDIAC AND RESPIRATORY EMERGENCIES

Respiratory failure, cardiac failure (also called cardiac arrest), or an airway obstruction may occur in the diagnostic imaging department without warning and when least expected. The radiographer may be the first health care worker to witness this event and thus will be the person to call the code and initiate emergency action. The human brain can survive without oxygen for only 2 to 4 minutes. This means that there is little time to ponder the situation before acting.

All health care staff must be prepared to perform basic CPR and the abdominal thrust maneuver. New basic life support guidelines have recently made early

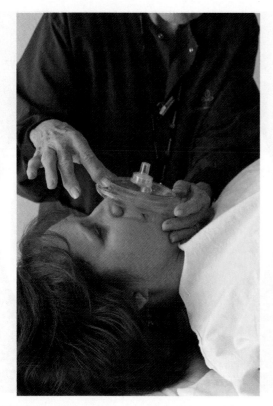

FIGURE 8-2 Disposable mask with a one-way valve.

cardiac defibrillation a high-priority goal and the ability to use an automatic external defibrillator (AED) a basic life support skill.

There are frequent changes in basic life support methods, and it will be the radiographer's responsibility to keep abreast of the changes and rules in the place of employment concerning responsibilities as a responder to a cardiac or respiratory type of emergency. The brief descriptions of CPR, the use of the AED, and the abdominal thrust maneuver do not prepare the technologist to administer these techniques. A complete Basic Life Support course for health care professionals is mandatory.

Any time the radiographer is working with a patient to open the airway, clean gloves must be worn. A disposable mask with a one-way valve is recommended when performing CPR (Fig. 8-2). This type of mask should be available in every diagnostic imaging room. A manual resuscitation bag may be used if available. AEDs must also be made available and ready for use for a health care worker who is competent to use them.

Cardiac Arrest

When the heart ceases to beat effectively, the blood can no longer circulate throughout the body, and the person no longer has an effective pulse. There are a number of possible causes of this type of event. The electrical activity of the heart may be disrupted, causing the

heart to beat too rapidly, as in ventricular fibrillation or ventricular tachycardia. The heart may beat too slowly, as in **bradycardia** or atrioventricular block. Pulseless electrical activity may also result from hypovolemic shock, cardiac tamponade, hypothermia, or a pulmonary embolism. In addition, drug overdoses, severe acidosis, or a severe myocardial infarction may cause this to occur. Irreversible brain damage and death result within minutes of a cardiac event, depending on the person's age and health status before the arrest.

Clinical Manifestations of Cardiac Arrest
- Loss of consciousness, pulse, and blood pressure
- Dilation of the pupils within seconds
- Possibility of seizures

Respiratory Dysfunction

Respiratory dysfunction may precede respiratory arrest. It can be the result of airway obstruction caused by positioning, the tongue falling backward into the throat of an unresponsive person, a foreign object lodged in the throat, disease, drug overdose, injury, or coma. Whatever the cause, gas exchange is no longer adequate to meet the needs of the body.

Clinical Manifestations of a Partially Obstructed Airway
- Labored, noisy breathing
- Wheezing
- Use of accessory muscles of the neck, abdomen, or chest on inspiration
- Neck vein distention
- Diaphoresis
- Anxiety
- Cyanosis of the lips and nail beds
- Possibly a productive cough with pink-tinged frothy sputum

Radiographer's Response to a Patient with a Partially Obstructed Airway
1. Call for assistance; do not leave the patient alone.
2. Assist the patient to a sitting or semi-Fowler position.
3. Attempt to relieve the patient's anxiety.
4. Prepare to administer oxygen.
5. Prepare to use the emergency cart.

Respiratory Arrest

Clinical Manifestations
- The patient stops responding
- The pulse continues to beat briefly and then quickly becomes weak and stops
- Chest movement stops, and no air is detectable moving through the patient's mouth

Radiographer's Response to Both Cardiac and Respiratory Arrest

1. If the patient is an adult and is found to be unresponsive, shake the patient and ask, "Are you all right?" If there is no response, call immediately for emergency medical services (call a CODE). If no one is near, shout for help, stating the location as well. "I need help STAT in Room 102." Do not leave the patient.

2. Assess the carotid pulse of an adult patient. Do not waste time taking the blood pressure or listening for a heartbeat.

3. If the patient is an adult with no pulse and the CODE has been called, place the patient in a supine position on a hard surface. If the patient is already on the radiographic table, leave the patient there, as this is a perfect place to perform CPR.

Begin Cardiopulmonary Resuscitation

1. Open the airway. Put on gloves; remove any obvious material in the mouth or throat. If the patient has dentures that are loose, remove them. Avoid pushing a foreign object farther back into the mouth or throat. Do not perform blind finger sweeps! Direct the chin up and back (Fig. 8-3). Never sweep the mouth of an infant or small child unless the object is visible and reachable.

2. Look, listen, and feel for airway movement. If there is nothing, tightly place the bag- or mouth-mask over the patient's mouth and nose. Take a deep breath and slowly, over 2 full seconds, with the least amount of air needed to make the chest rise, exhale into the mouth-mask. Allow the patient to exhale. Repeat the maneuver. This sequence reduces the amount of air that enters the stomach of the patient to prevent the complication of regurgitation, aspiration, and pneumonia.

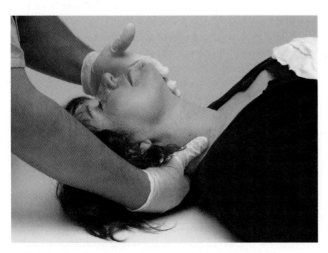

FIGURE 8-3 Direct the chin up and back.

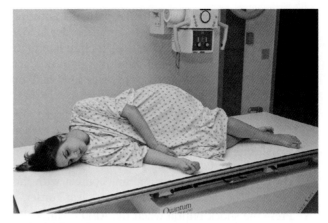

FIGURE 8-4 Patient in a recovery position.

3. If the patient is not breathing and initial ventilation attempts are not successful, assess for foreign body in airway. If rescue ventilations have failed and an obstructed airway is suspected, use abdominal thrusts to remove obstruction (as explained later in this chapter). Recheck for breathing.

4. If the patient is breathing, place him or her in a recovery position (Fig. 8-4).

5. Assess for signs of circulation by checking carotid pulse, and evaluate for coughing, movement, and breathing.

6. If no signs of circulation or breathing are present, the AED is not readily available, and the emergency team has not arrived, begin chest compressions.

Defibrillation

Cardiac arrest may precede or follow respiratory arrest. It may also occur when the electrical activity of the heart is present but not effective in delivering oxygenated blood to vital organs. When cardiac arrest occurs and the patient is being monitored or is immediately placed on a monitor, use the quick-look paddles found on most defibrillators to determine the presence of ventricular tachycardia or ventricular fibrillation. If these are not available, apply the AED as quickly as possible to analyze the patient's heart rhythm. For every minute that defibrillation is delayed, the patient's chances for survival decline by 10%. The AED procedure is briefly described below; however, all radiographers must be properly instructed in this procedure in a certified class with clinical practice.

1. Place the AED pack near the patient's left shoulder and open it. This should turn the power on automatically and initiate voice instruction from the pack. CPR may be continued until it is time to attach the electrodes.

2. Attach the electrodes onto the patient's anterior chest: one at the right upper sternal border below the clavicle and the other on the left chest lateral to the left nipple. Make sure there is a tight contact with the skin by removing any excessive hair or moisture that may be present (Fig. 8-5).

3. Press the analyze button to assess the need for defibrillation. The machine will state whether defibrillation shock is required.

4. If a shock is required, all persons must be totally clear of the bed or table and any contact with the patient. The machine will dictate a "clear" order.

5. Press the shock button when the AED dictates the order. Do not press the shock button before the order.

6. If the AED states that no shock is indicated and the patient remains without a pulse, resume CPR.

When the patient is a child, the cause of the arrest is frequently respiratory in nature. As a result, calling the emergency medical team should take place after CPR is administered for 1 minute unless another person is present who can call the CODE while the other person is administering CPR. The procedure is much the same for infants and children; however, there are some variations, which are listed in Display 8-3.

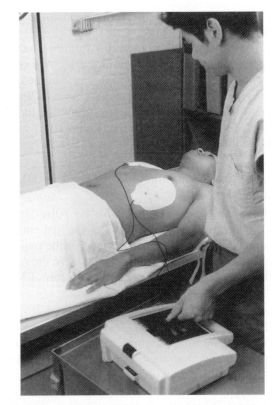

FIGURE 8-5 Attach one electrode at right upper sternal border below the clavicle and the other on the left chest lateral to the left nipple.

DISPLAY 8-3

Variations in CPR Techniques for Infants and Children

Neonate

- Head tilt, chin lift, (or jaw thrust if trauma is present)
- 2 effective breaths, then 30 to 60 breaths per minute
- Back blows or chest thrusts; no abdominal thrusts
- Compression landmark is the lower half of the sternum, 1 finger width below the intermammary line
- Use 2 fingers for compression at approximately ½ inch at about 120 compressions per minute or 90 compressions to 30 breaths

Infant under 1 year of age

- Head tilt, chin lift, (or jaw thrust if trauma is present)
- 2 effective breaths, then 20 breaths per minute
- Back blows or chest thrusts; no abdominal thrusts
- Brachial pulse checked

- Compression landmark is the lower half of the sternum, 1 finger width below the intermammary line
- Use 2 thumbs or 2 fingers for compression at approximately ½ to 1 inch at about 100 compressions per minute

Child ages 1 to 8 years

- Head tilt, chin lift, (or jaw thrust if trauma is present)
- 2 effective breaths in less than 10 seconds
- Check breathing by "look, listen, feel"
- Abdominal thrusts or chest thrusts
- The carotid pulse is checked
- Compression landmark is the lower half of the sternum with the heel of the hand; the compression depth of the chest is 1 to 1.5 inches at a rate of 100 per minute or 30 compressions to 2 ventilations

The use of a one-way mask on the infant or child for protection is desirable. If the radiographer has been trained in the use of a breather bag, it may be used. The equipment must be of a size to adequately fit the patient.

Take adequate time to determine the lack of a pulse (no more than 7 seconds). Performing cardiac compressions on a person whose heart is functioning is extremely dangerous to the patient. Once cardiac compressions have been started, interruptions should be avoided. In one-person rescue, this is not possible; therefore, the interruption in compressions should not last more than 7 seconds. Two-person CPR is not discussed in this text because it demands actual demonstration and return demonstration to be successful.

The rescuer's hands must be positioned correctly to prevent internal injury while the cardiac compressions are being performed. Do this in the following manner:

1. Find the lower margin of the patient's rib cage at the area where the ribs and sternum meet. Place the index finger above this junction and the heel of the other hand next to the finger. Place the second hand on top and interlace the fingers.

2. This should place the hands about 1.5 inches from the xiphoid tip toward the patient's head. The fingers should not touch the chest wall of the patient (Fig. 8-6).

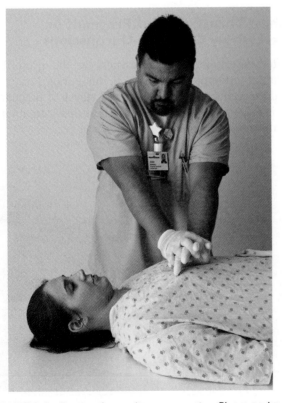

FIGURE 8-6 Position for cardiac compression. Place one hand on top of the other, keeping elbows straight.

3. Keep the elbows straight and use the body weight to help compress the sternum 1.5 to 2 inches directly downward; then release the compression completely.

4. Because it is more important to supply blood to the body, 30 compressions are given in a smooth, even rhythm before any ventilation. Do not rock during compressions. Make sure it is an up and down motion.

5. Inflate the patient's lungs two more times.

6. Reassess the patient's carotid pulse and respiratory status. If the patient has no pulse or respiration, continue with 30 compressions followed by 2 inflations until the emergency team arrives.

Radiographers and all health care personnel must guard against becoming infected by a communicable disease while performing lifesaving procedures by wearing disposable gloves and by learning to use a manual resuscitation bag or a one-way face mask. Education in the use of this equipment must be obtained before it can be used effectively; such education should be a part of CPR training.

■ AIRWAY OBSTRUCTION

A foreign body such as a piece of chewing gum or food may lodge in a patient's throat and produce respiratory arrest. This type of accident occurs most often in the elderly, the very young, or the intoxicated while eating. However, the radiographer must consider this possibility in any case of respiratory arrest.

When airway obstruction caused by a foreign object occurs, the patient usually appears to be quite normal, and then suddenly begins to choke. The patient grabs the throat and is unable to speak. If no one is present to observe this, the patient eventually loses consciousness. Unless the early signs are observed, it is impossible to know the cause of the unconscious state. Airway obstruction may occur with the patient sitting, standing, or lying down and must be dealt with initially in that position.

Radiographer's Response
1. If the patient does not respond and breathlessness is established as described in the preceding paragraphs, seal the patient's nose and mouth, and ventilate him or her as in the initial steps of CPR.

2. If the patient's chest rises and falls, proceed as for basic CPR.

3. If the patent's chest does not rise and fall, reposition the head using the head tilt, chin lift, or jaw thrust as indicated. Then attempt to ventilate again.

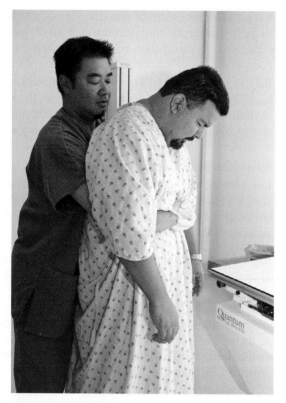

FIGURE 8-7   Abdominal thrust, standing.

4. If this is unsuccessful, assume that the airway is obstructed and use the abdominal thrust to attempt to remove the obstruction.

Abdominal Thrust: Patient Standing or Sitting

Stand behind the patient and grasp with both hands above the patient's umbilicus and below the xiphoid process of the sternum. Position the lower hand with the thumb inward; the other hand firmly grips the lower hand. Make a rapid upward movement that forces the abdomen inward and thrusts upward against the diaphragm (Fig. 8-7). This maneuver forces air up through the trachea and dislodges the foreign object. Never attempt to practice this maneuver on a person who is not in distress because of the possibility of serious injury. Be sure the hands are placed away from the xiphoid process to prevent internal injury.

Abdominal Thrust: Patient in Supine Position

Place the patient in a supine position. Kneel astride the patient's thighs and place the heel of one hand against the patient's abdomen above the navel and below the tip of the xiphoid process. Place the other hand over the first and quickly press the abdomen upward. Be

certain to direct the thrust directly up and not deviate to the left or right. This maneuver acts in the same way for the patient who is sitting or standing.

Chest Thrust: Patient Sitting or Standing

The chest thrust is used to dislodge a foreign object only if the patient is in the advanced stages of pregnancy or is excessively obese and the abdominal thrust cannot be used effectively.

Stand behind the patient with arms under the patient's armpits and around the chest. Place the thumb side of a fist in the middle of the sternum, avoiding the xiphoid process and the margins of the rib cage. Place the other hand on top and thrust backward. Repeat this maneuver until the object is dislodged.

If the patient is an infant and an obstructed airway is suspected, place the patient face down over the forearm with the infant's legs straddling the elbow. Support the infant's head and neck between the thumb and forefinger with the patient's head lower than the chest but not straight down. Deliver five sharp blows to the patient's back between the shoulder blades (Fig. 8-8). If this is not successful, perform chest thrusts with two or three fingers on the mid-sternum about one per second (Fig. 8-9).

The method of dealing with foreign body airway obstruction for infants and children also varies with their weight, age, and size.

Chest Thrust: Patient Pregnant or Excessively Obese or Unconscious

After determining breathlessness in the prescribed manner, attempt ventilation. If this is not successful and the patient is in the advanced stages of pregnancy or is excessively obese, use the chest thrust to attempt to dislodge the foreign object.

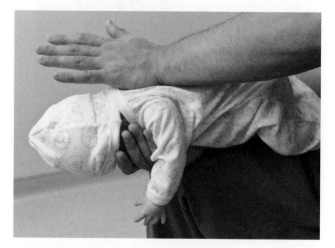

FIGURE 8-8   Be sure to support the infant's head between the thumb and fingers when delivering back blows.

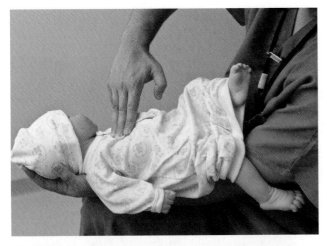

FIGURE 8-9 Chest compression on an infant to relieve complete foreign body airway obstruction.

Kneel beside the patient and place hands in the same position as with thrust for external cardiac compression. Make sure thrusts are slow and firm and performed as many times as is necessary to relieve the obstruction.

SEIZURES

A seizure is an unsystematic discharge of neurons of the cerebrum that results in an abrupt alteration in brain function. It usually begins with little or no warning and may last only seconds or for several minutes. A seizure is accompanied by a change in the level of consciousness.

Seizures themselves are not a disease, but are a syndrome or symptom of a disease. They may be caused by infections or disease, especially those that are accompanied by high fever. They may also be caused by extreme stress, head trauma, brain tumors, structural abnormalities of the cerebral cortex, genetic defects (epilepsy), birth trauma, vascular disease, congenital malformations, or postnatal trauma. Odors and flashing lights can cause a seizure in a person who is seizure prone.

There are basically two types of seizure: generalized and partial.

Generalized Seizures

Clinical Manifestations
- May utter a sharp cry as air is rapidly exhaled
- Muscles become rigid and eyes open wide
- May exhibit jerky body movements and rapid, irregular respirations
- May vomit
- May froth and have blood-streaked saliva caused by biting the lips or tongue
- May exhibit urinary or fecal incontinence
- Usually falls into a deep sleep after the seizure

Partial Seizures: Complex and Simple

The seizure activity depends on the area of the brain involved.

Clinical Manifestations of a Complex Partial Seizure
- Patient may remain motionless or may experience an excessive emotional outburst of fear, crying, or anger
- Patient may manifest facial grimacing, lip smacking, swallowing movements, or panting
- Patient will be confused for several minutes after the episode with no memory of the incident

Clinical Manifestations of a Simple Partial Seizure
- Only a finger or a hand may shake
- Patient may speak unintelligibly
- Patient may be dizzy
- Patient may sense strange odors, tastes, or sounds
- Patient will not lose consciousness

Radiographer's Response to a Patient Having a Seizure
1. Stay with the patient and gently secure him or her to prevent injury.
2. Call for assistance.
3. Do not attempt to insert anything into the patient's mouth.
4. Remove dentures and foreign objects from the patient's mouth if possible, but do not put fingers into the mouth.
5. Place a blanket or pillow under the patient's head to protect it from injury.
6. Do not restrain the arms or legs but protect them from injury.
7. Do not attempt to move the patient to the floor if he or she has not fallen there; if on a radiographic table, do not allow the patient to fall to the floor.
8. Observe the patient carefully and keep track of the time of the seizure to record later.
9. Provide the patient privacy.
10. After the seizure has ceased, position the patient to prevent aspiration of secretions and vomitus. Turn the patient to a Sim's position and put the face downward so that secretions may drain from his or her mouth.

SYNCOPE

Syncope, or fainting, is a transient loss of consciousness, which usually results from an insufficient blood supply to the brain. Heart disease, hunger, poor ventilation, extreme fatigue, and emotional trauma all are possible causes. The elderly patient who is asked to change positions from lying to standing too quickly may also have a syncopal reaction owing to orthostatic hypotension. Orthostatic hypotension is an abnormally low blood pressure occurring when a person stands up before the blood pooled in the extremities has time to circulate to the upper body.

Patients are frequently instructed not to eat breakfast before coming to the diagnostic imaging department from their homes or hospital rooms. Often they are ill, and lack of nourishment may increase the likelihood of fainting. The patient cannot choose the "proper" place in which to faint, so he or she may fall and cause injury to him or herself. The radiographer must be able to recognize and watch for the symptoms that indicate a patient is about to faint.

If it is suspected that the patient is in a weakened condition because of a recent traumatic injury or illness, do not allow the patient to stand for an upright image and then leave the patient to support him or herself while the exposure is obtained. Consider other methods of obtaining the exposure, or have an assistant stand beside the patient to support him or her, if necessary.

If caring for an elderly patient, allow the patient time to sit for several minutes before requesting that he or she stand or walk. Always be at the patient's side to protect him or her from falling.

Clinical Manifestations
- Pallor, complaints of dizziness and nausea
- Hyperpnea, tachycardia
- Cold, clammy skin

Radiographer's Response
1. If the patient complains of feeling dizzy or appears to be confused, have the patient lie down.
2. If the patient has actually fainted, place him or her in a supine position with legs elevated.
3. If the patient begins to fall, do not try to keep him or her standing. Support and assist the patient to the floor in a manner that prevents injury. Place a knee behind the patient's knee and an arm around the waist and assist the patient to the floor (Fig. 8-10).

THE RADIOGRAPHER'S RESPONSE TO THE PATIENT IN PAIN

In recent years, pain management has become a recognized health care problem that must be dealt with adequately and not left to the subjective judgment

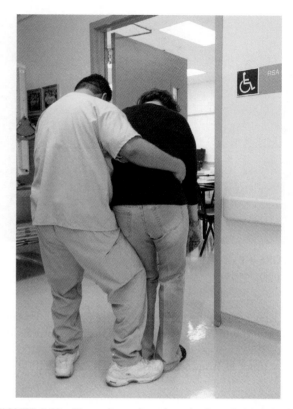

FIGURE 8-10   The radiographer places his knee behind the patient's knee to support her.

of health care workers as in the past. In 1999, The Joint Commission established standards for pain management for all patients. Pain control practice must be in compliance with those standards. Hospitals, long-term care facilities, home health care agencies, outpatient clinics, and managed care organizations must be knowledgeable in pain assessment and management. They must also have policies and procedures in place concerning use of analgesics and pain control therapies.

All accredited health care facilities must have a pain assessment tool with which to rate the degree of pain the patient is feeling. This tool must differ according to the patient's age, cultural background, and medical condition so that each patient can easily understand it. The scales used often are numerical in nature; that is, a scale from 1 to 10 with 10 being the most excruciating pain. Other facilities use faces that begin with a smile that progresses to tears for the most intolerable pain. When beginning to assess a patient, use the scale that is preferred in your institution as a guide.

Make sure that the patient remains as comfortable as possible while in the radiography department and never ignore a patient's complaint of pain. By using critical thinking skills when planning the patient's care, the radiographer can successfully plan pain control and maintain comfort and safety for the patient.

1. Carefully assess the patient's physical and emotional condition preceding the diagnostic imaging procedure.
2. Educate the patient concerning all aspects of the examination and what is expected of them during the examination.
3. Instruct the patient to inform someone if he or she feels any pain or abrupt changes in the general condition while the procedure is in progress.
4. Stop the procedure and immediately notify the physician if the patient complains of sudden pain or change in his or her condition during the procedure.
5. Confer with the patient's physician if the patient comes to the department in pain and, if possible, have the patient receive analgesic medication before working with the patient.

THE AGITATED OR CONFUSED PATIENT

Patients with emotional problems may come to the emergency suite for treatment that requires diagnostic radiographs, or patients who are hospitalized in mental health units may require diagnostic imaging procedures. These patients are frequently agitated or confused and may become combative.

Patients who react in a combative or aggressive manner usually do so because they are frightened or feel that they have no control over what is happening to them. They resort to violent behavior as a means of self-protection. This behavior may be caused by chemical abuse or by **psychosis** of varying causes. At times, the confused elderly patient forgets that he or she is not at home and mistakes others as intruders. Precautions to ensure safety must be taken when threatened with this type of behavior.

Patients that are more likely to demonstrate combative behavior are those who have a history of such outbursts or a history of growing confusion and disorientation. Other warning signals are increasing agitation demonstrated by rapid pacing back and forth across the room; a patient in animated and increasingly noisy conversation with a person who is not present; a demonstration of illogical thought processes; refusal to be cooperative; or distrust of the medical personnel and explanations of the procedure or fear of the examining room and equipment. Patients who are combative occasionally display no emotion at all.

Before approaching a patient who is not reacting in a rational manner, discuss the case with nursing personnel. If the patient is behaving in a combative manner or has a history of combativeness, request assistance with the examination. It is wise to trust first instincts about a patient's behavior. Do not become isolated with a potentially assaultive patient. Always leave a door open, and clear a direct path so leaving a room quickly is an option if necessary. Do not begin the procedure without assistance from security or some other protective personnel.

At times, patients who are agitated or confused react more favorably to persons of a specific gender. If this seems to be the case, having a radiographer of the preferred gender conduct the procedure will be helpful.

It is best to approach a patient who is agitated or confused from the side, not face to face. Never touch a patient who is behaving in this manner without first asking permission to do so and while explaining what is going to happen. Use simple, concise statements to explain the purpose of the procedure. Call the person by name. Give the angry patient an opportunity to express the anger, but make no attempt to defend or try to reason with the patient.

If a patient is speaking in a delusional or irrational manner, it is important not to become involved in the conversation. To do so might increase the patient's agitation. If the patient refuses to proceed, simply stop and return the patient to the area he or she originated from. Explain that the procedure will be continued at a later time. To continue to work with an agitated and confused person who is belligerent may cause injury to all persons involved.

If the radiographs are essential to the patient's treatment, the patient will have to be immobilized and supervised by persons in the hospital who are educated to care for such patients. Use of immobilizers is explained in Chapter 3.

If the situation escalates beyond control and the patient is actually prepared to strike out at those nearby, the radiographer should put as much distance as possible between him or her and the patient. Proceed as follows:

1. Speak in a calm but firm voice to the patient.
2. Let the patient know that he or she has created an uneasy environment and ask what can be done to overcome this.
3. Try to become an ally by making statements such as, "You must be really angry at the people here for putting you through all of these tests."
4. If this does not work, get out of the area and summon help. Do not approach the patient or make any effort to take anything out of his or her hands.

THE INTOXICATED PATIENT

Patients who are intoxicated are often involved in accidents that result in injuries to themselves and to others. When the intoxicated patient is brought to the emergency unit for care, he or she may be quarrelsome and reluctant to cooperate, may also neglect all rules of safety while being treated, and may inadvertently fall from a gurney or radiographic table.

The radiographer caring for an intoxicated patient must keep the communication simple, direct, and non-judgmental. Do not become involved in the patient's attempt to argue. If the patient refuses treatment or becomes increasingly difficult to manage, call for help immediately. Do not attempt to complete the assignment until adequate assistance has arrived. Do not leave the patient alone, and observe him or her at all times to prevent falls. More than one strong assistant may be required to complete the radiographic images of an intoxicated person.

Often, an intoxicated patient is accompanied by a person who is also intoxicated and belligerent. The companion may become aggressive and combative. In this instance, do not allow the companion to come into the examining room with the patient. Simply inform the companion that it is against the rules of radiation safety to be present and that he or she must wait outside. If the companion debates this request, stop the procedure and call for assistance. Note that under no circumstances should an intoxicated patient be allowed to leave the health care facility accompanied by an intoxicated companion. If necessary, notify the police to prevent this.

SUMMARY

Medical emergencies occur frequently in the radiographic imaging department. The radiographer may be the first or only person present at the onset of symptoms in a patient, so it is important to learn how to recognize an emergency situation and take the appropriate action if one occurs.

Assess the patient's levels of neurologic and cognitive functioning as he or she is prepared for the assigned procedure. It is at this time that changes in the patient's level of consciousness and mental status can be observed if they occur.

Shock is a common medical emergency. There are many causes of physiologic shock. Blood loss, infection, and cardiac failure are among the most common. Anaphylactic shock is caused by an allergic reaction and is the type that is most often seen in the radiography department. This is because iodinated contrast agents that are used for some radiographic imaging procedures and examinations may produce this reaction. Early symptoms of an anaphylactic reaction are nasal congestion, periorbital swelling, itching, dyspnea, tearing of eyes, and peripheral tingling, followed by flushing, urticaria, anxiety, and bronchospasm. If early symptoms of an anaphylactic reaction are suspected, the radiographer must stop the administration of the contrast agent immediately and initiate emergency action. If symptoms are not relieved, the patient may have seizures and respiratory arrest.

Pulmonary embolus is a medical emergency that may occur without warning. Patients who have had recent surgery should be watched more closely for this situation. Pulmonary emboli can be fatal if not treated immediately. Hypoglycemia, ketoacidosis, and hyperosmolar nonketotic syndrome may also be seen in patients who come into the diagnostic imaging department. Patients who have diabetes may come for examinations or procedures after having taken insulin or oral hypoglycemic medication and be without sufficient food intake to use the drug.

Cerebral vascular accidents are medical emergencies that must be recognized and dealt with immediately to prevent life-threatening consequences. The early signs and symptoms are often one-sided flaccidity of face and limbs, difficult or absent speech, eye deviation, dizziness, ataxia, possible neck stiffness, nausea, vomiting, and loss of consciousness.

Respiratory failure must be differentiated from cardiac failure. Respiratory failure is recognized by a lack of chest movement, absence of breath sounds, a diminishing pulse rate, and loss of consciousness. Cardiac failure results in an immediate cessation of the pulse and respiration and a loss of consciousness. Both call for immediate action if the patient's life is to be saved.

Airway obstruction by a foreign object should be suspected if a patient is feeling well and suddenly begins to demonstrate respiratory distress or is found unconscious and, when ventilation is attempted, the chest cannot be made to rise and fall, as it should during resuscitation. The abdominal thrust maneuver must be performed in response to this emergency.

Fainting and convulsive seizures may occur with little or no warning. The radiographer should be able to recognize these problems and protect the patient from injuries caused by aspiration of saliva or vomitus, by falls, or by hitting the head or extremities against hard surfaces.

The radiographer must be sensitive to the patient's need for pain management and control. Be able to assess the patient and plan his or her care in such a manner that the patient remains as comfortable and pain-free as possible. If the patient complains of pain or a change in his or her condition, stop the procedure and immediately notify the radiology nurse or the physician in charge.

Knowing where the emergency cart, oxygen, suction equipment, and other supplies are kept in the diagnostic imaging department is a must. Being able to offer assistance in emergency cases is critical to the patient's survival. It is the responsibility of all members of the health care team to be prepared to administer basic life support procedures to adults and children.

Working with patients who are agitated, confused, and potentially assaultive may occur. The cause may be chemical abuse, psychosis, or confusion due to stress, as is occasionally the case in the elderly patient. Be cautious in approaching these patients in order to maintain safety. If the patient refuses treatment, immediately comply with this refusal and return the patient to his or her quarters. If the radiographs are essential to the patient's treatment, get assistance from personnel who are educated in the care of mentally disturbed patients.

When caring for an intoxicated patient, it is important to behave in a nonjudgmental manner and address the patient simply and directly. If safety of any persons involved in this situation is threatened, do not continue, but get adequate personnel to help complete the assignment. If need be, contact security to remain present during the examination.

CHAPTER 8 TEST

1. List and describe the levels of neurologic functioning according to the Glasgow Coma Scale.
2. Explain the method of assessing mental status.
3. General signs and symptoms that the radiographer must learn to recognize as probable indicators that the patient is in shock include (circle all that apply):
   a. Strong, irregular pulse
   b. Hypertension
   c. Flushed face
   d. Respiration increases
   e. Skin is cold and clammy
   f. Acetone breath
   g. Mental status changes beginning with confusion and ending with coma
   h. Decreased temperature
   i. Weak, thready pulse
   j. Rapid heartbeat, hypotension
4. Why is anaphylactic shock the most frequently seen type of shock in the diagnostic imaging department?
   a. Patients who come for diagnostic imaging procedures are weak and debilitated
   b. Iodinated contrast agents are frequently used
   c. Patients here have more allergies
   d. X-radiation causes this problem
5. Early signs and symptoms of anaphylactic reaction are (circle all that apply):
   a. Itching at the site of injection
   b. Tearing of eyes
   c. Sneezing
   d. Feeling of warmth
   e. Anxiety
   f. Bronchospasm and edema of the airway
   g. Decreasing blood pressure
6. Myrtle Maywriter is a 43-year-old female who has come to diagnostic imaging this morning from her home for an upper GI series. After she has been in the room for a short time, she complains of a severe headache. Shortly after, you notice that she

has cold, clammy skin and speaks in a slurred manner. You suspect that Ms. Maywriter is:
   a. A diabetic and is having a ketoacidotic reaction
   b. Having a cardiac arrest
   c. An alcoholic and is drunk
   d. An epileptic and is having a seizure
   e. A diabetic and is having a hypoglycemic reaction
7. The immediate emergency treatment of Ms. Maywriter's problem in Question 6 is imperative. Place a "B" in front of the best answer, and place a "W" in front of the worst response.
   a. Prepare for oxygen administration and call the emergency team.
   b. Check for an identification of the patient as a diabetic, give her some form of concentrated sugar, and notify the physician in charge.
   c. Place the patient in a supine position, keep her warm, and call the emergency team.
   d. Continue with your work, but do not leave the patient alone.
8. Symptoms of a partially obstructed airway may include:
   a. Cold, clammy skin; pallor; weakness; anxiety
   b. Flushed, hot skin; hyperactivity; confusion; seizures
   c. Labored, noisy breathing; wheezing; use of neck muscles to assist with breathing
   d. Acetone breath, irregular pulse, noisy respiration, rapid heartbeat, flushed skin
9. A 16-year-old patient comes to the diagnostic imaging department for a CT scan. He is lying on the table in a supine position. He suddenly seems to lose consciousness and begins to move violently with jerking motions. You realize that he is having a generalized seizure. What is the best action to take? (Place a "B" in front of that answer.) What is the worst action to take? (Place a "W" in front of that answer.)
   a. Go to the patient immediately and restrain him or her with immobilizers.

b. Call for help and do not leave the patient.

c. Place the patient on the floor and begin CPR.

d. Call for help and make sure the patient does not injure himself.

10. Mrs. Gertrude Glucose, age 35, had an open reduction of her left femur 3 days earlier and has been transported to the diagnostic imaging department by gurney from her hospital room for radiographs. As you prepare the patient for the radiograph, she suddenly begins to complain of pain in her mid-chest and appears to be out of breath. You stop your preparation and take her pulse and blood pressure. You find out that her blood pressure is 120/80 and her radial pulse is 120 per minute and is very difficult to palpate because it is so weak and thready. You quickly notify the physician of the problem, and he directs you to call the emergency team. You do this and make other emergency preparations. You believe that this patient may be having:

a. A stroke

b. A seizure

c. A pulmonary embolus

d. An episode of syncope

11. Fainting is a common medical emergency in the diagnostic imaging department. If a patient appears to be fainting, what is the first thing to do?

a. Assist the patient to a safe position and then call for help.

b. Give smelling salts.

c. Get the emergency cart.

d. Prepare to administer oxygen.

12. Match the following:

a. Hypovolemic shock

b. CVA

c. Airway obstruction

d. Cardiogenic shock

e. Anaphylactic shock

i. Difficult speech, severe headache, one-sided, drooping eye and face, loss of consciousness

ii. Choking, inability to speak, eventual loss of consciousness

iii. Itching of eyes, apprehensiveness, wheezing, choking

iv. Loss of consciousness; decreased blood pressure; weak, rapid pulse

v. Pallor; thirst; cold, clammy skin; restlessness

13. List the questions that must be asked of a patient before receiving an iodinated contrast agent.

Trauma and Mobile Radiographic Considerations

STUDENT LEARNING OUTCOMES

After studying this chapter, the student will be able to:

1. List the general guidelines for radiographers to follow.
2. List members of the emergency room health care team.
3. List the basic rules in trauma radiography.
4. List common tubes and lines demonstrated with the mobile chest radiographic images.
5. List the basic supplies necessary when performing trauma and mobile radiographic procedures.
6. List the precautions a radiographer should take when the patient has a head injury.
7. List the precautions a radiographer should take when the patient has facial injuries.
8. List the precautions a radiographer should take if the patient may have a spinal cord injury.
9. List the precautions a radiographer should take if the patient may have a fracture.
10. List the precautions a radiographer should take when the patient has abdominal trauma or is in acute abdominal distress.

KEY TERMS

Abrasion: A scraping or rubbing away of the surface skin by friction

Cervical: Of or pertaining to the neck

Contusion: An injury that does not break the skin; caused by a blow to the body; characterized by swelling, discoloration, and pain

Ecchymosis: An oozing of blood from a vessel into tissues, forming a discolored area on the skin

Ectopic pregnancy: An abnormal pregnancy in which the embryo implants outside the uterine cavity

Gait: Manner of moving or walking

Hemiparesis: Paralysis affecting one side of the body

Hemothorax: Collection of blood in the pleural cavity

Hypovolemic: Abnormally decreased volume of circulating fluid (plasma) in the body

Lucidity: Clearness of mind

Paresthesia: An abnormal sensation such as burning, itching, tickling, or tingling

Pneumothorax: Accumulation of air or gas in the pleural cavity resulting in collapse of the lung on the affected side

Somatic: Pertaining to or characteristic of the body (soma)

Mobile or portable imaging procedures are performed on patients who cannot be transported to the imaging department because of a serious injury, illness, or condition. Therefore, many patients are imaged with the use of mobile radiography equipment in the emergency department, in special care rooms, in the patient's room, or in the operating rooms (Fig. 9-1).

The trauma patient may be strapped to a backboard with a cervical collar and splints in place. These patients commonly have oxygen, intravenous tubing, and life support equipment when the radiographer is to

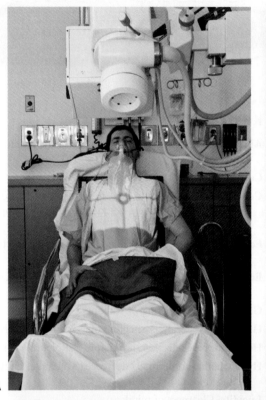

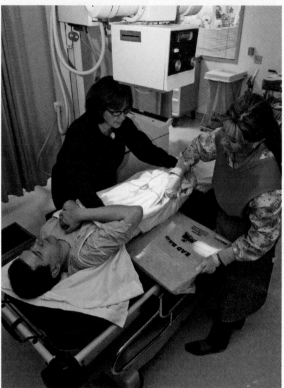

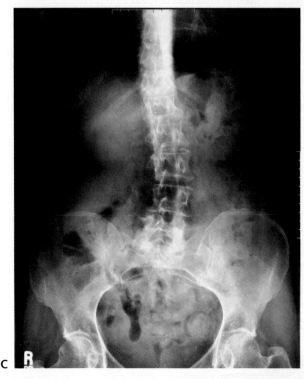

FIGURE 9-1 (A) Setting up for a portable AP chest semi-erect. (B) Setting up for a portable AP abdomen. (C) AP supine radiographic image of the abdomen.

perform trauma or mobile radiography. Since these patients cannot be transported to radiology, the radiographer must adapt his skills to achieve diagnostic images according to the patient's condition and needs. Specifically, a radiographer must adapt positioning and technical considerations during the course of performing trauma and mobile radiography. In addition, the radiographer must analyze each patient situation in relation to the procedures requested by the physician, while at the same time, keeping in mind general radiation protection measures. Pre-planning is essential for achieving diagnostic outcome images under trauma or mobile circumstances. This chapter introduces additional information that is needed in trauma and mobile radiography.

TRAUMATIC INJURIES

Traumatic injuries are caused by external force or violence (Fig. 9-2). Injury (trauma) is the leading cause of death among all persons under the age of 44. The injuries may be the result of:

- Motor vehicle accidents
- Pedestrian accidents
- Motorcycle accidents
- Falls from heights
- Assaults (stabbings and gunshot wounds)
- Blunt trauma
- Choking
- Industrial accidents
- Suicides
- Drowning
- Smoke inhalation
- Sports injuries

The trauma patient presents a wide variety of challenges for the radiographer. The nature of the injury to the patient and the patient's condition require the radiographer to use critical thinking and judgment of a knowledgeable radiographer. Technical knowledge combined with the ability to adapt creatively is required

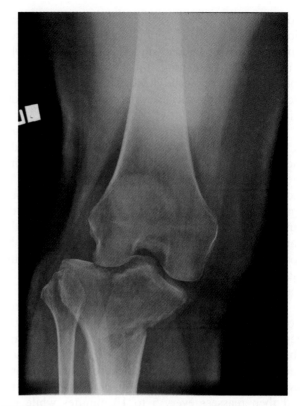

FIGURE 9-2   Traumatic injury caused by external force.

to provide the physician(s) with the necessary diagnostic information to treat the patient. In some cases, trauma radiographs are obtained rapidly to screen for life-threatening injuries.

The radiographer is one of the first members of the health care team to see the patient once he or she is admitted to the emergency room after traumatic injury or acute illness (Display 9-1). Trauma patients can have a single injury or multiple injuries. When the radiographer is called to the emergency room to perform diagnostic radiographic images, he must assume that he will be exposed to the patient's blood or body fluids. To avoid infecting oneself or the patient, always maintain standard precautions by having clean disposable

DISPLAY 9-1

Emergency Team Members

Emergency physician, attending physician, resident/medical student
General and/or specialty surgeon available if indicated
Two emergency registered nurses
Pediatric nurse (if required)
Radiology technologist

Respiratory therapist
Phlebotomist
Anesthesiologist
Admitting clerk
House supervisor

gloves available before beginning the procedure. Wear gloves, mask, goggles, and a protective gown or apron when caring for a patient who is hemorrhaging or who is nauseated and vomiting. If it is necessary to touch an open wound, wear sterile gloves. In addition, the image receptor must be protected with an impermeable covering or bag.

Many patients admitted to the emergency room are in severe pain. Depending on a patient's injuries, the radiographer will be required to assist in diagnosing the extent of injuries or illness by taking a series of radiographs. This requires patience and skill. The radiographer will need to accomplish the procedure without extending present injuries or increasing the patient's discomfort. Usually, time for achieving the goal is brief, since the patient's life is at risk. In trauma radiography, general radiation safety measures must be combined with speed and accuracy.

If the injured or acutely ill patient is transferred from the emergency room to the diagnostic imaging department for radiographs, the radiographer must observe the patient for symptoms of shock. The radiographer assesses the patient's neurologic status and level of consciousness before beginning any procedure, and then reassess every 5 to 10 minutes while the patient is in the department. If any changes in the patient's condition are observed, the physician and the emergency team are quickly alerted, and the radiographer prepares to assist with emergency measures as outlined in Chapter 7.

General Guidelines

General guidelines to follow when caring for a patient who has traumatic injuries are as follows:

1. Do not remove dressings or splints.
2. Do not move patients who are on a stretcher or backboard until ordered to do so by the physician in charge of the patient.

3. When performing an initial cross-table lateral **cervical** spine radiograph, never move the patient's head or neck or remove the cervical collar. The physician must interpret the radiograph and "clear" the cervical spine for injury before removing the collar or moving the patient.
4. Request direction from the emergency room team when planning moves, and assemble adequate assistance to move the patient safely and as painlessly as possible.
5. Do not disturb impaled objects. Support them so that they do not move as you image the patient.
6. Do not remove pneumatic antishock garments.
7. Have oxygen, suction equipment, and an emesis basin ready for use.
8. Work quickly, efficiently, and accurately to minimize repeat radiographs.

Basic Rules for Trauma Radiography

Basic rules to follow for trauma radiography are:

- Assess the situation and develop an action plan for the imaging procedure.
- Determine patient mobility, and explain the procedure to the patient.
- Predetermine equipment and accessories needed for the procedure (Display 9-2).
- Take at least two radiographs at 90-degree angles to one another for each body part (Fig. 9-3).
- Make sure the central ray and image receptor alignment approaches routine positioning applications, adapting to the patient's condition.
- Include all anatomy of interest.
- For long bone radiography, always include the joint nearest the trauma; if possible, also include the joint farthest from the trauma.

DISPLAY 9-2

Helpful Tips for Equipment and Accessories Needed

- Lead aprons & other protective apparel for the radiographer and others involved in the procedure
- Radiation detection monitoring dosimeter
- Universal precautions supplies (gloves, gown, mask as needed)
- Impermeable image receptor (cassette covers)

- Image receptors and grids (if required)
- Right or left markers and other markers to indicate whether x-ray beam is perpendicular or angled to the image receptor
- Mobile (portable) or C-arm unit

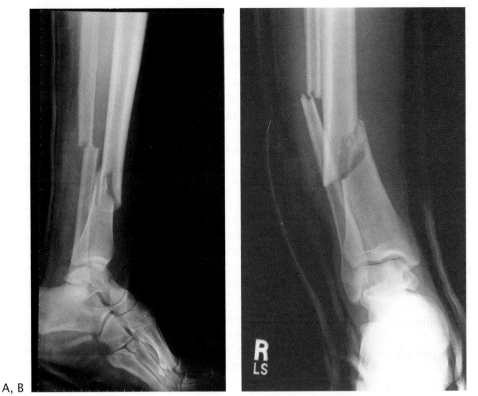

A, B

FIGURE 9-3   (**A**) Trauma to lateral right ankle. (**B**) Second projection 90 degrees from lateral ankle.

- Provide protective apparel for anyone who needs to be in the room caring for the injured patient.

A cooperative environment with all personnel involved in the emergency procedure will facilitate the proper care of the patient.

THE PATIENT WITH A HEAD INJURY

Injuries to the head are exceedingly common. Each year approximately 10 million head injuries are predicted to occur in the United States. The term head injury may refer to any injury of the skull, brain, or both that requires medical attention. Radiographers are not called as often as in past years to perform radiographic images because of the availability and effectiveness of computed tomography, which allows the physicians to diagnose head injuries (Fig. 9-4). All head injuries are potentially serious because they may involve the brain, which is the seat of consciousness and controls every human action.

The two basic types of head injury are open and closed. With an open injury to the skull or meninges, the brain is vulnerable to damage and infection because its protective casing has been broken. If the injury is closed (also called a *blunt injury),* the brain tissue may swell.

The swelling is limited by the confines of the skull, and the resulting pressure may cause extensive brain damage. The brain has little healing power, so any injury to it must be considered potentially permanent and serious.

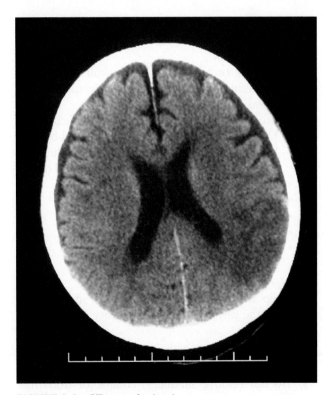

FIGURE 9-4   CT image for head trauma.

Fractures at the base of the skull *(basal skull fractures)* often have accompanying fractures of the facial bones. This type of injury may result in a tear in the *dura mater,* the outer membrane surrounding the brain and spinal cord, and a leakage of the cerebrospinal fluid may result.

Consider all patients with head injuries to have accompanying cervical spinal injuries until it is medically disproved. Take precautions to alleviate potential extension of these injuries as a matter of routine. It is vital as the radiographer to be knowledgeable in understanding the signs and symptoms of patients with a variety of injuries. It is important to report any observable changes in the patient's status to the emergency physician and/or team.

Clinical Manifestations of Head Injury
Closed Injury

- Varying levels of consciousness, ranging from drowsiness, confusion, irritability, and stupor to coma
- **Lucid** periods followed by periods of unconsciousness are possible
- Loss of reflexes
- Changes in vital signs
- Headache, visual disturbances, dizziness, and giddiness
- **Gait** abnormalities
- Unequal pupil dilation
- Seizures, vomiting, and **hemiparesis**

Open Injury

- **Abrasions, contusions,** or lacerations apparent on the skull
- A break or penetration in the skull or meninges apparent by inspection or on radiographic images
- Basal fractures resulting in leakage of cerebrospinal fluid, as demonstrated by leakage of blood on the sheet or dressing surrounded by a yellowish stain (the halo sign); cerebrospinal fluid may leak from the nose or ears or as a postnasal drip
- Varying levels of consciousness
- Subconjunctival hemorrhage
- Hearing loss
- Periorbital **ecchymosis** (raccoon's eyes)
- Facial nerve play

Radiographer's Reponse
1. Keep the patient's head and neck immobilized until the physician rules out injury to the spinal cord.
2. If possible, elevate the patient's head 15 to 30 degrees.
3. Do not remove sandbags, collars, or dressings. Take all radiographs with these in place.

4. Do not flex the patient's neck or turn it to either side. Rotation of the head may increase intracranial pressure.
5. Keep the patient's body temperature as normal as possible. Do not allow the patient to become chilled or overheated.
6. Check the patient's pulse and respirations frequently while performing the procedure.
7. Observe for airway obstruction.
8. Apply a sterile pressure dressing if bleeding becomes profuse, and call for emergency assistance.
9. Observe the patient for signs and symptoms of hypoxia and changes in level of consciousness. If a patient who is initially alert and cooperative suddenly appears to be drowsy or slow to respond, immediately notify the physician in charge of the patient.
10. Be prepared to assist with oxygen administration and other emergency treatment. Patients with head injuries must not be suctioned through nasal passages.

■ THE PATIENT WITH A FACIAL INJURY

Injuries to the facial bones are usually associated with injury to the soft tissues of the face. Often these injuries do not seem serious, but all are potentially disfiguring. Treat all patients who have serious facial injuries as if they also have basal skull fractures and injuries of the cervical spine (Fig. 9-5).

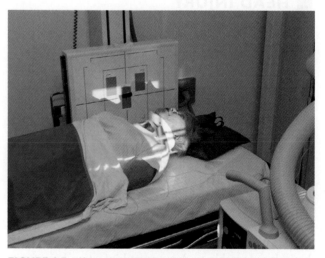

FIGURE 9-5   If a spinal cord injury is suspected, a horizontal beam lateral radiographic image is performed without moving the patient.

Clinical Manifestations

- Misalignment of the face or teeth
- Pain at the site of injury
- Ecchymosis of the floor of mouth and buccal mucosa
- Distortion of facial symmetry
- Inability to close the jaw
- Edema
- Abnormal movement of face or jaw
- Flatness of the cheek
- Loss of sensation on the side of injury
- Diplopia (double vision)
- Blindness caused by detached retina
- Nosebleed (epistaxis)
- Conjunctival hemorrhage
- **Paresthesia**
- Halo sign (indicates skull base fracture with leaking cerebrospinal fluid)
- Changes in level of consciousness; unconscious patient may have respiratory distress or failure caused by obstruction of tongue, loose teeth, bleeding, or other body fluids in airway

Radiographer's Response

1. Observe for airway obstruction. Watch for noisy labored respiration.
2. Do not remove sandbags, collars, or other supportive devices or move a patient unless supervised by the physician.
3. Apply a sterile pressure dressing if bleeding is profuse, and call for assistance.
4. Patients must not have suction through nasal passages performed on them.
5. Wear sterile gloves if in contact with open wounds.
6. If you find teeth that have fallen out, place them in a container moistened with gauze soaked in sterile water.
7. Be prepared to assist with oxygen and other emergency treatment, if necessary.
8. Observe for symptoms of shock; notify the physician in charge if condition of the patient or level of consciousness changes.

THE PATIENT WITH A SPINAL CORD INJURY

The spinal cord carries messages from the brain to the peripheral nervous system. It is housed in the vertebral canal, which extends down the length of the vertebral column. The spinal column is protected by the fluid in the canal and by the vertebrae—the bony structures encircling the canal. Motor function depends on the transmission of messages from the brain to the spinal nerves on either side of the spinal cord. Injury to or severing of the spinal cord causes message transmission to cease. The result is a cessation of motor function and partial or complete cessation of physical function from the level of damage to the cord to all parts below that level.

Most spinal cord injuries occur in the cervical or lumbar areas because these are the most mobile parts of the spinal column. The spinal cord loses its protection when there is injury to the protective vertebrae, and such an injury may result in compression or partial or complete severing of the cord. Spinal cord tissue, like brain tissue, has little healing power; injuries to it usually cause permanent damage.

The radiographer will be among the first of the health care workers to attend to the patient with a possible spinal cord injury so that he can assist in making the diagnostic assessment of the injury. If signs or symptoms of cervical spine injury are present, the patient will need a cervical spine series. Take great care in obtaining these radiographs to prevent extending the existing damage to the spinal cord. A portable cross-table lateral cervical spine radiographic image with a horizontal beam may be taken in the emergency suite without moving the patient or removing the backboard, collar, or sandbags used to immobilize the spine (Fig. 9-6). Remember that any movement can result in bone fragments or unstable

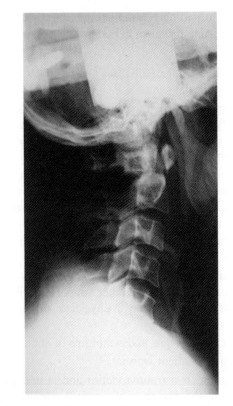

FIGURE 9-6 Portable cross-table lateral cervical spine radiographic image.

vertebrae compressing the spinal cord and extending the injury.

Clinical Manifestations

Complete Transection of Spinal Cord

- Flaccid paralysis of the skeletal muscles below the level of the injury
- Loss of all sensation (touch, pain, temperature, or pressure) below the level of injury; pain at site of injury possible
- Respiratory distress
- Bradycardia
- Loss of body temperature control
- Absence of **somatic** and visceral sensations below the site of the injury
- Unstable, lowered blood pressure
- Loss of ability to perspire below the level of injury
- Bowel and bladder incontinence
- Possible priapism in males

Partial Transection of Spinal Cord

- Asymmetrical, flaccid paralysis below the level of injury
- Asymmetrical loss of reflexes
- Some sensory retention: feeling of pain, temperature, pressure, and touch
- Some somatic and visceral sensation
- More stable blood pressure
- Ability to perspire intact unilaterally
- Possible priapism in males

Radiographer's Response

1. Monitor vital signs.
2. Maintain an open airway. If respirations change, notify the physician at once and call for assistance. If in respiratory failure, use jaw downward. Do not tilt the head.
3. Do not allow or request the patient to move when performing radiographs. Patient must be log rolled with a synchronized move supervised by the physician.
4. Do not move the patient's head or neck if position is awkward.
5. Do not remove sandbags, collars, antishock garments, backboard, or other supports until diagnosis is confirmed and a physician supervises the removal.
6. Observe for signs and symptoms of shock.
7. Keep the patient warm.
8. If patient is a trauma victim and is unconscious, assume the presence of a spinal cord injury and treat as such until directed to do otherwise by the patient's physician. All patients with head injuries

should be assumed to have cervical spine injuries and be treated as such.

IMAGING CONSIDERATIONS FOR THE MOBILE OR TRAUMA PATIENT

In the trauma patient, the cross-table lateral cervical spine radiograph, along with a chest radiograph, is commonly obtained immediately on the patient's arrival at the emergency department. The two diagnostic imaging exams are performed to screen for life-threatening injuries. Although injuries are better evaluated with other imaging modalities, the initial lateral cervical spine radiograph can allow early detections and intervention of many serious injuries in the severely injured patient. The lateral projection is considered adequate only when C1 to C7 has been imaged. An image that does not show the upper border of T1 should be supplemented with a swimmer's projection using a horizontal beam method (Fig. 9-7). The radiologist or other physician must carefully assess the image to evaluate the soft tissue structures for swelling, alignment injury, and possible fracture or subluxation. Since portions of the cranium are included, the lateral cervical spine radiograph may also verify proper endotracheal tube position and fracture of the face and skull. A sphenoid air-fluid level indicates a skull base fracture.

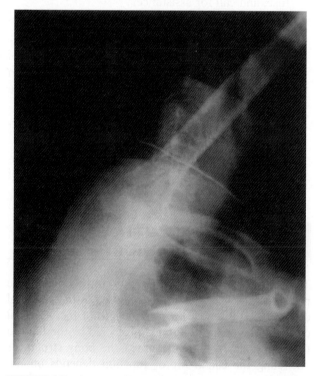

FIGURE 9-7 Swimmer's projection: horizontal beam lateral radiographic image.

Before moving the trauma patient, consider that injury to the cervical spine is present until the radiologist or physician has eliminated the possibility of an injury. The radiographer must be:

1. Aware of patient care through observation and analysis of the patient from the onset through the conclusion of the procedure.
2. Knowledgeable and use creative and accurate radiographic applications in positioning variations, adaptation of the equipment, image receptors, and technical factors to ensure a diagnostic image.
3. Prepared to perform exam(s) on patients with speed and have an action plan to facilitate several exams on one patient for the patient's comfort and overall flow of efficient imaging.
4. Aware and able to assess the presence of IVs, tubes, lines, and catheters as not to displace them during the imaging procedure.
5. Mindful of radiation protection practices especially the three cardinal principles of time, distance, and shielding during all trauma or mobile radiography.

Radiographer's Response
1. Monitor vital signs.
2. Maintain an open airway. If respirations change, notify the physician at once and call for assistance. If the patient is in respiratory failure, use jaw thrust maneuver to move jaw downward. Do not tilt the head.
3. Do not allow or request that the patient move for radiographs. Patient must be log rolled with a synchronized move supervised by the physician.
4. Do not move patient's head or neck if position is awkward.
5. Do not remove sandbags, collars, antishock garments, backboard, or other supports until diagnosis is confirmed and physician supervises the removal.
6. Observe for signs and symptoms of shock.
7. Keep patient warm.
8. If patient is a trauma victim and is unconscious, assume the presence of spinal cord injury and treat as such until directed to do otherwise by the patient's physician. All patients with head injuries should be assumed to have cervical spine injuries and be treated as such.

The mobile or portable chest x-ray is a mobile radiographic procedure frequently ordered for patients in the emergency room, surgery, recovery, intensive care units, cardiac care units, orthopedic wing, and general bedside. Chest images are performed for a variety of reasons (Display 9-3). A review of the chest image may reveal suspected and unsuspected pathology affecting the bony thorax, lung field, cardiac silhouette, or soft tissue.

DISPLAY 9-3

Mobile Chest Images Demonstrate and Verify Placement (with an increase of density) of the Following Tubes and Lines:

1. Tracheotomy tube (refer to Chapter 13) is a curved tube used to keep the opening free after tracheotomy to provide or protect an airway.
2. Swan-Ganz catheter is inserted into the subclavian vein, the internal or external jugular vein, or in a large peripheral vein to provide an accurate and convenient means of hemodynamic assessment; obtain blood pressure readings to introduce medications and intravenous fluids.
3. Central venous pressure (CVP) catheter is inserted into the subclavian, basilic, jugular, or femoral vein and advanced to the right atrium by way of the inferior or superior vena cava depending on the site of insertion to monitor the amount of blood returning to the heart.
4. Hickman catheter is inserted into the superior vena cava and is used for monitoring, providing nutrition, administering medications, and for drawing blood.
5. Peripherally inserted central catheter (PICC) is inserted into the subclavian vein to the superior vena cava; commonly used for prolonged antibiotic therapy, nutrition, and to draw blood.
6. Temporary or permanent pacemakers are artificial devices that can trigger mechanical contractions of the heart by emitting periodic electrical discharges, which regulates the heart rate by assisting or taking over for the heart's natural pacemaker.
7. Chest tubes are large catheters placed in the pleural cavity to evacuate fluid and air; commonly inserted in the sixth intercostal space in the mid or posterior axillary line (Fig. 9-8).

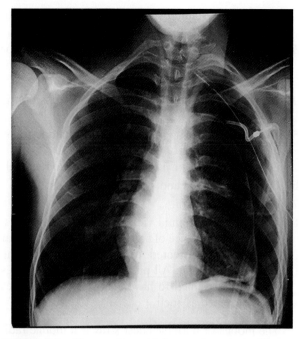

FIGURE 9-8   Chest radiographic image of a patient with a chest tube (left lung pneumothorax).

A portable chest image is obtained to demonstrate tube or line placement. In order to evaluate proper placement of the tubes or lines, the lungs may have to be slightly overexposed to clearly delineate the proper placement.

Mobile Radiography Helpful Tips

1. Verify the request for the radiographic procedure whether orders are verbal or written.
2. If assistance is required to hold the patient during the procedure, ask another radiographer, the attending nurse, or other appropriate member of the health care team to wear a lead apron during the x-ray exposure.
3. Verify the patient's identification with at least two patient identifiers.
4. Call the patient by his or her preferred name.
5. Introduce yourself to the patient.
6. If family members are present, explain the need for them to leave the room for the procedure, unless their assistance is needed.
7. Explain the procedure and check for understanding.
8. Visually inspect the room for mobile x-ray unit placement, IVs, oxygen, tubes, lines, catheters, and other medical equipment.
9. Use universal precautions.
10. Position the mobile unit, set the technique on the control panel, and position the x-ray tube over the anatomy part of interest.
11. Place the image receptor under the patient's anatomy of interest and collimate.
12. Call out "x-ray" to give individuals in close proximity time to leave the area.
13. Wear protective apparel and initiate the x-ray exposure using the maximum distance.
14. Leave the patient's room in order by arranging the sheets, blankets, and pillows.
15. Reposition any medical equipment to the original state.
16. Assure patient safety before leaving the bedside.

THE PATIENT WITH A FRACTURE

A fracture may be defined as a disturbance in the continuity of a bone. Fractures can be classified simply as open or closed. An open fracture indicates a visible wound that extends between the fracture and the skin surface. The broken bone itself often breaks through the soft tissue, making the fracture clearly visible.

A closed fracture may not be obvious to the untrained eye. Often there is swelling around the injured areas, pain, and deformity of the limb. All or some of these symptoms may be absent, and a closed fracture still may be present.

Internal injuries caused by fractures of the pelvic bones are a leading cause of death after motor vehicle accidents. While caring for trauma patients, always consider the possibility of a fractured pelvis when caring for patients with multiple traumatic injuries. Use extreme caution when making initial diagnostic radiographs because the slightest movement may initiate hemorrhage or irreparable damage to a vital organ. Patients with suspected pelvic fractures may be on a backboard or in pneumatic antishock garments. These are radiolucent and must remain in place during initial assessment radiographs. At times, it may be feasible to move the patient to the radiographic table on the backboard that has been placed by the emergency team, since this device allows the patient to remain immobilized.

A large number of trauma deaths result from blunt or penetrating trauma to the thorax. Multiple rib fractures can cause a flail chest, which in turn may result in **pneumothorax** (air or gas in the pleural space that collapses the lung) (Fig. 9-9) or **hemothorax** (blood in the pleural space). Fractured ribs are extremely painful and can be life-threatening. Stab and gunshot wounds can also cause fractures to the ribs and hemorrhage into the pleural cavity. When working with patients who have suffered this type of trauma, work quickly while observing the patient for symptoms of shock due to hemorrhage. Also avoid causing further pain or extending injuries.

Hip fractures and fractures of the femur are common among elderly patients as a result of bony changes

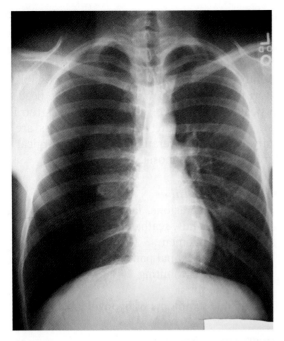

FIGURE 9-9 Chest radiographic image of a patient with a right pneumothorax.

related to age and disease (Fig. 9-10). These fractures are a common result of home accidents in elderly patients, and patients must be treated with utmost care to prevent extension of the injury.

Clinical Manifestations
- Pain and swelling
- Functional loss
- Deformity of the limb
- Grating sound or feel (crepitus) if moved
- Discoloration of surrounding tissue caused by hemorrhage within tissue (closed fracture)
- Overt bleeding (open fracture)
- Possible signs and symptoms of shock

In patients with trauma, images to rule out fractures or dislocations may be taken with mobile equipment in the emergency department; or, if the patient's condition permits, images may be taken in the radiology department.

Radiographer's Response
1. Keep affected limb or body part immobilized.
2. Any patient movement must be directed by the physician in charge of the patient.
3. Inform the patient of any intended moves and enlist his support.
4. Do not remove splints or other supportive devices.
5. In moving a splinted limb, support the joint and support the limb both above and below the fracture. Move the limb with one person at the distal end and one at the proximal end. On a specified signal, move the limb as a single unit (Fig. 9-11).

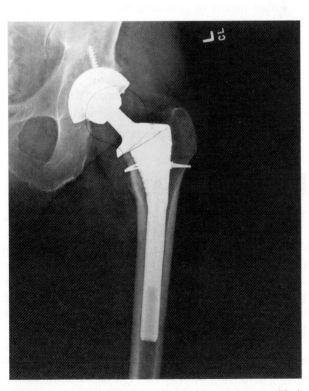

FIGURE 9-10 Hip prosthesis radiographic image on an elderly patient.

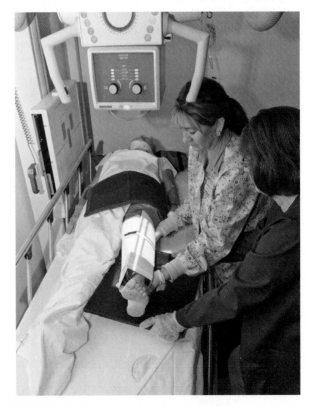

FIGURE 9-11 Proper moving of a splinted limb.

6. If the patient has an open fracture, wear sterile gloves if in contact with the wound, and use standard precautions measures.

7. Observe the patient for signs and symptoms of shock, and be prepared to act if such an emergency occurs.

Follow-up studies ordered on patients following the initial exam are usually performed in the radiology department, but may also be performed as a mobile procedure. In some cases, the patient may require surgery after initial exam. Therefore, you will be required to go to surgery during various procedures. In addition to the conventional portable mobile x-ray equipment, a radiographer must be prepared to use the C-arm fluoroscopic mobile unit for a wide variety of procedures as part of the health care team in the operating room. The radiographer's role during operating room procedures is to provide the physician or physicians with images of the site of interest for determining the exact location, position, and alignment for the appropriate fixation or approach for the patient treatment and care.

THE PATIENT WITH ABDOMINAL TRAUMA OR ACUTE ABDOMINAL DISTRESS

There are a number of causes of acute abdominal distress, many of which are life-threatening. Among them are blunt or penetrating trauma, resulting in internal and possibly external hemorrhage, appendicitis, bleeding ulcers, **ectopic pregnancy**, cholecystitis, pancreatitis, and bowel obstruction (Fig. 9-12). Whatever the cause of the distress, the symptoms are somewhat similar and, for the radiographer's purpose, may be grouped together. It is the responsibility of the radiographer to take the diagnostic images as quickly and efficiently as possible and with the least possible discomfort to the patient. An assistant may be needed to help position and move the patient who is too ill to assist. Patients in acute abdominal distress are frequently sent to the operating room for a surgical procedure following diagnosis.

Clinical Manifestations
- Possible abrasions, lacerations, entry and exit bullet wounds, seatbelt contusions
- A rigid abdomen
- Severe abdominal pain
- Nausea and vomiting
- Extreme thirst
- Possible symptoms of **hypovolemic** shock

Radiographer's Response
1. Do not remove antishock garments.
2. If the patient has open wounds, wear gloves; sterile gloves are indicated if in direct contact with the wound.
3. Call for assistance if the patient is too ill to help you move him or her.
4. If the patient is unable to stand for upright exposures or maintain the position on a tilt table, use other means of obtaining necessary radiographic images.
5. Transport the patient by gurney.
6. Have an emesis basin and tissues prepared in case the patient vomits.
7. Do not give the patient anything to drink or eat.
8. Observe for symptoms of shock, and be prepared to call the emergency team.

THE PATIENT AT HOME

The home is rapidly becoming one of the major areas for health care. As the cost of hospital care increases, the patient is being discharged from the hospital, in many instances, while still acutely ill. This change requires members of the health care team to go to the patient in the home to continue care. Therefore, you may be required on occasion to go to a patient's home to take portable radiographs.

For a patient to be eligible for health care in the home, he must be acutely ill, homebound, and in need of skilled nursing care. The cost of home health care is usually paid for by Medicare, Medicaid, or private health care insurance, although it may be paid for by

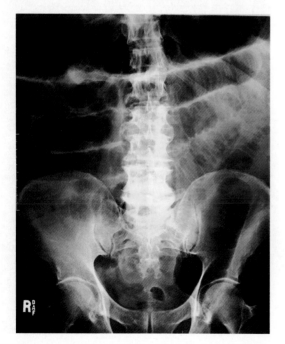

FIGURE 9-12 Bowel obstruction, AP projection of the abdomen.

the individual recipient. Most home health care visits are paid for by Medicare, since the greatest need for home care is for the elderly patient.

Radiography in the home must be ordered by the patient's physician and, if the patient has private health care insurance, approved by the insurance carrier as well. When going to a private home, expect some differences in methods of delivering care. There is little control of the work environment; the cleanliness, organization, and general environment may add to the challenges of the patient's care during the imaging procedure. The practice of sound medical aseptic technique, patient safety, and radiation safety procedures must be adhered too regardless of the environmental restrictions. In addition, patient confidentiality and standard of patient care must never be compromised.

Use of therapeutic communication techniques to establish rapport with the patient and the patient's caregivers is the first step toward a successful home visit. Prepare the patient for the prescribed radiographic imaging procedures by explaining to him what is to be done and by providing effective instructions during the procedure with the patient. If the patient is unable to cooperate during the procedure, ask the caregiver for assistance during the radiographic examination. Instruct the patient and/or the caregiver as to the radiation safety requirements in terms of use of protective apparel. When the exam is complete, double check to be certain that the patient is safe and that the caregiver understands that the visit is over and that the patient's physician will inform the patient and caregiver of the results of the radiographs.

SUMMARY

As a radiographer, follow the general precautionary guidelines when assigned to care for patients with traumatic injuries. Remember to follow universal blood and body fluid precautions when called to the emergency room department.

Patients with a spinal cord injury must be moved in a specific manner and only with specific directions from the physician in charge. Do not remove supportive devices without physician's orders.

Treat patients with head injuries and facial injuries as if they also have spinal cord injuries until it is verified that they do not. Also, consider basal skull fractures if the patient has injuries to the facial bones. Patients with these injuries should not be moved for initial diagnostic radiographic films without orders from the physician in charge of their care or without the physician's supervision.

When working with trauma patients, observe for changes in the level of consciousness, mental status, hemorrhage, shock, and respiratory distress. Patients with fractured extremities should also be moved with great care and under their physician's supervision so

that movement does not increase their pain or extend their injury. If splints or antishock garments are in place, do not remove them. Use strict aseptic practices for patients with open fractures to prevent infection.

Abdominal trauma and acute abdominal distress also are emergencies. Patients with acute abdominal pain are often very ill and are unable to assist the radiographer. Take radiographic images as quickly and gently as possible. An assistant should be on hand to help move the patient who is in severe pain or unable to cooperate. Some patients may not be able to be placed in an upright position while the exposures are being made. If this is the case, use alternative approaches for obtaining the necessary images to provide diagnostic information. These patients should be transported by gurney.

Home health care is increasingly common. If assigned to make a home radiographic imaging visit, remember that the work environment may not be as clean or orderly as in a diagnostic imaging department. However, adhere to the same standards of patient care, radiographic imaging, radiation safety, and medical asepsis that apply in the diagnostic department.

CHAPTER 9 TEST

1. When called to the emergency room, supplies needed may include:
   a. Gloves
   b. A mask
   c. A protective gown
   d. Goggles
   e. a, b, c, and d
2. List the guidelines that you should follow when caring for a patient with a traumatic injury.

3. List possible members of the emergency room health care team.
4. A radiographer must consider that all patients with head injuries may also have:
   a. Fractures
   b. Seizures
   c. Shock
   d. Cervical spine injuries
   e. Changes in vital signs

5. What precaution(s) must be followed when taking radiographic exposures of a patient who has a head injury?
   a. Keep the head and neck immobilized until the physician in charge rules out cervical spine injury.
   b. Wear sterile gloves if the patient has open wounds.
   c. Check the patient's vital signs frequently.
   d. a and b
   e. a, b, and c
6. What precaution(s) must a radiographer take when caring for a patient with a fractured extremity?
   a. Support the joint above and below the fracture and at the joints if moving a splinted limb.
   b. Do not remove splints without the direction of the physician in charge.
   c. Inform the patient before moving the fractured limb.
   d. None
   e. a, b, and c
7. You have been assigned to radiograph Mr. J. J. He has been transported by the local police to the emergency room of the hospital in which you are employed. He is complaining of severe pain in his right leg. As you approach the patient, you notice that he is walking rapidly up and down the corridor. His head is bent and he is talking rapidly to persons who are not present. He occasionally stops, looks up at the ceiling, and shouts that he

has to "get them." Your best manner of dealing with this situation would be to do what?
   a. Walk directly up to the patient, introduce yourself, and explain your purpose in being there.
   b. Get an assistant, approach the patient from his or her side, stop slightly away from the patient, and explain your purpose.
   c. Tell the emergency room nurse to forget it.
   d. Have the male orderlies restrain the patient.
8. List three factors that you must consider when caring for the patient with acute abdominal distress.
9. Special care is necessary when caring for a patient whose brain or spinal cord might be injured because:
   a. Extreme pain may result from the movement
   b. This type of injury heals slowly
   c. The incidence of infection is high
   d. These tissues have very little ability to heal
10. What is the leading cause of death for all persons under 44 years of age?
    a. Cancer
    b. Stroke
    c. Trauma
    d. Drowning
11. List some causes of injuries.
12. List the basic rules in trauma radiography.
13. Explain the change in patient care emphasis if the patient is to be radiographed at home.
14. Explain when the cervical collar may be removed on a trauma patient.

Pediatric Radiographic Considerations

STUDENT LEARNING OUTCOMES

After studying this chapter, the student will be able to:

1. Define the pediatric patient.
2. Discuss professional, appropriate, age-specific, and effective communication strategies for pediatric patients, parents, and guardians during radiographic procedures.
3. Discuss transporting infants and children.
4. Demonstrate safe methods of immobilizing a pediatric patient with commercial available devices and other positioning aids.
5. Describe proper radiation protection and safety measures, techniques, and practices used in pediatric radiography (ALARA principle).
6. Discuss your role as the radiographer in a suspected child abuse procedure.
7. Discuss administering medication to the pediatric patient in radiographic imaging procedures.

KEY TERMS

Adolescent: The period of life beginning at puberty and ending with physical maturity

Child abuse: The psychological, emotional, and sexual abuse of a child

Disinfectant: A solution capable of destroying pathogenic micro-organisms or inhibiting their growth

Enhance: Increase

Hand hygiene: Handwashing with soap and water or the use of alcohol-based products that do not require water

Hypothermia: Significant loss of body heat below 98.6°F

Immobilization: The act or process of fixing or rendering immobile

Infant: Newborn baby or a child under the age of 1 year

Isolette: A type of bed used in the newborn intensive care unit to keep babies warm and protected from the environment

Neonate: Newborn infant up to 1 month of age

NICU: Neonatal intensive care unit

Pigg-O-Stat: Commercial mechanical immobilizer device

Preschooler: A child who is not old enough to attend kindergarten

School age: Age at which the child is considered old enough to attend school

Toddler: Young child learning to walk

THE PEDIATRIC PATIENT

Pediatric patients range in age from infancy to 15 years. Children in this broadly defined group require special care, depending on their age and ability to comprehend the radiographic procedures. In order to be both sensitive and effective in performing the imaging procedure, radiographers must use age-appropriate methods of communication and execution of the required procedure according to a child's age. Caring for infants and children demands special safety and effective communication techniques and approaches that are different from adult radiography. It also requires a sensitive approach toward the accompanying parents or guardian. Display 10-1 outlines developmental approaches to be taken with children. In addition to imaging pediatric patients in the diagnostic imaging department, mobile procedures are performed on pediatric patients in the hospital room, emergency room, operating room, and neonatal intensive care nursery.

The pediatric patient includes: **neonates** in neonatal intensive care unit **(NICU), infants, toddlers, preschoolers,** and **school age** children. The immaturity of the neonatal immune system, in particular, dictates adherence of health care personnel to infection control practices. Infection control precautions are described in Chapter 4. Preventative measures to reduce infections in the pediatric patient begin with basic practices such as proper handwashing and hygiene to prevent the spread of infections.

Children of all ages respond in a positive manner to honesty and friendliness. A small child may be very frightened when entering the radiographic imaging department and seeing the darkened rooms and massive equipment. If the radiographer spends a few moments establishing a rapport with the child and acquainting the child with the new environment, the procedure will proceed more smoothly in a non-threatening manner and the child will leave the department with a positive attitude about the imaging process.

Most children resist immediate close contact with strangers. Therefore, it is best to talk to the child from a comfortable distance and allow the child to become accustomed to one's presence before approaching him. The radiographer must explain what is going to happen during the procedure to the child who is old enough to understand. The radiographer should also give the child an estimate of how long the procedure will last and what will be expected of him or her. The child should be prepared for any discomfort that he or she may feel. If the child is to receive contrast media or medications, the method of administration needs to be explained. Explanations to children are most effective if they are brief, simple, and to the point. The child should not be given choices when it is not appropriate because it may be confusing (Display 10-2).

The radiographer should speak to the child face to face even if he must sit or kneel on the floor to do so. To avoid misunderstandings, only one person should explain and direct the child. It may therefore be necessary to reach an agreement with the accompanying adult about who is going to assume this responsibility. Using a soft tone of voice and speaking in terms that are simple and familiar will **enhance** communication. The radiographer must be certain that the child understands what is being said. If the child wishes to

---

DISPLAY 10-1

Developmental Approaches by Age

Age	Developmental Approach
Birth to 6 months	Symbiotic—not fearful of strangers
6 months to 3 years	Separation-individualization—fear of strangers initially, followed by the toddler clinging to the parent
3 to 6 years	Preschool—age of initiative; a period of fantasy play and increasing verbal activity
6 to 12 years	Age of industry—a period of cognitive growth; growing interest in and ability to understand cause and effect
12 to 19 years	Adolescence—age of identity; heightened awareness of the body and its perceived effect on others

From Dixon SD, Stein MT: *Encounters with Children: Pediatric Behavior and Development,* 3rd ed. St. Louis: Mosby-Year Book, 2000.

DISPLAY 10-2

Caring for Children during Radiographic Procedures

Infants (Birth–12 Months)

Identify the patient. Educate by explaining the procedure to the parents or guardians. Maintain trust, assess need, maintain safe surroundings, and never leave unattended.

Toddlers (1–3 years)

Identify the patient. Educate by explaining the procedure to the parents and patient, assess needs and level of independence, have concern for privacy, maintain safe surroundings, and never leave unattended.

Preschooler (3–5 years)

Identify the patient. Educate parents and patient, assess needs, support independence, have concern for privacy, maintain safe surroundings, and never leave unattended.

School Age (6–12 years)

Identify the patient. Educate parents and patients, assess needs, and have concern for privacy.

---

carry a toy or security item to the radiographic room, he or she should be allowed to do so if at all possible. If it is not practical, explain to the child that the toy will be placed so the child can see it during the procedure. Return the toy to the child immediately after the procedure.

When explaining a procedure to a child, tell him what part of the body will be examined, why, and who will be performing the procedure. Also explain how the examination will proceed, what part of the child's body must be touched to accomplish the procedure, and why he must hold still during the process.

Some children are very modest. If a child's body must be exposed for an examination, only the necessary part should be exposed. The radiographer must guard against allowing the child to become chilled while in his care. This is particularly important for infants, because they lose body heat rapidly and **hypothermia** may occur.

Parents or guardians who accompany the child will feel less anxious if they are given an explanation of the procedure. Enlist their cooperation by encouraging them to explain the child's special needs and sensitivities. If the adult can be allowed to remain with the child during the procedure without jeopardizing the child's safety or the successful completion of the procedure, provide the appropriate protective apparel and other radiation protective measures. Also, give parents or guardians specific instructions about what is expected of them during the procedure. It is important to follow the department policies and procedures addressing the parents' or guardians' role during the radiographic examinations.

Explicit instructions must be provided for the adults involved in the exam in all aspects. The adult holding the child must assure the child will not fall from the x-ray table. If the parents are holding the child during the imaging procedure, they must wear the proper protective apparel, which includes a lead apron and possibly lead gloves. In addition to explaining the importance of wearing the protective apparel, the radiographer should explain how to secure the apron and assist them with the garments. Make sure that the child is not left unattended while this is being done. The radiographer must never assume that the parent is watching the child on an x-ray table and must instruct parents in the exact measures they need to take. For instance:

RADIOGRAPHER: *I would like you to stand on this side of the table with your hands on your child [use child's name] at all times. It will be necessary for you to wear this lead apron while I am x-raying your child as a radiation protective measure. I will hold the child while you put on the apron. The apron fastens with Velcro attachments on the sides. Now, if you will please keep your hands on the child at all times.*

If the child refuses to follow directions and is emotionally distraught, it may be necessary for the accompanying adult to leave the room. In this case, the child must be made to understand that the doctor and his or her parents want the examination to be done and that it will be done. Then, repeat the directions and proceed. Do not belittle or criticize the child's behavior; remain nonjudgmental and matter-of-fact and accomplish the

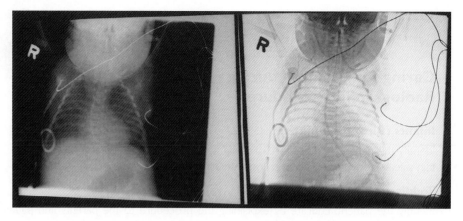

FIGURE 10-1 Chest images of a newborn infant with tubes.

task as quickly as possible. Display 10-2 summarizes the steps in caring for children during radiographic procedures.

The High-Risk Newborn Infant

Many hospitals have special care units for high-risk newborn infants. In many areas of the United States, infants are transported to such facilities for special care from the hospital in which they were born. Infants may be considered to be at high risk for life-threatening problems if they are of low birth weight or if they have other perinatal problems.

Infants whose lives are at risk require special care considerations in highly specialized neonatal intensive care units (NICU). Here they are protected from threats to their nutritional status, environmental problems such as changes in their body temperature, and infection by being placed in **isolettes** with environmental and thermal control and by the practice of meticulous infection control measures.

Infection prevention and control practices are the responsibility of all health care personnel, including the radiographer. The NICU patient in particular has an immature immune system and therefore is more susceptible to infection. The radiographer must follow and adhere to the pediatric unit standard precautions policies and procedures. **Hand hygiene** is the basic important practice that reduces the risk of infection transmission. A surgical scrub, or a 2-minute scrub as for medical asepsis, may be required of all health care personnel entering these nurseries. Protective gowns are worn over scrub uniforms. Gowns, gloves, mask, and eye protection may be required. The radiographer must have the proper education and training on pediatric standard precautions for the prevention of the transmission of infection. The prevention of infection includes cleaning the x-ray equipment, which includes the mobile x-ray machine, the image receptors, gonadal shielding, and right or left markers. The mobile machine must be wiped clean with a **disinfectant** solution and

must be free of dust before entering the nursery. Specific procedures must be followed addressing the radiographic equipment and accessories.

Consult with the nurse in charge of the infant's care. The nurse will assist by positioning and immobilizing the infant. Take care to prevent chilling the infant or dislodging any catheters or tubing while performing the radiographic procedure (Fig. 10-1). Provide a protective apparel apron to the nurse who is assisting to hold the infant (Fig. 10-2); provide the infant with gonadal shielding when appropriate.

If the radiographer has any sort of respiratory infection or infected cuts on his hands, another radiographer should be asked to take the NICU assignment to prevent introduction of infectious microorganisms into the protective environment of the NICU.

The Adolescent or Older Child

The older child or early **adolescent** is often expected to act as an adult would act under similar circumstances. This is

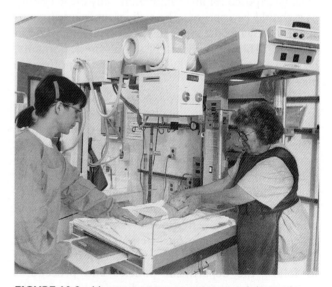

FIGURE 10-2 Nurse wearing protective apparel during the imaging of an infant in the neonatal intensive care unit.

not a fair expectation, since children of this age are not yet adults. When they are threatened by illness or injury, they return to the more familiar role of being a child.

The teenager is apt to be perceived as hostile and self-centered. Communication will cease if a health care worker conveys a feeling of disapproval. The radiographer can overcome this behavior by conveying a nonjudgmental attitude and using the therapeutic communication technique described in Chapter 2. Communication strategy approaches appropriate to the comprehension level of the patient must be modified according to the patient and or the parent needs. The interview with the teenager must include the following basic points:

- Identify the patient
- Explain the procedure
- Educate the patient
- Maintain the patient's concern for privacy
- Provide after care directions

When caring for the older child, the radiographer should be as direct and as honest as possible in explanations of what will occur during the procedure. Use simple terms and allow the patient to ask questions and express fears and apprehension. If the child feels more secure with a parent accompanying him or her, this should be allowed, if it is permitted under hospital policy. If not, the adult may stay close by and be with the child between radiographic images or as often as is appropriate and safe. The child's privacy must be respected. No part of the child's body should be exposed without an explanation of the necessity for doing so. If the patient can be allowed to make choices, let him or her do so. This gives the older child a feeling of having some control of the situation.

TRANSPORTING INFANTS AND CHILDREN

The radiographer may be responsible for transporting infants and children from one area to another area in the radiographic imaging department in addition to transporting them to the radiology department from the hospital rooms. Additional safety measures to prevent injuring the very young patient are required. In addition, standard precautions must be followed during the transporting of the pediatric patients in all circumstances.

Take care to ascertain the identity of the patient using at least two patient identifiers; the type of procedure that the child is to receive must be verified and confirmed, and the appropriate gowning and removal of artifacts must be considered. The identification band

on the wrist or ankle must be checked with the nurse in charge of the patient before the child is taken from their room and checked again against the patient chart or the requisition for the procedure when the child arrives in the department.

The method of transfer depends on the child's size and the nature of the illness or injury. Under most circumstances, it is safe to carry infants and very small children for short distances (e.g., from one diagnostic imaging room to another). For longer distances, it is necessary to place the child in a crib with all sides up and locked.

Some cribs come with tops to prevent the active child from climbing over the crib rails. Crib rails must never be placed in a half-raised position because an active child can climb over them and will fall from a greater height than if the rails had not been raised at all.

Older children may be transported on a gurney with the side rails up and locked and a safety belt securely fastened. Some older children may prefer to be transported in a wheelchair. If this means of transportation is appropriate, make sure that the safety belt is securely fastened for the entire time that the child is seated in the wheelchair. Children must never be left alone while in diagnostic imaging. If they are placed on a radiographic table, an attendant must be at their side until the procedure is completed and they are taken from the procedure room. If children must wait in an outside corridor, they must be attended at all times.

Infants or small children must have back support if they are being held or carried. This can be done in a horizontal hold with the child supported against the body and the head supported on the arm at the elbow with a hand grasping the patient's thigh (Fig. 10-3). Another method of holding an infant or small child is holding the child upright with the buttocks resting on the arm with the other arm around the infant supporting the back and neck.

When a child is returned to a hospital room, the radiographer must be certain that the side rails of the crib are up, and must check to be certain that they are locked. The bedside stand should not be at close range to prevent the child from using it as a stepping place to climb out of the crib. No unsafe items or liquids should be within reach of the child's crib. The nurse in charge of the child must be notified that the child has been returned to the room.

IMMOBILIZATION AND THE ANXIOUS CHILD

Occasionally, the very anxious or frightened child is not able to stay quietly in one place long enough for a successful diagnostic procedure to be completed; therefore, careful **immobilization** methods must be initiated. In some situations, a child may not be able to be held in

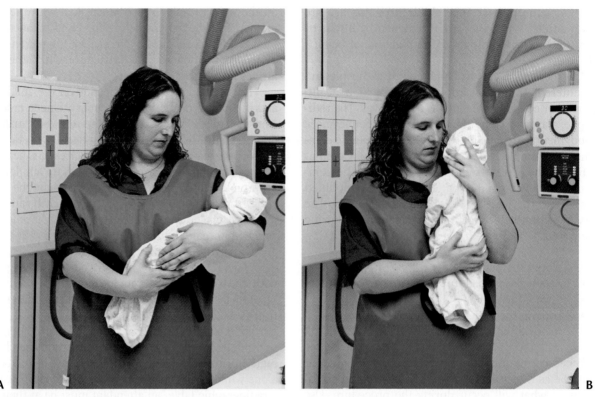

FIGURE 10-3   (**A**) Mother holding and supporting infant's back and head. (**B**) Mother holding infant upright supporting the back and head.

position for an examination and safe immobilization devices will be necessary. Immobilizers should be used only when no other means are safe or logical and should be of a quality that will not cause injury to the patient or compromise the outcome of radiographic images.

There are several methods of immobilizing children. An immobilizer can be made by folding a sheet in a specified manner or may be a commercial immobilizer. The child may also be held in position by one or two assistants, provided they are given the proper radiation protective apparel. There are several commercial immobilizers available that are safe and effective for specific procedures. Whatever type of immobilizer is chosen, the child who is old enough must be made to understand, before the immobilizer is applied, that this is not a method of punishment and that it will be removed as soon as the procedure is completed.

The **Pigg-O-Stat** is commonly used during chest radiography. It is important to prepare the parents and the child prior to beginning the procedure. Effectively informing the parent of the use of the immobilizer and the reason for it will reduce the anxiety associated with observing their child in the device.

RADIOGRAPHER: *It is important to immobilize your child [use child's name] during the x-rays. (At this time explain and demonstrate how the child will be immobilized without actually plac-*

ing the pediatric patient in the device. Explain that the unit will not hurt the child.) (1) By safely and carefully placing your child in the unit, we will obtain diagnostic images and eliminate the need for repeat exposures due to motion. (2) If your child cries, the chest x-rays will be of better quality for the Radiologist to evaluate, since the lungs will fill with air. (3) I will perform the x-rays as efficiently and quickly as possible. (4) If department protocol allows, invite the parent to wear a lead apron and stand next to the child while in the Pigg-O-Stat.

Ask the parent or guardian if he or she has any questions before proceeding with the immobilization technique. Some department protocols provide the parent with protective apparel allowing the parent to stand close to the child in the Pigg-O-Stat, which provides reassurance for both the parent and the child and lessens anxiety and fear. If a child must be physically immobilized by an assistant during the examination, it is important to follow the department's pediatric immobilization protocol. Under no circumstances should anyone use undue force when immobilizing the child; take care not to pinch or bruise the child's skin or interfere with circulation. It is better to use a sheet or commercial immobilizer than to have the assistant use force because the former is an acceptable practice

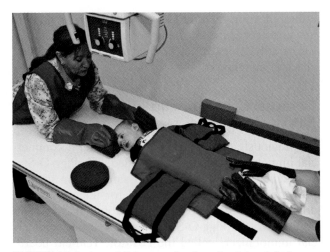

FIGURE 10-4 Immobilizing a pediatric patient's head during skull radiography.

and less threatening and frightening to a child. To prevent a small child from rolling his head from side to side during skull radiography (Fig. 10-4), the person holding the child should stand at the head of the table and support the child's head with sponges between the hands, making sure to exert no pressure on the child's ears or fontanels. When imaging infant's and toddler's upper or lower extremities, it is important for the parent or the assistant to use lead gloves in addition to the lead apron when holding an extremity (Fig. 10-5).

As with any radiographic procedure, the pediatric patient must be provided with appropriate gonadal shielding.

Sheet Immobilizers

Sheet immobilizers are effective and can easily be formed into any size or fashion desired. To make a sheet immobilizer, fold a large sheet. Then place the top of the sheet at the child's shoulders and the bottom at the child's feet. Leave the greater portion of the sheet at one side of the child. Bring the longer side back over the arm and under the body and other arm. Next, bring back the sheet over the exposed arm and under the body again. This method of immobilization keeps the two arms safely and completely immobile and leaves the neck exposed as for a soft tissue lateral neck image (Fig. 10-6).

Mummy-Style Sheet Wrap Immobilizer

Another method of immobilization is the mummy-style sheet immobilizer approach. It is accomplished by folding a sheet or a blanket into a triangle and placing it on

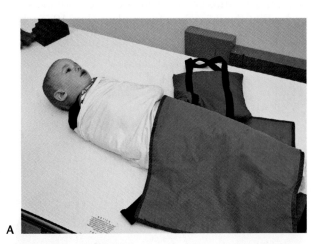

A

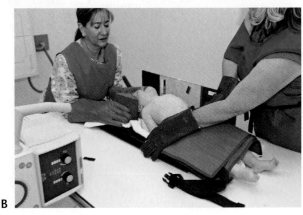

B

FIGURE 10-6 **(A)** Pediatric patient wrapped in a sheet for immobilization. **(B)** Pediatric patient unwrapped for a soft tissue lateral neck image with shielding.

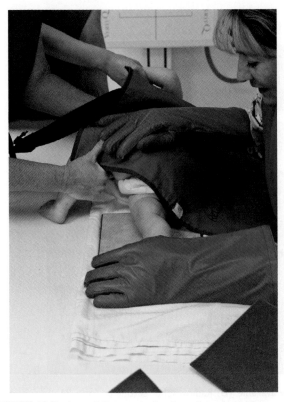

FIGURE 10-5 Immobilizing a pediatric patient during lower limb imaging.

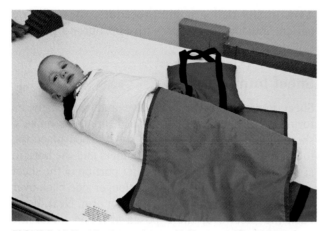

FIGURE 10-7 Mummy-style immobilization with shielding.

the radiographic table. The distance from the fold to the lower corner of the sheet should be twice the length of the child. Then place the child onto the sheet, with the folds slightly above the child's shoulders, making sure that the child's clothes are loosened or removed before being placed on the sheet if necessary. Bring one corner of the sheet over one arm and under the child's body. If both arms are to be immobilized, turn the sheet and repeat the procedure for the legs (Fig. 10-7). This

immobilization method can be used for radiographic imaging procedures of the upper or lower extremities. Kerlix or roller gauze can be used to immobilize an arm or leg of an infant.

Commercial Immobilizers and Other Positioning Aids

As previously mentioned, there are several commercial immobilizers also recommended. The Pigg-O-Stat is excellent for holding a child safely in an upright position (Fig. 10-8). It is useful for imaging procedures of the chest or upright abdominal exams. In addition to the Pigg-O-Stat, there are other commercial immobilizers called the Posi-tot, Tam-em board, and Infantainer. Each of the commercially available units facilitates pediatric exams by reducing the need for repeat exposures due to motion, therefore decreasing the patient dose. Other positioning aids and devices are available that aid in immobilization such as the device used in Figure 10-9. Creativity and patient safety are limitations for positioning aids which include the use of sandbags, plexiglass, tape, Velcro, lead, and lead aprons.

Radiation protection is a priority for infants and children because of the radiosensitivity of their rapid

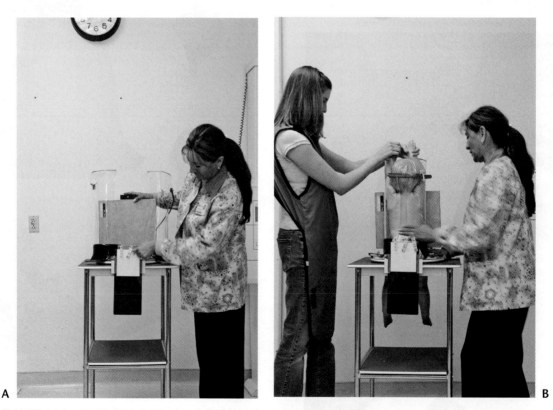

A   B

FIGURE 10-8   (A) The Pigg-O-Stat immobilizer is commercially available. **(B)** Radiographer setting up for a PA chest with the mother assisting.

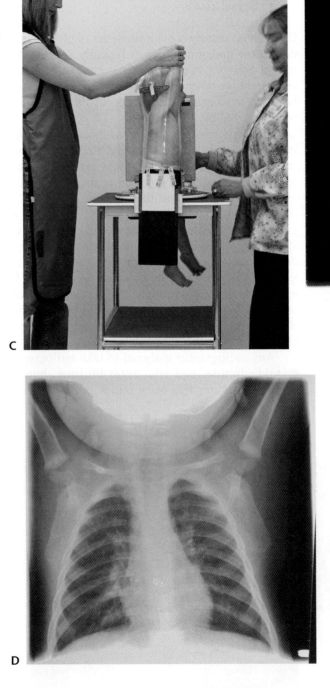

C

E

D

FIGURE 10-8 (Continued) (**C**) Radiographer setting up for a lateral chest with the mother assisting. (**D**) PA chest image performed on a pediatric patient with a Pigg-O-Stat. (**E**) Lateral chest image performed on a pediatric patient with a Pigg-O-Stat.

and changing cell growth. The radiographer is responsible for using effective radiation protective measures during pediatric imaging procedures. The ALARA (As Low As Reasonably Achievable) concept should be practiced in all aspects of the various procedures. Gender- and examination-appropriate shielding reduces radiation exposure to the patient. In particular, gonadal shielding, either the contact or the shadow type, reduces patient dose of radiation. The departmental protocol regarding shielding should be implemented for all pediatric procedures. In addition, fast speed imaging systems, short exposure times, and proper collimation greatly reduce the patient's radiation exposure (Fig. 10-10).

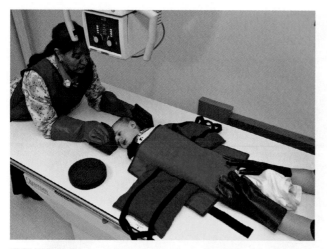

FIGURE 10-9   Immobilization with sandbags, shielding, and sponges.

CHILD ABUSE

Child abuse is any act of omission or commission that endangers or impairs a child's physical or emotional health and development. Unfortunately, the incidence of child abuse has increased in recent years. Child abuse includes:

- Physical abuse and neglect
- Emotional abuse
- Sexual abuse

Child abuse usually is not a single act of physical abuse, neglect, or molestation, but is typically a repeated pattern of behavior. A child abuser is most often a parent, stepparent, or other caretaker of a child. He or she can be found in all cultural, ethnic, occupational, and socioeconomic groups.

The radiographer may be assigned to radiograph injuries that are the result of child abuse. It will be the radiographer's ethical and perhaps legal obligation to report child abuse to the person at the institution who makes the inquiries and the required reports in such cases. In some states, all health care personnel are obligated to report suspected cases of child abuse. In other states, designated health care providers are obligated to do so. A radiographer must learn the legal parameters of this obligation in the state in which he practices. Each institution also has a protocol that dictates the method of processing suspected cases of child abuse, which a radiographer is also obliged to know and use if the situation arises.

Any radiographer assigned to take radiographs of a child's injuries and who notes bruising, burns, or possible fractures that seem out of proportion to the

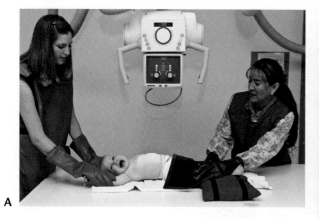

FIGURE 10-10   (**A**) Use of collimation and gonadal shielding during an AP abdomen. (**B**) Pediatric radiographic image: AP abdomen.

DISPLAY 10-3

Indicators of Physical Abuse

History

- The child states the injury was caused by abuse.
- Knowledge that a child's injury is unusual for a specific age group.
- Parent is unable to explain the cause of injury.

Behavior Indicators (the following behaviors may result from child abuse)

- Child is excessively passive, compliant, or fearful.
- Child is excessively aggressive or physically violent.
- Child or caretaker attempts to hide injuries.
- Child makes detailed and age-inappropriate comments regarding sexual behavior.

report of how the injury occurred may need to consider abuse.

Perhaps an older child will tell a story about how the injuries occurred that does not correspond to what the caretaker has related. A child may report not having eaten for an inordinately long time because his or her parents have not provided food. Whatever form the suspected abuse takes, the radiographer must report it to the designated person in the workplace. In most states, the health care worker who reports suspected child abuse is protected from legal action if the report proves to be false; however, take care to refrain from false accusations. Often children misjudge what is a safe action and suffer accidents because of their own mistaken judgment. Display 10-3 outlines common indications of abuse.

ADMINISTERING MEDICATION TO THE PEDIATRIC PATIENT IN RADIOGRAPHIC IMAGING

Administering medications to children in diagnostic imaging is a sensitive issue. The medical care of children is most frequently the role of physicians and registered nurses who have specialized education in pediatrics. Medicating children can be life threatening and must not be undertaken by the radiographer. However, if a registered nurse is not available to administer the contrast media to patients under 18 years of age, with proper education and certification, the radiographer may administer the contrast media. Drug absorption, biotransformation, distribution, use, and elimination are different in infants, children, and early adolescents compared with adults. For this reason, knowledge of

pediatric medication administration is required to administer drugs accurately and safely to patients in these age groups.

The radiographer must be aware of the potential for overmedication or for an adverse reaction to a drug or contrast agent in children. Before an infant or child receives medication or a contrast agent, the child must be assessed. Questions for the child's parents or caregiver are:

1. Does the child have allergies to any foods or medicines?
2. How does the child respond to medicines?
3. In what form are medicines administered to the child at home?
4. Will a parent be able to supervise the child after he or she is discharged from this department following this procedure?
5. Are there any unusual circumstances concerning this child and his or her ability to take medicines that the physician should know about before administering a drug?
6. Is the parent educated in the action, purpose, and potential side effects of the drug being administered?

After gathering this data, pass the information on to the physician who will prescribe the drug or contrast media and to the nurse who will administer it.

As the radiographer, make certain that the child who is receiving drugs or contrast media in the department is carefully monitored and is not released from the department until there is no risk of complications. The assessment and care of the child are usually performed by a registered nurse who works in diagnostic imaging; however, if a nurse is not present, the radiographer and the physician must ensure that they are done properly. Before the child who received a contrast agent or sedating medication is discharged, he must be assessed by a physician and given authorization to leave with a parent or guardian. If the child is sleeping, he or she must remain hospitalized until awakening.

CATHETERIZATION OF PEDIATRIC PATIENTS

The pediatric patient may require catheterization in the radiology department for a cystographic procedure, which may include a voiding cystourethrography (Fig. 10-11). Catheterization of pediatric patients is recommended by registered nurses or physicians who have specialized education in pediatrics. Refer to Chapter 12 for general patient education about, care during, and the procedure for catheterization.

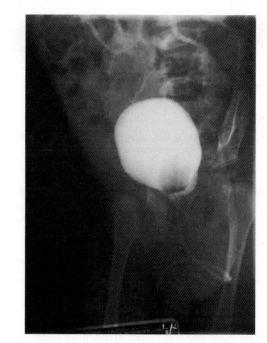

FIGURE 10-11   Cystogram radiographic image on a pediatric patient.

SUMMARY

The pediatric patient ranges in age from newborn to 15 years of age. The radiographer must relate to all patients in an appropriate and specific manner, regardless of age. The infant is usually accompanied by parents. The radiographer should attempt to ease the parents' anxiety by giving them an explanation of the procedure to be performed and the approximate amount of time it will take.

If it is necessary to immobilize the child, the radiographer should explain the reasons for this procedure to the child, if he or she is old enough to understand, as well as to the parents. If it is necessary to immobilize a child, an immobilizer made of soft material such as a sheet may be used. If the child is to be immobilized by being held, it should be done in a firm, safe non-threatening manner to prevent injury or unnecessary repeat radiographs. One's body should never be placed over a child as an immobilizer. A sheet immobilizer or one manufactured commercially may be less traumatic for

the patient and more effective. Protective apparel and shields should be worn by persons immobilizing a child to prevent exposure to radiation.

Child abuse usually is not a single act of physical abuse, neglect, or molestation, but is typically a repeated pattern of behavior. A child abuser is most often a parent, stepparent, or other caretaker of a child. He or she can be found in all cultural, ethnic, occupational, and socioeconomic groups. The radiographer must pay close attention to the child and parent or caregiver for behavior clues or red flags if child abuse is suspected.

Medicating children can be life threatening and must not be undertaken by the radiographer. However, if a registered nurse is not available to administer the contrast media to patients under 18 years of age, with proper education and certification, the radiographer may administer the contrast media.

CHAPTER 10 TEST

1. List four considerations the radiographer must incorporate into communication with a child.
2. Describe the variations in communication a radiographer must use in communicating with an adolescent.
3. Describe symptoms that a child may display that may indicate abuse.

4. When caring for a pediatric patient, the best method of transport is always:
   a. A gurney
   b. Carrying the child
   c. A crib
   d. Depends on the distance involved and the age of the child

5. When caring for a 6-year-old child, the radiographer should:
   a. Explain the procedure to the patient in great detail
   b. Tell the patient that there will be no pain or discomfort, regardless of the type of examination
   c. Be friendly, honest, and concise in your explanation to the child
   d. Routinely immobilize the child to be examined
6. At what age is a child considered an infant, toddler, preschooler, and school age?
7. When interviewing the teenager, list the main points that should be included.
8. Name two commercially available immobilizers.
9. List other supplies or devices that may be used to immobilize pediatric patients.
10. Why must radiation protection measures be applied, especially during pediatric radiography?
11. What are the radiographer's responsibilities when child abuse is suspected?

Geriatric Radiographic Considerations

STUDENT LEARNING OUTCOMES

After studying this chapter, the student will be able to:

1. Discuss the special considerations while imaging geriatric patients and describe their special care needs.

2. Discuss normal changes associated with aging for the integumentary, cardiovascular, pulmonary, hepatic, gastrointestinal, genitourinary, and musculoskeletal systems.

3. Explain the precautions to take for a patient who has had an arthroplasty.

4. Discuss cultural considerations when caring for the geriatric patient.

5. Discuss the radiographer's role in a suspected elder abuse procedure.

KEY TERMS

Actinic keratosis: A slow, localized thickening of the outer layers of the skin as a result of chronic, excessive exposure to the sun

Adduct: To draw toward a center, or median, line

Alzheimer disease: An illness characterized by dementia, confusion, memory failure, disorientation, restlessness, speech disturbances, and an inability to carry out purposeful movements; onset usually occurs in persons aged 55 or older

Arthroplasty: Plastic repair of a joint

Baroreceptor: A sensory nerve terminal that is stimulated by changes in pressure

Dementia: Organic mental syndrome characterized by general loss of intellectual abilities involving impairment of memory, judgment, and abstract thinking

Depression: A morbid sadness, dejection, or melancholy

Geriatrics: The branch of medicine that deals with all aspects of aging, including pathological and social problems

Hallucination: A sensory impression (sight, sound, touch, smell, or taste) that has no basis in external stimulation

Kyphosis: An abnormal condition of the vertebral column in which there is increased convexity in the curvature of the thoracic spine

Lentigines: Round, flat, brown, highly pigmented spots on the skin caused by increased deposition of melanin; often occurs on the exposed skin of the elderly

Macule: A small, flat blemish or discoloration that is flush with the skin surface

Polypharmacy: Administration of excessive medications or of many drugs together

Presbyopia: Loss of ability to focus on near objects

Prosthesis: An artificial substitute for a missing part

Urinary incontinence: Inability to control urinary functions

THE GERIATRIC PATIENT

The number of people over 65 years of age in the United States is predicted to be more than 70 million people by the year 2030. At the present time, one in every eight persons falls into this category. With 85 million baby boomers, the largest population reaching 60 years of age, one out of every five Americans is projected to be over 65 by 2030. Persons over 85 years of age constitute one of the fastest-growing portions of the population (Display 11-1). For health care workers, this means that most of their patients will be 65 years of age or older; therefore, they must understand the changes that occur as one ages. The radiographer must understand that age 65 is an arbitrary age that has been designated for convenience as the age at which a person is eligible for Medicare benefits, Social Security benefits, and retirement from many positions. Many persons at this age are still quite youthful and productive; therefore, all persons must be assessed on an individual basis, not merely by their chronological age (Display 11-2).

The human body undergoes normal physiologic and anatomic changes as it ages. These changes do not occur uniformly in all people, so it is not correct to say that all persons begin to demonstrate the changes of age at the same time. Lifestyles, culture, and hereditary factors contribute to the aging process. When an elderly patient is admitted to the radiographic imaging department, the radiographer must be able to differentiate between the normal changes of aging and deficits resulting from a disease process.

The elderly person is more frequently burdened with major illnesses that are chronic rather than acute in nature. Heart disease, cancer, and strokes are the cause of 80% of deaths in persons over age 65. Hypertension, arthritis, diabetes mellitus, pulmonary disease, and visual and hearing impairments are also common conditions requiring long-term care. These conditions result in a great deal of physical discomfort and a multitude of social and psychological problems.

Large numbers of medications are prescribed and consumed by the elderly. Many of these medications affect the patient's response level. Often, problems attributed to the aging process are the result of multiple medication consumption, which is frequently called **polypharmacy.**

Depression is a common and debilitating emotional problem of the aged person. The threat of becoming a burden to one's family, the fear of losing one's good health, or the necessity of giving up an independent lifestyle owing to chronic disease result in feelings of helplessness and hopelessness that can give rise to a major depressive episode. Symptoms of depression in the elderly person are often confused with **dementia.** Symptoms of dementia, including disorientation, confusion, gross memory deficits, paranoid ideation, **hallucinations**, and depression, are not part of the normal aging process. When these symptoms are present in an

---

DISPLAY 11-1

Aging Americans

The Geriatric Patient

Number of people 65 or older	35 million	Percentage of the population 65 or older	13% (2000 projection)
Number of people 85 or older	4 million	Percentage of the population 85 or older	2% (2000 projection)
Life expectancy	% of people age 65 expected to reach age 90: 26%		
Those with moderate or severe memory impairment	Men, 65-69: 5% Women, 65-69: 4% Men, 85 & up: 37% Women, 85 & up: 35%		
Those who consider themselves in good to fair health	65-74: 9% 85 & up: approximately 4%		

Excerpted from the Census Bureau; Centers for Disease Control and Prevention; Federal Interagency Forum on Aging Related Statistics, "Older Americans 2000: Key Indicators of Well-Being."

DISPLAY 11-2

Categories of Persons 65 Years and Older

Young-old	65 to 75 years
Old	75 to 85 years
Old-old	85 to 100 years
Elite old	Over 100 years

elderly patient, the radiographer must remember that they are indicative of a disease process. Persons with **Alzheimer disease** present with symptoms of dementia, which usually occur in persons over age 65, although it may occur at an earlier time. Persons with Alzheimer disease or other diseases that produce symptoms of dementia are frequently seen for a radiographic imaging examination. Recent studies have indicated that of people over the age of 85 years about 50% suffer from Alzheimer disease at various stages.

When caring for a patient who exhibits symptoms of dementia, remember that the person may not be able to understand or retain directions. The radiographer will have to explain to the patient what is to be done and then assist him or her in following the directions. The patient who is confused or has a paranoid ideation may become frightened when confronted by the forbidding atmosphere of the radiographic imaging department. Allowing a familiar person to be present in the examination room to assist the patient may make the patient feel more secure and allow the procedure to be accomplished more effectively.

Persons who are depressed may be so preoccupied that they do not respond to outside stimuli. It may be necessary to give the same instructions a number of times to a depressed person and then to assist the patient in following directions.

When an examination of the **geriatric** patient is complete, the radiographer must assist him or her to return to the dressing room or lavatory, because the stress of the procedure may result in forgetfulness. Make certain that the patient is attended before leaving him or her. The elderly patient must not be left alone in the radiographic imaging room, because he or she may become confused and may be in danger of falling from the examining table.

CHANGES ASSOCIATED WITH AGING

Older adults may not have the same symptoms of a disease as a younger adult. They may have nonspecific symptoms such as dizziness, falls for no apparent reason, infections without fever, or **urinary incontinence**, to name a

few. These are symptoms of disease and not a part of the normal aging process. The radiographer must be able to differentiate what is normal from what is pathological. As aging progresses, the body systems change in a gradual manner. A brief overview of how the body systems change with normal aging, as well as the precautions the radiographer must consider because of these changes, follows.

Integumentary System

Normal Changes of Aging
- The skin wrinkles, becomes lax, and loses turgor.
- The vascularity of the dermis decreases, and the skin of white people begins to look paler and more opaque.
- Skin on the back of the hands and forearms becomes thin and fragile.
- Areas of skin lose pigment; purple **macules** and senile purpura may appear as a result of blood leaked through weakened capillaries.
- Brown macules called senile **lentigines** appear on the backs of the hands, on the forearms, and on the face.
- Seborrheic keratoses and **actinic keratoses** may develop.
- Nails lose their luster and may yellow and thicken, especially the toenails.
- Hair loses its pigment and begins to gray.
- Hair patterns change and the hair becomes thin and more brittle.
- There is hair loss on the scalp and other body areas.

Many skin changes listed above occur only in white ethnicities and are not normal in persons of dark-skinned ethnicities.

Implications for the Radiographer The skin of the geriatric patient is more fragile than that of a younger person and is thus more easily traumatized. Ensure that the skin

CALL OUT!

Lying on a hard radiographic table may be especially painful for the geriatric patient; use a full table pad.

of the elderly patient is not damaged. The preventive measures listed in Chapter 3 must be followed at all times.

Changes in the Head and Neck

Normal Changes of Aging

- There is mild loss of visual acuity, particularly **presbyopia**.
- The light-sensing threshold is affected, and adaptation from light to dark and color perception diminish.
- Tear production is either reduced or increased.
- The skin of the eyelid loosens and the muscle tone decreases.
- Sensory, neural, and conductive changes occur in the ear.
- Hearing loss is common.
- There is loss of muscle mass in the neck.
- There is an accentuated forward upper thoracic curve, which may result in **kyphosis** (Fig. 11-1).
- The senses of taste and smell decrease.

CALL OUT!

Assess the patient's condition frequently; ask the patient if he or she feels dizzy or feels like falling. Ensure and protect the patient from injury during radiographic examinations.

Implications for the Radiographer Rapid changes in lighting, such as moving from a brightly lighted waiting room into a darkened examining room, may cause

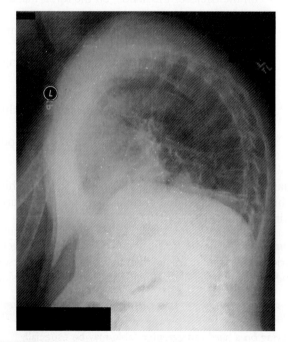

FIGURE 11-1   Lateral chest radiographic image demonstrating kyphosis.

the elderly patient momentary blindness. Offer patients assistance so that they do not fall.

Loss of sense of smell and hearing loss must be considered. The radiographer must ascertain that the patient is able to hear directions and must speak loudly enough for the patient to understand what is being said. Do not assume, however, that all older persons have a hearing deficit and need to be spoken to in an abnormally loud voice.

During fluoroscopic examinations, background noise from the equipment may prevent the patient from hearing the instructions. Be especially careful to clearly state instructions and check for understanding.

Pulmonary System

Normal Changes of Aging

- Pulmonary function changes with age; lung capacity diminishes owing to stiffening of the chest wall, among other changes.
- The cough reflex becomes less effective.
- The normal respiratory defense mechanisms lose effectiveness.

Implications for the Radiographer The patient becomes breathless and fatigues more easily. Because of the decreasing effectiveness of the cough reflex, the patient is more apt to aspirate fluids when drinking. There will be an increased risk of pulmonary infections resulting from the loss of respiratory defense mechanisms. A patient with chronic pulmonary disease cannot be expected to lie flat for more than brief periods of time, since this position increases dyspnea.

During chest radiographic examination, when possible, ask the geriatric patient to hold his or her breath on the second full inhalation to ensure full lung expansion (Fig. 11-2).

The radiographer must instruct the patient to drink slowly to avoid choking when drinking the contrast media for an upper gastrointestinal examination. Position the patient in an upright sitting position to prevent aspiration.

The Cardiovascular System

Normal Changes of Aging

- Structural changes occur in the heart as aging progresses.
- The coronary arteries calcify and lose elasticity (Fig. 11-3)
- The aorta and its branches dilate and elongate; the heart valve thickens.
- There is a decline in coronary blood flow.

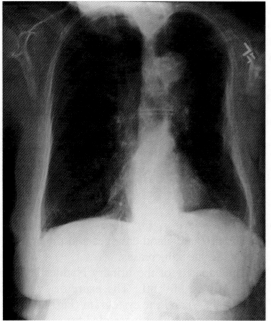

FIGURE 11-2   PA chest images of a geriatric patient with full lung expansion.

- The **baroreceptors** in the aorta and internal carotid arteries become less sensitive to blood volume and pressure changes.

Implications for the Radiographer   Owing to normal cardiovascular changes of aging, the elderly patient tires more easily; imaging examinations and procedures should be conducted in as efficient a manner as possible to avoid fatigue. If a procedure is unavoidably lengthy, the patient must be allowed to rest at intervals.

Hypothermia and complaints of feeling cold are common problems for the elderly patient because of decreased circulation; therefore, it is important to avoid chilling.

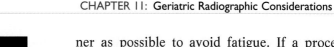

CALL OUT!

Additional blankets may be helpful to prevent discomfort or, in extreme cases, hypothermia during and between radiographic examinations.

One fourth of people over age 65 have postural hypotension (a drop in systolic blood pressure of 20 to 30 mm Hg) for 1 to 2 minutes after changing from a prone to a standing position. Rapid position changes result in a feeling of dizziness and the patient may fall. The radiographer must always assist the elderly patient to a sitting position for a short time before he or she stands and steps off the radiographic table. This allows the patient to adjust to the new position before walking.

The Gastrointestinal System

Normal Changes of Aging
- Gastric secretion, absorption, and motility decrease.
- There is a predisposition to dryness of the mouth, and the swallowing reflex becomes less effective.
- The abdominal muscles weaken.
- Absorption of iron, vitamin B_{12}, and folate decreases, with resulting potential for anemia.
- Many elderly patients are edentulous (without teeth), or the teeth present are decayed or gums diseased. Many have full dentures or partial plates.
- Esophageal motility declines.
- The tone of the internal anal sphincter decreases.

Implications for the Radiographer   If the patient is required to fast before a diagnostic examination, schedule the examination for the early morning so that the patient can have breakfast close to the usual time.

Medications may not be dissolved and absorbed from the stomach as effectively or as they are meant to be. Therefore, the ability to swallow is also affected. This may impair the elderly patient's ability to drink liquid contrast agents. Instruct the patient to drink slowly to avoid choking. The patient who must drink liquid in

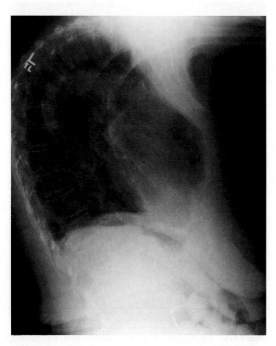

FIGURE 11-3   Lateral chest demonstrating calcified aorta.

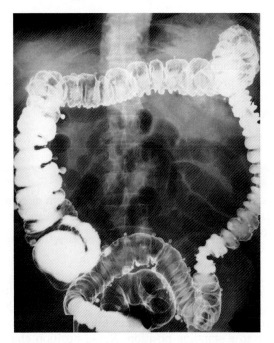

FIGURE 11-4 Double contrast enema radiographic image of an elderly patient; diverticula present.

the imaging department must be positioned in an upright sitting position to prevent aspiration.

Caution must be exercised when dealing with the patient's dentures or partial plates in terms of secure placement. If they must be removed for some reason, place them in a plastic denture cup and in a secure location where they will not be broken or lost. Return them to the patient as soon as it is possible to do so safely.

The elderly patient may have a difficult time retaining the contrast media (Fig. 11-4) during a lower gastrointestinal examination because of loss of sphincter control. This potential problem must be considered when planning for the procedure.

> ### ◀))) CALL OUT!
> The use of an enema tip with an inflatable cuff will facilitate the lower gastrointestinal examination in patients with loss of sphincter control.

The Hepatic System

Normal Changes of Aging
- Liver size decreases.
- Enzyme activity and the synthesis of cholesterol decrease.
- Bile storage is reduced.

Implications for the Radiographer The elderly person has an increased potential for drug toxicity, since most drugs are metabolized in the liver. Be alert for adverse drug reactions in the elderly patient.

The Genitourinary System

Normal Changes of Aging: Women
- Muscle tone and bladder capacity decrease.
- Pubic hair becomes sparse.
- Vaginal atrophy occurs.
- Involuntary bladder contractions increase.

Normal Changes of Aging: Men
- The prostate gland enlarges and the tone of the bladder neck increases.
- The capacity of the urinary bladder is reduced by 500 to 900 mL. The excretory urographic (Fig. 11-5) and the cystogram (Fig. 11-6) exams demonstrate the urinary bladder.
- The size of the penis and testes is decreased, owing to sclerosis of blood vessels.

There is a change in sexual response in men and women, but both can remain sexually active, if they are healthy, into the seventh or eighth decade of life.

Implications for the Radiographer Loss of muscle tone in the female genitourinary system may make the patient more susceptible to urinary incontinence in

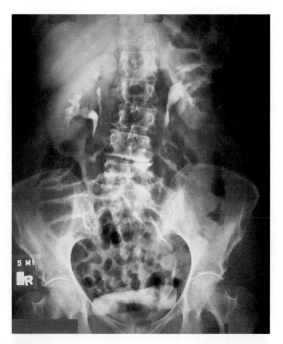

FIGURE 11-5 Excretory urogram radiographic image of an elderly patient.

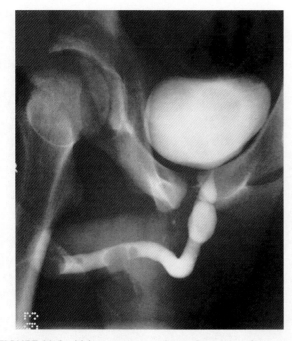

FIGURE 11-6 Male cystogram radiographic image of an elderly patient.

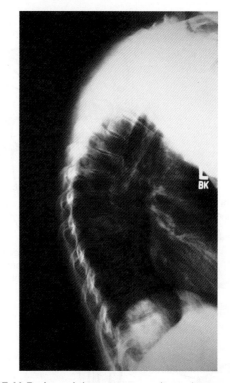

FIGURE 11-7 Lateral thoracic spine radiographic image of an elderly patient.

stressful situations. Both the elderly male and female patient may have a limited bladder capacity and may need to urinate more frequently. Have a bedpan and urinal available for elderly patients who cannot use the lavatory easily.

Musculoskeletal System

Normal Changes of Aging

- Bone mass is reduced and bones become weaker.
- Muscle mass decreases. Muscle cells decrease in number and are replaced by fibrous connective tissue.
- Muscle strength decreases.
- Intervertebral discs shrink and vertebrae collapse, resulting in shortening of the spinal column (Fig. 11-7).
- Articular cartilage erodes.
- The normal lordotic curve of the lower back flattens.
- Flexion and extension of the lower back are diminished.
- Placement of the neck and shaft of the femur changes.
- Posture and gait change. In men, the gait narrows and becomes wider based. In women, the legs bow and the gait is somewhat waddling.

Implications for the Radiographer Increased muscular weakness increases a patient's discomfort when

he or she is expected to assume positions necessary for imaging procedures. Painful joints and deformities accompanied by decreased tolerance for movement also increase discomfort. The radiographer must assist the patient to the required position and then support him or her with positioning sponges to facilitate maintaining that position. The risk of falling is greater when caring for elderly patients owing to musculoskeletal changes. It is the radiographer's obligation to assist patients in positioning and in getting on and off the radiographic table to prevent falls.

The Patient Who Has Had Arthroplastic Surgery

Total joint replacement has become a common procedure in hospitals throughout the United States. The joints of many elderly persons become very painful because of degenerative joint disease, and an operative procedure is done to replace the diseased joint with a **prosthesis. Arthroplasty** is also indicated for persons with joint diseases such as rheumatoid arthritis or for persons with joint deformities due to injury. Although knee and hip arthroplasty are the most common, almost any joint that is malfunctioning can be replaced (Fig. 11-8).

Radiographs are frequently requested several days after arthroplastic surgery to determine the rate of the healing process and the ability of the patient to return

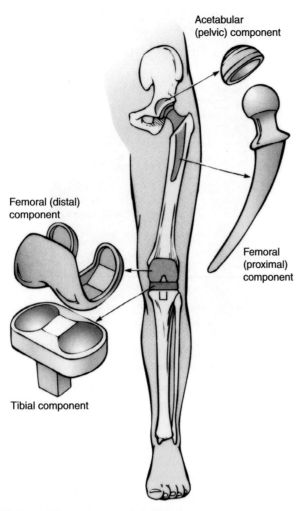

FIGURE 11-8 Hip and knee replacement.

Acetabular (pelvic) component

Femoral (distal) component

Femoral (proximal) component

Tibial component

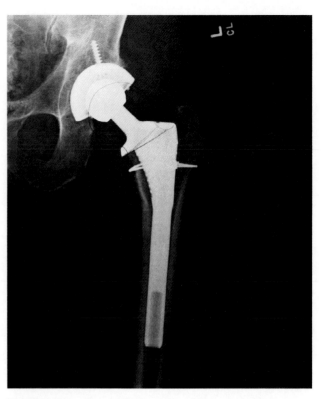

FIGURE 11-9 Hip prosthesis radiographic image: AP projection.

to daily activities (Fig. 11-9). There are restrictions on movement and positioning ordered postoperatively by the patient's surgeon that must be followed by all health care workers involved in the patient's care to prevent damage to the new joint.

The most common complication after hip replacement is dislocation of the prosthesis. Correct positioning following surgery is necessary to prevent this. The affected leg must be prevented from **adducting** and the operative hip must be kept in extension. A special pillow is sometimes used for this purpose; at other times, a regular, large pillow is used. When the patient is sitting in a chair, the legs must remain uncrossed and the hips must not be flexed more than 90 degrees. Weight bearing on the affected side is restricted for varying lengths of time depending on the type of prosthesis chosen. The radiographer must understand the needs of the patient who has had an arthroplasty so that he or she will not be injured while being cared for in radiographic imaging.

After knee arthroplasty, the patient is sometimes placed on a continuous passive motion device. Weight bearing is restricted and restored gradually. The knee should not be hyperflexed and the patient should not kneel. For shoulder and elbow arthroplasty, protocols for postoperative care are variable. Ankle replacement has not achieved widespread use at this time. Whatever the arthroplasty, the radiographer must understand the restrictions on weight bearing and movement for each patient and adhere to them to prevent irreparable damage to the joint involved.

Radiographer's Response

1. When the patient with a recent arthroplasty comes to the radiographic imaging department, the radiographer must understand and adhere to the limits that have been placed on the patient's weight bearing and mobility of the restricted joint.

2. Move patients who have had hip, knee, or ankle arthroplasty to and from the department by gurney. They cannot get onto and off the radiographic table without placing weight on the affected limb. Move patients toward their affected side in this situation.

3. After hip arthroplasty, do not allow the patient's affected leg to adduct (move toward the center of the body). Keep a pillow or block between the legs to prevent this.

4. Do not position the patient with weight on the surgical incision site.

5. Do not hyperflex affected joints.

The Neurologic System

Normal Changes of Aging
- Brain weight changes, which may be due to reduced size of neurons (Fig. 11-10).
- The ability to store information changes very little in the absence of disease; however, some short-term memory loss occurs.
- Sensorimotor function decreases.
- Reaction time to both simple and complex stimuli decreases.
- The time needed to perform activities increases.
- The lens of the eye thickens, making the pupils of the eye appear smaller.
- There is a decrease in postural stability that is greater in women than in men.
- A decrease in proprioception creates problems with spatial relations.
- There is loss of sensitivity to deep pain.

Implications for the Radiographer Remember that the elderly patient is less responsive to painful stimuli and is not aware of a painful stimulus until an injury has occurred. The radiographer must increase awareness of potential for patient injury.

The elderly patient may have visual problems in the dimly lit radiographic imaging rooms. He or she may also need guidance to avoid colliding with objects

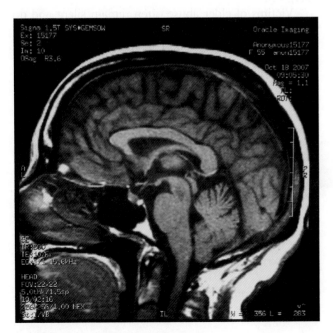

FIGURE 11-10 MRI image of the brain.

that are not seen easily. For example, the patient may not see the stool to determine where to place the feet to step down from the radiographic table.

The elderly person processes information and direction in a slower fashion. The radiographer must be certain that the patient understands directions and allow him more time to execute moves.

CALL OUT!

The radiographer is responsible for preventing accidents.

CULTURAL CONSIDERATIONS AND AGING

Radiographers are aware of the challenges that may be experienced when imaging the elderly due to physicals limitations such as impaired vision, hearing, and or limited mobility. Equally important is the need for the radiographer to develop cultural knowledge, awareness, and sensitivity when imaging the elderly in order to provide the best care. The word culture defines human behavior and beliefs, which include thoughts, communicated words, actions, and customs of various social, ethnic, religious, and economic groups. The importance of respecting the patient's beliefs and values will improve patient care and provide a positive outcome for the imaging procedure. Otherwise, cultural insensitivity and intolerance may have an adverse effect on patient care.

The culture of the patient is reflected in an attitude toward aging, illness and its treatment, pain, death, and dying. Some elderly patients are accepting of whatever treatment the physician and other health care workers offer. Others require a detailed explanation and reassurance at every step. The relationship between the patient and the caregiver also varies with the cultural beliefs of the patient and his or her family. Some caregivers are highly solicitous and anxious concerning the treatment that their relative is to receive. Others leave the patient in the health care worker's hands and attend to other affairs.

Radiographers must perform the procedure by following an approach with sensitivity to the patient's cultural differences. In some societies, it is understood that the adult child who is the caregiver will attend to every detail of a parent's medical treatment, while in other cultures the patient is expected to know and understand how to conduct his or her own care. If a caregiver is to oversee the patient's care, the radiographer should include them in the procedure based on their appropriate expectations to engage in the imaging procedure according to the departmental protocol. If

DISPLAY 11-3

Recognizing the Warning Signs of Abuse

Physical abuse: Injuries are incompatible with the explanations; bruises, scratches or other injuries; inappropriate use of physical restraint or medication.

Sexual abuse: The elder patient communicates act of sexual abuse; bruising on the breast or genital areas with or without bleeding.

Emotional or psychological abuse: Elderly person or dependent adult is withdrawn or secretive or is hesitant to talk freely around caregiver; family members or caregivers isolate the elder, restricting contact with other family members or friends; the elder verbally reports mistreatment.

Neglect: Poor hygiene; dirty or torn clothes or lack of appropriate shelter; medical conditions that go untreated; malnutrition or dehydration.

Financial abuse: Unusual bank account activity; unpaid bills, eviction notices, or discontinued utilities; changes in spending patterns often accompanied by the appearance of a new "best friend"; the elder reporting financial abuse in various forms.

---

this is not the case, the patient will need careful and complete direction appropriately and effectively communicated. Whatever the culture of the patient, one must be sensitive and take differences into consideration to provide the best possible patient care. The examination or procedure will be more comfortable for the patient, which will facilitate the procedure for the elderly patient as well as the health care provider.

ELDER ABUSE

It is estimated that one out of every 20 seniors experiences elder abuse; the abusers are family members, caregivers, strangers, men, and women. Elder abuse is the neglect, mistreatment, or exploitation of anyone age 65 or older (or any disabled dependent adult). Unfortunately, the prevalence and reporting of elder abuse have increased in recent years. Elder abuse can involve:

- Physical abuse or violence: the use of physical force that may result in bodily injury, physical pain, or impairment

- Sexual abuse: nonconsensual sexual contact of any kind with an elderly person
- Emotional or psychological abuse: the inflicting of anguish, pain, or distress through verbal or nonverbal acts
- Isolation or caregiver's neglect or self-neglect: the refusal or failure to fulfill any part of a person's obligations or duties to an elder or self
- Financial abuse: occurs when anyone takes or keeps an elder's property with the intent to defraud (Display 11-3)

There are three subcategories of elder abuse: (1) domestic elder abuse, (2) institutional elder abuse, (Display 11-4) and (3) self-neglect or self-abuse.

Display 11-5 lists indications of elder abuse by a caregiver.

Victims of elder abuse often remain silent and do not report incidences of abuse. They may fear retaliation or do not wish to report an abusive family member to protect the abuser from legal consequences.

Implications for the Radiographer The radiographer may be assigned to image a geriatric patient and

---

DISPLAY 11-4

Avoiding Elder Abuse or Neglect during Imaging Procedures

1. Avoid pinching patient's skin, rough handling, or shoving while transferring the geriatric patient from a gurney or wheelchair onto the radiographic table.
2. When immobilizing elderly patients, utilize the standards of care for immobilizing the geriatric patient as prescribed by the institution during radiographic procedures.
3. Assist geriatric patients when they ask for help.

DISPLAY 11-5

Caregiver Indicators of Elder Abuse

- Caregiver responds for the elder, preventing the patient from responding.
- Caregiver is flirtatious in an inappropriate sexual approach to the patient.

- Caregiver lacks affection toward patient.

---

suspect abuse. It will be the radiographer's ethical and legal obligation to report elder abuse to the person at the institution who makes the inquiries and the required report in such cases. In some states, all health care personnel are obligated to report suspected cases of elder abuse. In other states, designated health care providers are obligated to do so. The radiographer must learn the legal parameters of this obligation for the state in which he or she practices. Mandatory reporting laws, including penalties for not reporting abuse, exist in most states. Each institution has a protocol that dictates the method of reporting and processing suspected cases of elder abuse, which the radiographer is obliged to know and use if the situation arises.

SUMMARY

Health care workers must assess each elderly patient to determine any special needs. The imaging technologist must understand that one cannot generalize concerning the disabilities of aging because they vary in each individual. The imaging technologist must be able to distinguish the physical limitations that are part of the normal aging process from those resulting from a disease process or abuse. The incidence of elder abuse has increased in recent years. In some states, health care workers are required to report suspected cases of elder abuse.

Patients who have had joint replacement surgery have specific postoperative orders for care. The radiographer is obligated to inquire about the patient's restrictions concerning mobility and weight bearing. Patients who have had a knee, hip, or ankle arthroplasty must be transferred to and from the radiographic imaging department by gurney, because they are not able to get on and off the radiographic table without placing weight on the affected joint. Patients who have had hip arthroplasty must not adduct the affected leg and, when sitting, must not flex the hip more than 90 degrees. Patients who have had knee arthroplasty must not flex their affected joint more than 90 degrees.

Whatever the culture of the elderly patient, one must perform the imaging procedure with an approach involving sensitivity to the patient's cultural differences. The examination will be more comfortable for the patient. The importance of respecting the patient's beliefs and values will improve and provide a positive outcome for the imaging procedure. Otherwise, cultural insensitivity and intolerance may have an adverse effect on patient care.

CHAPTER 11 TEST

1. Describe the normal changes of aging as related to the following body systems
   a. Integumentary system
   b. Cardiovascular system
   c. Pulmonary system
   d. Hepatic system
   e. Gastrointestinal system
2. Confusion and other symptoms of dementia are to be expected in an elderly patient, since they are part of the normal aging process.
   a. True
   b. False

3. Eighty percent of deaths in persons over age 65 are due to:
   a. Trauma, peritonitis, and emphysema
   b. Fractures, chemical abuse, and schizophrenia
   c. Cancer, heart disease, and strokes
   d. Diabetes mellitus, arthritis, and hypertension
4. When the radiographer must schedule an elderly patient for a difficult diagnostic examination, it is best to schedule the examination for:
   a. Evening hours so that the patient has the day to rest

b. Early morning hours so that the patient can have breakfast as close to the usual time as possible
c. In the middle of the day so that traffic is less hectic
d. At a time that is convenient for the radiographer

5. Physiologic changes that come with aging that the radiographer should consider as he works with the elderly patient include:
a. Loss of the sensation of pain
b. Loss of sensitivity to heat or cold
c. Diminishing cough reflex
d. Loss of the sense of humor
e. a, b, and c

6. Assessment of the elderly should include:
a. Ability to see and hear
b. Ability to move without assistance
c. Level of understanding
d. a and b
e. a, b, and c

7. When is arthroplasty indicated?
8. Which joints are most commonly replaced?
9. What is the outcome of cultural sensitivity when imaging the elderly patient?
10. What are two caregiver indicators of elder abuse?
11. What are the warning signs of abuse?

Patient Care during Urologic Radiographic Procedures

STUDENT LEARNING OUTCOMES

After studying this chapter, the student will be able to:

1. Explain the need for infection control when working with patients who have urologic diagnoses.

2. Demonstrate the correct method of inserting a straight catheter and a retention catheter into the adult urinary bladder.

3. Explain the correct method of transporting a patient who has a retention catheter in place.

4. Demonstrate the correct method of removing an adult retention catheter from the urinary bladder.

5. Describe the patient care precautions that must be taken by the radiographer when a patient is undergoing cystography, retrograde pyelography or placement of a ureteral stent.

6. Describe alternate methods of catheterization of the adult urinary bladder, and explain patient care responsibilities of the radiographer when these catheters are in place.

7. Describe how to assist in the catheterization of a pediatric patient using an infant feeding tube.

KEY TERMS

Cystography: Radiographic imaging of the urinary bladder

Cystoscope: An instrument used for examining the urinary bladder and ureters that is equipped with a light, a viewing obturator, and a lumen for passing catheters

Incontinence: The inability to refrain from yielding to the normal impulse to defecate or urinate

Lithotomy position: A posture in which knees are flexed and thighs abducted and rotated externally

Penoscrotal junction: The area of the male penis that meets the scrotum

Perineal: Pertaining to the area between the anus and the scrotum in the male and the vulva and the anus in the female

Reflux: Backward flow; usually unnatural, as when urine travels back up the ureter

Retrograde: Moving in the direction that is the opposite of what is normal

Sphincter: A circular band of muscle constricting an orifice, which contracts to close the opening

Ureteral catheter: A firm catheter inserted into the ureter attached to a cystoscope

Void: The action of emptying urine from the bladder

Infections of the urinary tract are the most common nosocomial infections. A common cause of these infections is poor infection control practices by health care workers during placement of catheters in the urinary bladder or during care for patients who have indwelling catheters in place. Radiographers frequently work with patients who have urinary catheters in place. In some institutions, radiographers are responsible for inserting a catheter into the patient's urinary bladder before radiographic imaging procedures take place.

Catheterization of the urinary bladder refers to the insertion of a plastic, silicone, or rubber tube through the urethral meatus into the urinary bladder. Catheters are inserted into the urinary bladder for a number of reasons: to keep the bladder empty while the surrounding tissues heal after surgical procedures; to drain, irrigate, or instill medication into the bladder; to assist the **incontinent** patient to control urinary flow; to begin bladder retraining; or to diagnose disease, malformation, or injury of the bladder.

Cystography, retrograde pyelography, and placement of ureteral stents all involve radiographic imaging. These procedures are performed frequently in the special procedures area of the radiographic imaging department or in the cystoscopy laboratory. As part of the health care team, radiographers actively participate in these diagnostic examinations and treatments because fluoroscopy and radiographic images are required while they are in progress.

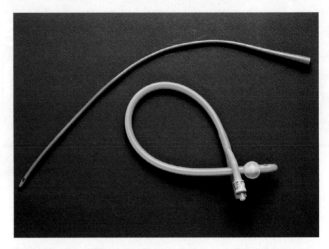

FIGURE 12-1   The top catheter depicts a straight catheter.

PREPARATION FOR CATHETERIZATION

The urinary bladder is sterile; therefore urinary catheterization requires sterile technique. Since the urinary bladder is easily infected, any object or solution that is inserted into it must be free of bacteria and their spores. Infection or injury may result when the technique used in the performance of the catheterization of the urinary bladder is poor or when caring for a patient.

Catheterization is not performed without a specific order from the physician in charge of the patient. It is less stressful for some patients if male technologists catheterize male patients and female technologists catheterize female patients.

When a physician requests catheterization of a patient, it must be established which type of catheter is to be used. Depending on the reason for the radiographic procedure, a straight catheter or an indwelling catheter (usually a Foley) is chosen. A straight catheter is used to obtain a specimen or to empty the bladder and is then removed. An indwelling catheter is inserted and left in place to allow for continuous drainage of urine. Most hospitals provide prepared sterile trays for catheterization with the desired type and size of catheter and the necessary equipment included. A tray set is chosen according to the type of catheter to be inserted. The equipment needed to perform catheterization is listed in Table 12-1.

The antiseptic solution most frequently used for cleansing the penis or the female perineum before catheterization is a povidone-iodine solution. For cleansing purposes, the patient must be assessed for allergic response to iodine before this solution is used. A drape sheet and an extra means of casting light on the **perineal** area are also needed. Do not attempt to catheterize a female patient unless adequate lighting is provided. Catheter size and tips vary and are graded according to lumen size, usually on the French scale.

TABLE 12-1	Equipment Needed to Perform Catheterization		
Straight or indwelling catheter	Antiseptic solution	Cotton balls for cleansing	Water-soluble lubricant
Specimen bottle	Receptacle for draining urine for a straight catheter	Closed-system drainage set for indwelling catheter	Sterile gloves Sterile drape Sterile forceps

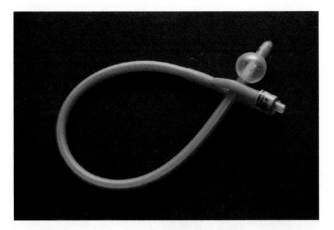

FIGURE 12-2   A Foley catheter with the balloon inflated.

The size of the catheter is listed on the prepared catheterization set.

A straight catheter is a single-lumen tube (Fig. 12-1). Indwelling catheters have a double lumen with an inflatable balloon at one end. One lumen is attached to a urinary bag to allow for continuous urinary drainage; the other lumen is a passageway controlled by a valve that serves as a portal for instilling sterile water into the balloon. The balloon holds the catheter in place after it is inserted into the bladder (Fig. 12-2). A third type of catheter, known as the Alcock catheter, may occasionally be seen. This type of catheter has three lumens in which the third lumen provides a passage for irrigation solution and is used for patients in need of continuous bladder irrigation.

PROCEDURE

Female Catheterization

The female urethra is usually 3 to 5 cm (1½ to 2 inches) in length and smaller in diameter than the male urethra. A smaller catheter than that used for male catheterization is necessary for the female patient. Catheters are sized by the French scale. The smaller the number listed on the catheter package, the smaller the lumen size of the catheter. A 14F (used for an adult female) is smaller in diameter than a 20F (used for an adult male).

When a radiography request for a procedure that requires catheterization is received, the technologist first determines what type (straight or indwelling) of catheter to choose. Next, all equipment is assembled and the technologist washes his/her hands. Patients are often embarrassed and apprehensive about this procedure, so a good explanation and reassurance that there will be little, if any, pain is vital to the success of the procedure. This explanation should be completed once the patient has been seated on the radiographic table and prior to placing the patient in position for the catheterization. Inform the patient that there will be a slight sensation of pressure when the catheter is inserted. Provide privacy for her by using a screen or by closing the door from the radiography room to the work area. Assess the patient's ability to maintain a position that allows for adequate exposure of the perineum. Assess the perineal area for soiling at this time. If the perineum is soiled, obtain washcloths, soap, warm water, and clean disposable gloves and cleanse the area before beginning the procedure. Then proceed with the steps for catheterization.

1. Position the patient on her back; have her flex her knees and relax her thighs so as to externally rotate

them. This is called the *dorsal recumbent* (**lithotomy**) position.

2. Drape the patient with a sheet so that only the perineum is exposed. If she is disabled and cannot maintain this position, be prepared to assist her to maintain adequate exposure for the catheterization procedure to continue.

3. Adjust the light so that it shines directly on the perineal area (Fig. 12-3A). It is difficult to locate the urinary meatus in many women unless adequate lighting is available.

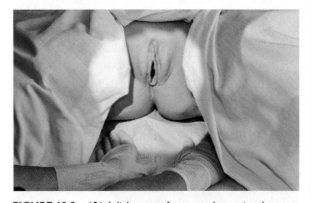

FIGURE 12-3   **(A)** A light must focus on the perineal area.

4. Open the sterile pack, which may be conveniently placed between the patient's legs if she is cooperative and will not contaminate the sterile field. If this is not the case, open the tray on a Mayo stand at the side of the radiographic table. The outer plastic veering of the pack may be used as a waste receptacle or provide an

(continued)

impermeable waste bag. Place it in a convenient spot away from the sterile field and in a place where the sterile field will not be crossed as contaminated items are placed into the bag.

5. Put on sterile gloves. The gloves are usually the uppermost item in the sterile pack and are cuffed for putting on by means of the open-gloving technique for sterile gloving.

6. Pick up the first sterile drape. With both hands covered with this drape, place it slightly under the patient's hips extending it to the front of the buttocks to cover the table.

7. Place the second drape, which is a fenestrated drape allowing for only perineal exposure (Fig. 12-3B). This drape may be omitted from the pack. If this is the case, sterile towels should be placed on either side of the perineal area.

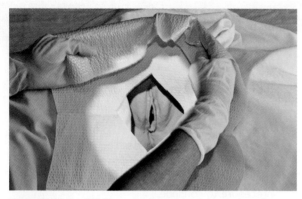

FIGURE 12-3   (B) Place the fenestrated drape over the perineal area.

8. If the catheterization to be done is an indwelling type, the syringe containing sterile water will be attached to the inflation valve at this time. Test the balloon by pushing the plunger down and instilling 2 or 3 mL of solution to be certain that the balloon will not leak (Fig. 12-3C). After determining this, withdraw the water leaving the syringe tip connected to the valve to be used later.

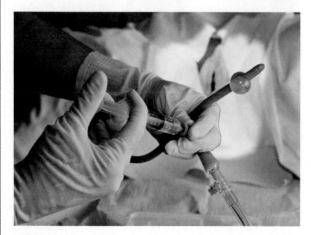

FIGURE 12-3   (C) Test the balloon to assure it will inflate.

9. Open the container of sterile, water-soluble lubricant, and lubricate the catheter tip about ½ inch (1.2 cm) (Fig. 12-3D).

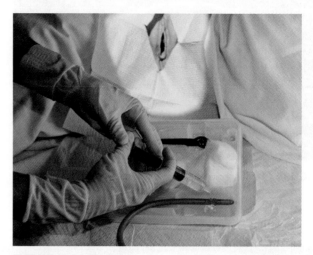

FIGURE 12-3   (D) Lubricate the tip of the catheter.

10. An iodophor solution is usually included in the sterile catheterization set. Open it at this time. If the kit contains solution and cotton balls, pour the solution over all except two of the cotton balls. Keep one or two cotton balls dry to wipe away the excess antiseptic. If the kit contains swabs, tear open the top of the package and set it aside in the upright position.

11. Inform the patient that she is about to have her perineum cleansed with a solution that is slightly cold and wet.

12. With the nondominant hand, separate the labia minora until the urethral meatus is clearly visible (Fig. 12-3E). This glove is now contaminated and will be maintained in this position to allow exposure of the area until the procedure is complete.

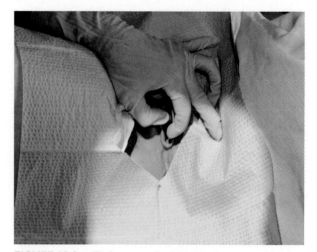

FIGURE 12-3   (E) Separate the labia minora.

(continued)

13. With the forceps, pick up one of the antiseptic-saturated cotton balls. If using swabs, pull one out of the package, leaving the rest in place.

14. Cleanse the distal side of the meatus with a single downward stroke (Fig. 12-3F). Drop the contaminated cotton ball (swab) into the waste receptacle prepared earlier. Be careful not to cross over the sterile field with the contaminated article.

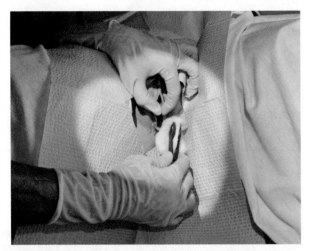

FIGURE 12-3   (F) Cleanse the meatus with a single downward stroke.

15. Pick up a second cotton ball (swab) that is saturated with antiseptic solution and wipe down the proximal side of the labia and meatus. Discard this appropriately. Next, using the third saturated ball (swab), wipe down the center directly over the meatus. Discard this without crossing the sterile field. If there is excess solution, use one of the dry cotton balls or one of the provided dry cotton swabs to make a single downward stroke over the center of the meatus.

16. Inform the patient that the catheter is about to be inserted, and ask her to take a deep breath while the catheter is being inserted.

17. Keep the contaminated, nondominant hand in place, while the dominant hand, which is sterile, picks up the lubricated catheter and inserts it into the urethra (Fig. 12-3G). As the patient exhales, the **sphincter** will relax, allowing the catheter to pass unobstructed into the bladder. If a definite resistance despite slight pressure on the catheter is felt, do not continue with the procedure. When urine begins to flow from the catheter, the catheter has passed through the sphincter and into the bladder. When this occurs, insert the catheter about 1 inch more, and then remove the hand holding the perineum down to the catheter to hold it in place until the bladder is emptied.

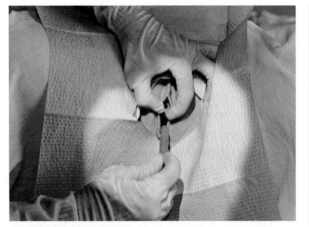

FIGURE 12-3   (G) Insert the lubricated catheter into the urethral meatus..

18. If a straight catheter is being used, place the drainage basin so that it will catch the urine. If a urine specimen is required, allow a small amount of urine to pass through the catheter. Clamp the catheter, remove the drainage basin and replace it with the specimen container. Release the clamp and allow approximately 30 mL of urine to drain into the sterile specimen container. Reclamp the catheter so that the lid of the specimen container can be closed. After removing the specimen, allow the remaining urine to drain into the drainage basin.

19. If an indwelling catheter is being used, a drainage tube may be attached at the distal end of the catheter. The urine will flow into the tubing and into the drainage bag that is attached. Insert the catheter 1 inch more (2.5 cm) before releasing hold of the perineum with the nondominant hand to hold the catheter in place.

20. If the catheter is to be indwelling, pick up the syringe that is attached to the valve and push in the plunger until all of the water in the syringe has been injected into the balloon. It is most often filled with 5 to 10 mL of sterile water (Fig. 12-3H). Pinch the valve portal with the nondominant hand while removing the

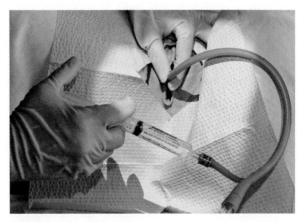

FIGURE 12-3   (H) Instill the water from the syringe into the balloon of the indwelling catheter.

(continued)

syringe from the valve. Most indwelling catheters valves are self-sealing, so when the syringe is removed, the procedure is complete.

21. Gently tug on the indwelling catheter to be certain that it will be retained (Fig. 12-31). If resistance is felt, the balloon is properly inflated and seated against the urethral opening inside the bladder.

22. Remove the soiled equipment and gloves. Allow the patient to return to a comfortable position. The technologist should now wash his/her hands.

23. If the catheter is to remain in place for some time, tape it to the patient's inner thigh to prevent it from becoming dislodged. Make certain that there is no tension placed on the catheter as it is taped. Arrangement for urinary drainage must be made, depending on the procedure that is to follow.

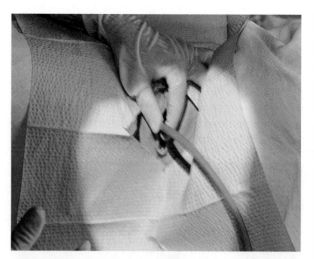

FIGURE 12-3 **(I)** Gently tug on the catheter to seat it in place.

PROCEDURE

Male Catheterization

The equipment needed for catheterizing male patients is similar to that used for female patients; however, because the male urethra is considerably longer than the female's, a slightly larger catheter is usually required. The male urethra is 5.5 to 7 inches (14 to 18 cm) in length; therefore, a 16F to 20F catheter is required. The patient is placed in a supine position with his legs slightly abducted. His torso and legs are covered to the pubis so that exposure is minimal. Make certain that the patient's pubic area is clean. If he is not circumcised, put on clean, disposable gloves, withdraw the foreskin of the penis, and clean the urethral meatus. Remove the gloves on completion and complete a 30-second hand wash. To begin, have good lighting available.

1. Open the sterile pack on a Mayo stand beside the patient or between the patient's thighs if he can be depended on not to contaminate the sterile field.

2. Prepare the pack as in Steps 4 through 10 for female catheterization. Place the first sterile drape over the thigh up to the scrotum and the fenestrated drape over the pubic area, leaving the penis exposed.

3. Pick up the catheter and lubricate it heavily from the tip down about 7 inches, since more lubricant is required to facilitate passage of the catheter for males than for females.

4. Inform the patient about cleaning the penis with an antiseptic solution, then grasp the penis firmly at the shaft with the nondominant hand, retract the foreskin (if applicable) and keep it retracted until the procedure is complete. Slightly spread the urinary meatus between the thumb and forefinger. If the penis is not firmly held, an erection may be stimulated. The hand holding the penis is now contaminated and must remain in position until the procedure is complete.

5. Pick up the forceps and a cotton ball saturated with antiseptic solution (or a swab). Cleanse from the urethral meatus to the glans using a circular motion. Do not go over an area already cleaned. Drop the cotton ball (swab) into the waste receptacle.

6. Repeat this procedure two more times.

7. Inform the patient that the catheter is about to be inserted. Pick up the lubricated catheter with the sterile hand. Ask the patient to bear down as if he were trying to urinate, since the action will relax the sphincter.

8. With the nondominant hand only, extend the penis forward and upward. Stretching the penis into a slight angle will straighten the urethra and make insertion of the catheter into the bladder easier.

(continued)

9. Using gentle, constant pressure, insert the catheter (Fig. 12-4). Too much force may cause a spasm of the sphincter and delay insertion. Do not try to proceed if there is an obstruction; withdraw the catheter and notify the physician.

10. When the urine begins to flow, the catheter is in the bladder; insert the catheter about another ½ inch (1.2 cm).

11. Depending on the type of catheter used for the procedure, follow Steps 16 through 20 as for female catheterization listed previously. Replace the foreskin over the glans.

12. If the indwelling catheter is to be in place for some time, tape it to the lower abdomen using non-allergenic tape, with the penis directed toward the patient's chest. Allow slack so that there is no tension on the catheter. This position minimizes trauma to the urethra by straightening the angle of the **penoscrotal junction.**

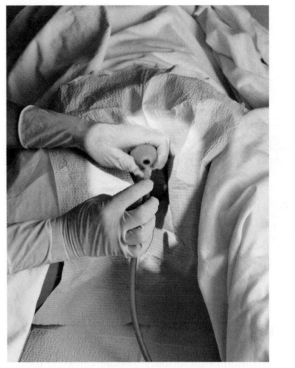

FIGURE 12-4 Using gentle constant pressure, insert the catheter into the penis.

REMOVING AN INDWELLING CATHETER

A physician's order is needed before an indwelling catheter may be removed. Equipment needed to remove a catheter is listed in Table 12-2. Usually, the radiographer is required to remove an indwelling catheter from a patient only after it was inserted in the department for a procedure. There is little, if any, discomfort with this procedure.

1. Uncover the patient just enough to see the insertion point of the catheter. Ask the female patient to separate her legs slightly. Remove any tape that holds the catheter in place. Put on clean disposable gloves and place paper toweling under the catheter.

2. Insert the tip of the syringe into the valve port and pull back on the plunger until all the sterile water from the retention balloon is removed (Fig. 12-5).

3. When the water is completely removed from the balloon, wrap the paper toweling around the catheter and gently withdraw it from the bladder. If any resistance is felt, stop the procedure and try to remove any water that may be remaining in the balloon. If continued resistance is felt while trying to remove the catheter, stop and notify the physician or radiology nurse. The catheter should come out easily.

4. Wrap the catheter in the toweling and place the entire contents into a non-permeable waste bag.

5. If urine output measurement is required, do this after removing the catheter to allow urine to drain from the catheter and tubing into the bag. Record the total amount of urine in the chart.

6. Once all the soiled equipment has been placed into a waste receptacle, remove the gloves and complete a medically aseptic handwash.

7. Return to the patient to assure that he or she is comfortable.

> **⚠ WARNING!**
>
> When removing an indwelling catheter, remember to deflate the balloon.

TABLE 12-2　Equipment Needed for Removal of an Indwelling Catheter

| 10-mL syringe | Paper towels | Nonpermeable disposable bag | Clean disposable gloves | Waste receptacle |

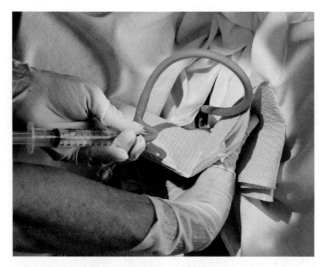

FIGURE 12-5   After removing the water from an indwelling catheter, withdraw the catheter into a paper towel.

PEDIATRIC CATHETERIZATION

Catheterization of the urinary bladder can be emotionally and physically traumatic for the child and his or her family. If there has been a traumatic catheterization attempt previously, the child is almost never willing to fully cooperate in the future. Therefore, it is imperative that only the most experienced radiographer or radiology nurse perform catheterization on pediatric or infant patients. The parents and age-appropriate child must have the procedure fully explained to them in language that is understood. The child should be positioned comfortably with the parents by his or her side or at the end of the table by the head of the child. For female children, a relaxed "frog-leg" position is optimal. A second radiographer may be necessary to help hold the child's legs in this position if the parents are not present.

Sterile technique and nonlatex gloves and catheters should be used. Children require a much smaller size catheter. If the child is less than 5 years of age, a 5F to 8F is usually small enough to be used. Infants may require the use of an infant feeding tube. Children under the age of 3 may be catheterized with a 5F feeding tube for short-term catheterization procedures.

The sterile field may be limited to the immediate perimeatal area. As in the adult patient, once the non-dominant hand touches the patient's skin, that hand must remain in place for the remainder of the procedure.

For female children, only the perimeatal area should be cleansed because the labia might become slippery and difficult to hold apart. The cleaning solution should be rinsed off with sterile saline-soaked cotton balls that have been warmed to body temperature to lessen discomfort.

The urethral meatus must be identified prior to catheterization to avoid unnecessary recatheterization due to contamination. Usually gentle downward pressure on the upper portion of the hymen with a cotton ball will allow visualization of the urethral meatus. If the catheter is inadvertently inserted into the vagina, leave it there as a landmark. Use a second sterile catheter and insert it above the first one.

For the male child, the foreskin should be gently retracted as applicable. However, it should be removed only until the urethral meatus is visualized to avoid damage to the penis. The penis should be gently extended in the horizontal plane with the penis pointed toward the feet. After placing the tip in the urethral meatus, the catheter should be gently and slowly advanced until resistance is felt. This resistance is the external urethral sphincter (EUS) and is an indication that the catheter is about to enter the bladder. It may take up to 1 to 2 minutes for the EUS to relax and allow passage of the catheter.

> ⚠ **WARNING!**
>
> Do not attempt to force a catheter through a closed EUS. The use of a repeated back and forth movement of the catheter can result in urethral injury.

The cuff of an indwelling catheter should not be inflated unless the radiographer is certain that the catheter is in the bladder. Once the catheter is situated, hypoallergenic or paper tape should be used to secure the catheter in place.

In instances where the child is completely unable to cooperate, sedation may be administered. Children who receive sedation should be carefully monitored and discharged only after the effects of the sedation have worn off and discharge criteria have been met.

CATHETER CARE IN THE RADIOGRAPHIC IMAGING DEPARTMENT

Often patients must be transported to the diagnostic imaging department with indwelling catheters in place. If this is the case, the drainage bag must be kept below the level of the urinary bladder. This maintains gravity flow and prevents contamination due to backflow of urine. If urine is allowed to flow back into the bladder or if drainage is obstructed, a urinary tract infection may result (Fig. 12-6). The drainage tubing must be placed over the patient's leg and coiled on the gurney or tabletop, not below the level of the patient's hips. If the drainage bag is to be lifted above the patient during a move, the drainage tubing should be clamped.

If the patient with an indwelling catheter is transported by wheelchair, attach the drainage bag to the underside of the wheelchair. The tubing must be coiled at the level of the patient's hips. Take care not to allow the

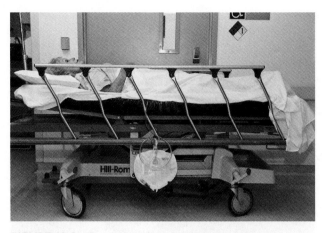

FIGURE 12-6   The drainage bag from an indwelling catheter must be placed below the level of the urinary bladder.

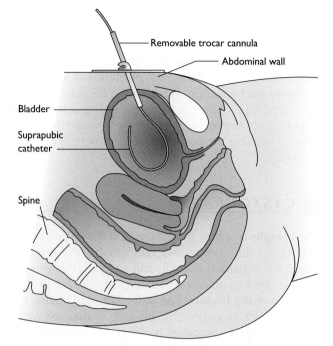

FIGURE 12-7   Suprapubic bladder drainage (From *Brunner & Suddarth's Textbook of Medical-Surgical Nursing,* 11th ed. Philadelphia: Lippincott Williams & Wilkins, 2008).

tubing or drainage bag to become entangled in the wheels of the chair or to touch the floor. Never place a drainage bag on the patient's lap or abdomen during transport because this may cause a **reflux** of urine into the bladder.

Avoid disconnecting the catheter from its closed drainage system. Maintenance of a closed urinary drainage system is essential if infection is to be prevented. Once the closed drainage system has been invaded, it should not be reconnected. The patient must have a new catheter with new closed-system drainage reinserted if catheter drainage of the bladder is to be continued. The radiographer should never take it upon himself or herself to disconnect the catheter from the drainage system; nor should the radiographer empty the drainage bag without a physician's request to do so. If this becomes necessary, a nurse should be consulted to determine if urinary output is being monitored or if the urine is being saved for laboratory testing purposes.

> ## 📢 CALL OUT!
> The radiographer should never disconnect a catheter from the closed drainage system, nor should he or she empty the drainage bag.

Alternative Methods of Urinary Drainage

There are two common methods of dealing with urinary drainage on a temporary or permanent basis, the suprapubic catheter (also called a cystocatheter) and the condom, or Texas, catheter. The *suprapubic catheter* is placed directly into the bladder by means of an abdominal incision. This method is sometimes chosen to divert the flow of urine from the urethral route after gynecologic surgery, urethral injuries, or prostatic obstructions or for chronic **incontinence** or loss of bladder control. Suprapubic catheters are believed to reduce the risk of infection as a long-term method of bladder drainage and to facilitate normal urination after surgical procedures. The catheter is attached to a

closed urinary drainage system and is secured with sutures, tape, or a body seal system (Fig. 12-7).

When caring for the patient with a suprapubic catheter, the radiographer must be careful not to put any tension on the catheter. The same rules of asepsis as for patients with other closed-system urinary drainage, such as keeping the bag below the patient's bladder level at all times, must also be followed.

The *condom catheter* is an externally applied drainage device used for male patients who are susceptible to urinary tract infections or are incontinent or comatose and whose bladder continues to empty spontaneously (Fig. 12-8). If the patient is not prone to urinary tract infections, a Foley indwelling catheter is most likely to be used.

The condom catheter is a soft rubber sheath that is placed over the penis and secured with a special type of adhesive material. The distal end of the condom has an opening that fits onto a drainage tube and

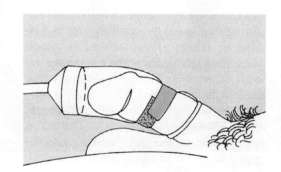

FIGURE 12-8   A condom catheter.

terminates in a drainage bag that attaches to the patient's thigh. The drainage bag can be emptied easily when necessary.

The condom catheter is changed every 24 to 48 hours. This helps to reduce the possibility of acquiring a urinary tract infection. When caring for patients who have condom catheters in place, the radiographer must guard against dislodging the catheter from the drainage tube or twisting the condom and causing pain or skin irritation.

CYSTOGRAPHY

Cystography is radiographic imaging of the urinary bladder. Using fluoroscopy and radiography, the urinary bladder is visualized as it fills and empties. This procedure is done to diagnose pathological changes in the function of the bladder. The pathology may be due to tumors inside or outside the bladder, trauma, or vesicoureteral reflux (abnormal backflow of urine into the ureters). Cystography also demonstrates anatomic changes in the bladder floor, the posterior urethrovesical angle, and the angle of the urethra in female patients when stress is applied to the bladder wall. It also determines cystoureteral reflux due to incompetent ureteral valves.

Cystographic procedures that may be scheduled are cystourethrography (radiography of the urinary bladder and urethra) (Fig. 12-9), voiding cystography (radiography of the patient's ability to empty the urinary bladder) (Fig. 12-10), and voiding cystourethrography (the urethra is studied as the patient voids upon removal of the catheter). The patient may be scheduled for any one or a combination of these procedures.

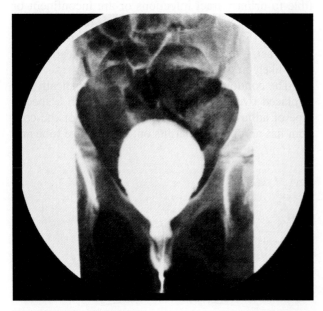

FIGURE 12-9 Cystograph.

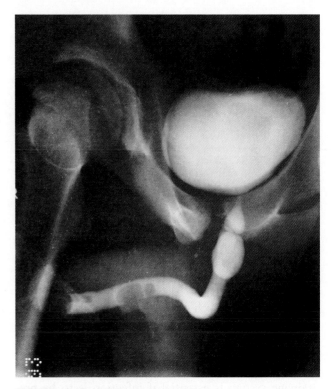

FIGURE 12-10 Voiding cystourethrogram.

Patient Education before Cystography

The patient is usually advised to restrict intake of liquids for several hours before the procedure. This helps to prevent the dilution of the contrast by urine in the patient's bladder. Inform the patient that he or she will be catheterized and an iodinated contrast agent and possible air will be instilled into the bladder. The patient should be prepared to expect some discomfort and a feeling of the need to void. Instruct the patient not to move unless directed to do so during the examination. Assess the patient for allergic reactions to drugs and iodinated contrast agents, as well as for other health problems. However, note that the incidence of anaphylactic reaction to an iodinated contrast medium is not as great in this examination, since the contrast agent is administered into the bladder, not intravenously. Pregnancy is generally a contraindication to having this procedure, and patients with urinary tract infections must have special consideration. It is possible to spread the infection to other pelvic organs in inserting the catheter and instilling a contrast medium. Usually, a signed informed consent is required.

Many times, patients undergoing this procedure are pediatric patients. The parents must be consulted for allergic history and any possible contraindications that may be present. Obtaining the cooperation of children may be facilitated by the presence of at least one parent in the room during the examination. Proper radiation protection procedures must be observed for the parent staying with the child. Gonadal shielding for the patient is not possible since the lead shielding would obscure the bladder. Making the child feel comfortable by dimming the lights may help in allowing the child to void on the radiographic table for cystourethrography.

Patient Care during Cystography

When the patient arrives in the radiography department, instruct him or her to disrobe and put on a patient gown. The patient should also be instructed to urinate before the catheterization to empty the bladder as much as possible. The patient is placed in a supine position, and preliminary (scout) images are taken. The patient is then catheterized with a retention catheter as describe earlier in this chapter. In some institutions, the radiographer will be responsible for the catheterization procedure.

All patients are draped to maintain privacy. To prevent infection, follow strict surgical aseptic technique while the examination is being performed.

The bladder is filled with a contrast agent (200 to 300 mL for an adult; 50 to 100 mL for a child). Air may be used to provide contrast on some occasions. Images are taken of the patient in varying positions. The bladder is drained or the patient is asked to urinate so that his or her ability to empty the bladder in a normal manner can be examined. In other instances, the catheter is removed, and images may be taken as the patient **voids** while on the radiographic table and the contrast agent passes through the urethra. This is called a *voiding cystourethrogram*. This procedure may cause a great deal of stress and embarrassment for the patient. The radiographer must be cognizant of this and preserve the patient's dignity and privacy while it is in progress.

Patient Care following Cystography

After cystography, the patient is told that he or she may resume normal activities as the physician prescribes. Instruct the patient to immediately report any symptoms of chills, fever, excessive blood in the urine, any changes in the ability to urinate, or pain on urination to the referring physician.

Also instruct the patient to increase fluid intake for 24 hours to aid in elimination of contrast agent from the bladder. Inform him or her that some burning may occur on urination and that there may be a small amount of pink-tinged urine for a few hours after the examination.

Cystourethrography may be performed on patients who are paralyzed owing to spinal cord injury or disease. These patients are susceptible to a condition called autonomic dysreflexia. This is a condition in which a stimulus, such as a full rectum or an overdistended bladder, creates an exaggerated response by the sympathetic nervous system. In such cases, the patient may complain of a sudden, severe headache that results from

hypertension. Other symptoms include: sweating and flushing of the face, while other areas of the body may be cold and pale; tachycardia or bradycardia; nasal stuffiness; and a feeling of apprehension.

If a patient with paraplegia or quadriplegia is being cared for and complains of a sudden headache, the following action must be taken:

1. Stop the procedure and notify the physician; prepare to call the emergency team and have the emergency cart at hand.
2. Place the patient in a Fowler's position.
3. Monitor the patient's blood pressure and apical pulse.
4. Remove the source of the stimulus; if the bladder is distended with contrast agent or urine, empty it immediately.
5. Propantheline bromide may be administered to prevent or treat nausea.

Failure to respond to these symptoms may result in myocardial infarction or cerebral hemorrhage.

RETROGRADE PYELOGRAPHY

Retrograde pyelography is a radiographic technique performed to visualize the proximal ureters and the kidneys after injection of an iodinated contrast agent (Fig. 12-11). This procedure is usually performed in a cystoscopy suite, routinely located in the surgery area

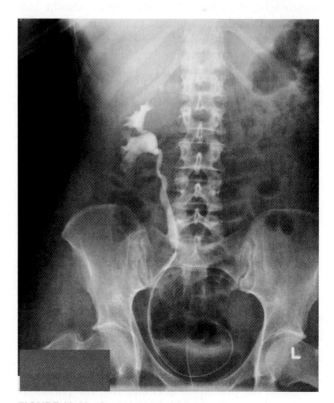

FIGURE 12-11   Retrograde pyelogram.

under the direction of a urologist. The radiographer must be present to take the necessary radiographic images and to provide fluoroscopic examinations of the patient as ordered. Retrograde pyelography is performed to assess the ureters for obstruction resulting from strictures, tumors, stones, scarring, or other pathological processes when other methods are contraindicated. Since this procedure is a filling of the renal collecting system through a catheter, renal function is not studied.

Patient Education and Preparation

To ensure adequate visualization during this procedure, the patient may be instructed to have enemas to clear the bowel just before the procedure is to be performed. The procedure may be performed under a light general anesthesia or under local anesthesia. If general anesthesia is to be given, the patient will be instructed to have no food or fluids by mouth after midnight the night before the procedure. For local anesthesia, the patient may have a liquid breakfast. The patient must be informed that he or she may receive a mild sedative and a drug to reduce the bladder spasm during the procedure. An informed consent must be signed, and the patient must be screened for pregnancy and allergies to drugs and iodinated contrast media. Because of the nature of the procedure, the preparation of the patient is generally the responsibility of the surgery staff, the urologist, and the anesthesiologist; however, the radiographer should still make sure that the radiology request and informed consent are in order.

The Procedure

The patient may be placed in a modified lithotomy position. To prevent impaired circulation, take care to keep pressure off the legs while the patient is in this position. The radiographer is responsible for fluoroscopy and radiographs during this procedure, and a nurse and the physician will monitor the patient.

A contrast medium is injected through a catheter inserted into the ureter (ureteral catheter) from the bladder by means of a **cystoscope**. Retrograde pyelography is normally performed on one side. However, it is possible that both kidneys must be studied. When this is the case, each side is catheterized and examined independently of the other. Images are taken to demonstrate the proximal ureters and the structure of the renal pelvis. The catheter is withdrawn, and more contrast agent is injected to visualize the remaining portion of the ureter. The procedure takes approximately 1 hour.

After the procedure is completed, the patient is instructed to notify the physician if he or she observes

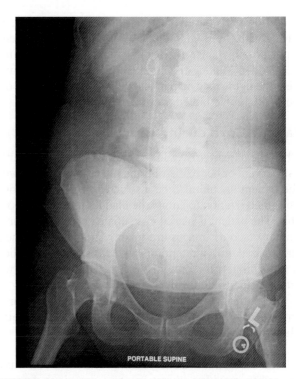

FIGURE 12-12   Ureteral stent. The double pigtail on the patient's right is shaped to resist migration. The proximal end is in the renal pelvis, and the distal curls are in the bladder.

bleeding, fever, chills, or other signs of infection. If the patient has had a general anesthetic, he or she will be observed in a recovery area until awake and alert and the vital signs are stable. The patient may resume a regular schedule as soon as the physician gives permission. Fluids should be increased for 24 hours to aid in elimination of the contrast agent. Again, the after care instruction of the patient is usually the responsibility of the surgery staff.

Ureteral Stents

If the patient has an obstructed ureter due to a stricture, edema, or an advanced malignant tumor, a stent may be inserted into the ureter on a temporary or permanent basis to relieve the problem (Fig. 12-12). Stents are made of soft, pliable silicone and may be placed surgically or during a retrograde pyelogram.

There are complications associated with the presence of any foreign body in the ureter, including stents. Complications are infection and obstruction from encrustation and clot formation. The radiographer is responsible for the radiographic aspects of this procedure, and patient care and instruction will be the responsibility of the physician and the nurse. The patient usually receives a general anesthetic for this procedure and is allowed to recover in the recovery suite.

SUMMARY

All health care workers have the responsibility to practice infection control when inserting catheters into the urinary bladder and caring for patients with catheters in place. The radiographer works with patients who have catheters in place, as well as being responsible for performing the catheterization procedure itself. Surgical aseptic technique must be maintained when performing this procedure, and the appropriate catheter care must be learned to care for patients with a retention catheter.

Catheterization of the urinary bladder is the process of inserting a plastic, rubber, or silicone tube through the urethral meatus into the urinary bladder. There are two types of catheters: the straight catheter and the indwelling catheter. Catheter insertion and removal require a physician's order (in the form of a radiographic examination request).

The same type of equipment is required for catheterization of both female and male patients, although the procedure varies slightly because of anatomic differences. A larger catheter is required for the adult male. Before a catheterization procedure, the patient must be given adequate explanation, reassurance, and privacy to reduce embarrassment and anxiety. Pediatric and infant catheterization must be performed only by the most competent in catheterization. Children are not as cooperative as adults, and once a child has a bad experience with catheterization, it is almost impossible to gain confidence and trust to make a future catheterization an

easy procedure. Children require a small size catheter, and infants may need an infant feeding tube.

Correct care of the indwelling catheter while the patient is being transported to the diagnostic imaging department is necessary for the prevention of urinary tract infection or injury. The drainage bag must remain lower than the level of the urinary bladder to ensure gravity flow of urine. Closed-system drainage of the urinary bladder should not be broken and tension of the catheter must be avoided. The urinary drainage bag should not be emptied unless under specific orders to do so by the physician.

Radiographers are responsible for the radiographic images taken during cystography, retrograde pyelography, and placement of ureteral stents. The radiographers' obligation to maintain infection control and patient safety while these procedures are in progress must be learned.

Alternative methods of urinary drainage are by suprapubic catheter and external condom catheter. Patients who have these types of urinary drainage require precautionary care to prevent urinary tract infections and injury.

Caution should be used when cystourethrograms are performed if the patient is paralyzed. Autonomic dysreflexia, a life-threatening complication, may result from the stimulus of a full urinary bladder. The symptoms of this problem must be learned, and the radiographer must be ready to respond if these symptoms occur.

CHAPTER 12 TEST

1. The most common nosocomial infections are
   a. Bloodborne infections
   b. Respiratory tract infections
   c. Wound infections
   d. Urinary tract infections
2. The best way to prevent urinary tract infections during catheterization of the urinary bladder is
   a. By maintaining strict surgical aseptic technique
   b. By increasing the patient's fluid intake
   c. By requesting that the physician initiate antimicrobial therapy
   d. By keeping the patient isolated
3. How will the radiographer know that the catheter has entered the bladder of the patient?
4. Place the following in the order to be followed if a retention catheter is inserted.
   _____ Drape the patient with the fenestrated drape
   _____ Cleanse the meatus with antiseptic solution
   _____ Put on sterile gloves
   _____ Inflate the balloon on the cuff of the catheter
   _____ Insert the catheter
   _____ Prepare the lubricant
   _____ Tug gently to seat the balloon against the meatus
5. What is the most important consideration when removing a retention catheter?
6. When transporting a patient with a retention catheter and closed-system drainage in place, which of the following must be observed? Circle all that apply.
   a. Empty the drainage bag
   b. Disconnect the drainage bag
   c. Raise the bag quickly above the legs
   d. Lay the bag on the patient's lap
   e. Coil the extra tubing at the level of the patient's hip
   f. Clamp the drainage tube if it must be raised above the hip level

g. Hang the drainage bag alongside the patient below the hip level

7. The radiographer should empty the drainage bag if he or she sees that it is full. True or false?

8. Mr. Sherman Alonzo has been admitted to the surgery suite for retrograde cystography. Mr. Alonzo was paralyzed several years ago in a motocross accident and is recently experiencing some emptying difficulties. While the contrast agent is being instilled and halfway through the study, he begins to complain of a sudden headache and nausea. He begins to move and moan from the pain. From the responses below, place a "B" in front of the best response and a "W" in front of the worst response.

a. _____ Take the patient's vital signs

b. _____ Tell the patient that you need one more image and to hold still

c. _____ Assess the patient for hives and call the nurse

d. _____ Stop the procedure and allow the surgery staff to take over

9. During cystography, what is the radiographer's role? (circle all that apply)

a. Perform vital signs to assess the patient's stability

b. Assure that the radiographic equipment is working

c. Make sure that the informed consent has been signed and is with the radiographic request

d. Assist the fluoroscopy of the patient

e. Provide after care instructions to the patient

10. Which of the following procedures is performed to visualize the proximal ureters and the kidneys but will not demonstrate function?

a. Cystography

b. Cystourethrography

c. Retrograde pyelography

11. List two alternative methods of urinary drainage.

12. Why is the patient instructed to increase fluid intake for 24 hours following any study that involves contrast media in the bladder?

Patient Care during Gastrointestinal Radiographic Procedures

STUDENT LEARNING OUTCOMES

After studying this chapter, the student will be able to:

1. Explain the radiographer's teaching responsibilities before, during, and after radiographic imaging examination of the gastrointestinal (GI) system.

2. Explain the correct order of scheduling radiographic imaging examinations if multiple examinations are ordered.

3. Differentiate between positive and negative contrast agents.

4. List the potential adverse effects of positive and negative contrast agents when they are used in imaging examinations of the GI system.

5. Explain the precautions the radiographer must take during administration of a barium enema in an adult and pediatric patient.

6. Describe the patient care considerations for a patient with an ostomy who is having a barium enema.

7. Demonstrate the correct method of administering a barium enema in the school laboratory.

KEY TERMS

Adverse effects: The development of undesired side effects or toxicity caused by the administration of drugs

Alimentary canal: The organs of digestion; the digestive tract

Colostomy: An artificial opening (stoma) created in the large intestine and brought to the surface of the abdomen for the purpose of evacuating the bowels

Diverticulitis: Inflammation of a sac or pouch protruding from the walls of the intestines, especially the colon

Flatus: Gas expelled from the digestive tract through the anus

Ileostomy: An artificial opening (stoma) erected in the small intestine (ileum) and brought to the surface for the purpose of evacuating feces

Nasogastric tube: A thin tube that is inserted through the nose and into the stomach for the purpose of instilling substances or for the removal of substances

Ostomy: General term for an operation in which an artificial opening is formed

Peritonitis: Inflammation of the serous membrane lining the abdominal cavity and surrounding the abdominal organs

Stoma: An opening in the body created by bringing a loop of bowel to the skin surface

Radiographic imaging procedures of the upper and lower gastrointestinal (GI) system are done in relatively large numbers. While the radiographer may consider some of these procedures as routine duties, the patient receiving them may not consider it as a routine experience. They can be stressful and uncomfortable examinations that may place the patient in physical and emotional jeopardy. This is particularly true for the very young and the very old patient.

Contrast studies that include the use of high-density barium and air are effective methods of detecting conditions of the upper and lower GI system. When imaging of the GI tract using barium is contraindicated, an iodinated contrast agent may be prescribed.

Several methods of imaging the liver, the gallbladder, and the biliary tree are available. These can involve the use of iodinated contrast agents given by the oral or intravenous route. Ultrasound and radionuclide studies are other methods used to visualize particular areas of the GI system. These special methods of imaging are discussed in Chapter 16.

When working with contrast media, the radiographer must know the indications and contraindications for their use, the potential adverse reactions of each, safe method of patient care, and the patient teaching that must accompany their use. Most patients have had no experience with these procedures and the preparation that is required. The radiographer is responsible for educating the patient in these areas. There may be hesitation, and perhaps even revulsion, with the technical aspects of enema administration. Dietary restrictions and medication prescribed before these procedures is not unusual. A matter-of-fact, professional manner when instructing the patient will alleviate patient anxiety.

TYPES OF CONTRAST MEDIA

There are two types of radiographic contrast agents: negative and positive. Negative contrast agents decrease organ density to produce contrast. The most commonly used negative agents are carbon dioxide and air. Positive contrast agents are used to increase organ density and improve radiographic visualization. Positive contrast agents are barium sulfate and iodinated preparations. Contrast agents are discussed in Chapter 15.

Negative Agents

Carbon dioxide and air are the most frequently used negative contrast media. They may be used singly or in combination with a positive contrast medium for studies of the GI system. Complications associated with the use of negative contrast agents can result from inadvertent injection of air into the bloodstream, producing an air embolus. Although the injection of negative contrast agents into the bloodstream during GI procedures is unlikely, it is important to remember the complications associated with this.

Positive Agents

Positive contrast agents create a density difference by attenuating and absorbing the ionizing radiographic beam. This reduces or stops the x-ray beam from hitting the image receptor, thereby creating a white or opaque area on the image. There are two types of positive contrast agents: barium and iodinated contrast. While barium is relatively nontoxic, iodinated contrasts present a greater danger to the patient. The choice of which positive contrast agent to use is generally the decision of the radiologist; however, the radiographer must be familiar with all types of positive contrasts and their use.

Barium Sulfate

Barium sulfate is the most frequently chosen contrast medium for radiologic examination of the GI tract. It is a white, crystalline powder that is mixed with water to make a suspension. It may be administered by mouth for examination of the upper GI tract, by rectum for examination of the lower GI tract, or by infusion of a thin suspension through a duodenal tube to visualize the jejunum and ileum. The use of high-contrast barium solution in the **alimentary canal** reveals organ outlines and demonstrates pathologic conditions of the visceral walls. By using double contrast of barium and air, the ability to detect small lesions is improved.

The toxic effects of barium are negligible if the suspension remains within the GI tract; however, if there is a break in the gastric mucosa caused by injury or disease, the barium sulfate may pass into the peritoneal cavity or into the bloodstream and result in **adverse effects**. If barium leaks into the peritoneal cavity, **peritonitis** may result. This possibility increases if the barium is mixed with fecal material. Fibrosis or formation of a barium granuloma may be a further complication. The possibility of leakage of the barium into the venous circulation through a perforation in the gastric mucosa as a result of trauma or disease must also be considered. This would produce an embolus that might be fatal. When perforation of the GI tract is suspected, an absorbable water-soluble iodinated contrast medium is used in place of barium.

Barium sulfate is often constipating. If the patient is not properly instructed following a procedure that involves its use, he or she may ignore the condition rather than have it treated, and fecal impaction or a bowel obstruction may result.

If the patient reports that a previous administration of oral barium suspension produced a sensation of nausea, the radiologist should be notified before it is administered again, because if the patient vomits, aspiration of barium may result. While barium itself is rarely a cause for nausea, the patient may convince himself or herself that it is the barium that is causing the nausea.

SCHEDULING DIAGNOSTIC IMAGING EXAMINATIONS

Patients often present for medical treatment with vague symptomatology that requires multiple imaging and direct-view examinations before an accurate diagnosis can be made. During the medical diagnostic process, one patient may have a series of examinations, some of which are performed in the radiographic imaging department and some elsewhere.

If the radiographer is responsible for scheduling radiographic imaging examinations, inquiries regarding other examinations that the patient may be expected to undergo must be made. Critical thinking and thoughtful planning are required to facilitate the patient's speedy diagnosis.

1. Procedures that require fasting must be done in the morning. This is especially important when scheduling diabetic, elderly, or pediatric patients.
2. All radiographic examinations or procedures that do not require contrast media should be scheduled first.
3. Ultrasonography and nuclear medicine procedures must be scheduled prior to contrast studies so that the contrast will not interfere with these examinations.
4. Iodinated contrast studies must be performed prior to barium studies, as the barium is denser and will obscure the iodinated contrast.
5. When a patient is scheduled for both upper and lower GI systems with barium, the lower GI series should be scheduled first, as barium clears quickly from the lower bowel.

PATIENT PREPARATION FOR STUDIES OF THE LOWER GI TRACT

Correct preparation of the patient for barium studies of the lower GI tract is essential and may seem relatively complex to the patient. This preparation varies across health care facilities and with each patient's special needs. The radiographer's responsibility is to learn the specific procedure in his or her place of employment. If the patient is an outpatient, the radiographer may be responsible for giving the patient the appointment for the examination and the instruction for its preparation.

The following directions generally apply at most institutions, with modifications for particular patients.

Pediatric and infant patient preparation is much less complex than for the adult patient. From the age of newborn to 2 years, usually no preparation is necessary. Up to the age of 10 years, the child should be on a low residue meal the evening before.

If the appointment is made far enough in advance, the adult patient is instructed to eat foods low in residue for 2 to 3 days prior to the procedure. A low-residue diet excludes tough meats; raw, cooked, and dried fruits; raw vegetables; juices containing the pulp of fruits or vegetables; whole-grain breads and cereals, especially bran and cracked wheat types; nuts, peanut butter, and coconut; olives, pickles, seeds, and popcorn; and dried peas and beans. The patient should take no more than two cups of milk each day and avoid strong cheeses. The patient should be encouraged to increase fluid intake (water) for 2 to 3 days before the examination to assist in clearing the lower bowel of waste.

Twenty-four hours before the examination, a clear liquid diet is usually prescribed for all 3 meals. A clear liquid diet may include coffee or tea with sugar but no milk, clear gelatin, clear broth, and carbonated beverages. The patient should be instructed to drink five 8-ounce glasses of water or clear liquids during these 24 hours.

The afternoon preceding the examination, 10 ounces of magnesium citrate or its equivalent is prescribed. The evening before the examination, another laxative may be ordered. Laxatives must never be given to a patient without the physician's order. They can be harmful to persons with bowel obstructions and other pathologic conditions of the GI tract.

Patients with insulin-dependent diabetes mellitus and non-insulin-dependent diabetes mellitus require special pre-examination orders and instruction. The radiographer must ascertain the patient's medical status before giving instruction in preparation for any GI series. Patients with diabetes mellitus must also be instructed concerning administration of morning insulin or other antidiabetic medications. Usually these medications are postponed until the examination is complete and the patient is able to eat.

Cleansing enemas are generally prescribed the night before or early in the morning of the examination. Since there are several types and variations of cleansing enemas, the radiographer must become familiar with all of them and must be able to administer one of them, if necessary. Occasionally, a patient comes to the radiographic imaging department poorly prepared for a radiographic study of the lower bowel, and the radiographer has to complete the preparation in the department by administering an additional cleansing enema. By learning the procedure, the radiographer is able to give clear, concise directions to the patient who needs instruction.

Cleansing Enemas

The type of cleansing enema to be used is always ordered by the physician. The most frequently used cleansing enemas include the saline enema, the hypertonic enema, the oil-retention enema, the tap water enema, and the soapsuds (SS) enema.

Cleansing enemas can influence fluid and electrolyte balance in the body to varying degrees because they each have a different degree of osmolarity, which influences the movement of fluids between the colon and the interstitial spaces beyond the intestinal wall. This means that, in the presence of some cleansing solutions that are instilled into the lower bowel, the bowel extracts fluid from the surrounding interstitial spaces. This happens because the higher osmolarity of the cleansing solution (hyperosmolar) induces the fluid to move across the semi-permeable membranes of the intestinal wall. The body fluid that has moved into the large intestine is then excreted from the body along with the enema solution. Dehydration occurs if an excess of body fluid is excreted. This situation can be reversed.

Another situation occurs when an excess of fluid with low osmolarity (hypo-osmolar) may be instilled into the lower bowel and absorbed into the interstitial spaces surrounding the colon, thus creating fluid excess in the body. This is called fluid toxicity. These potential hazards must be considered when the physician orders a particular solution for use as a cleansing enema.

> ### ⚠ WARNING!
>
> Hyperosmolar fluids can create dehydration.
> Hypo-osmolar fluids can create fluid toxicity.

Saline Enemas

There are two types of saline enemas: normal saline and hypertonic saline. Normal saline is the safest solution to use for a cleansing enema because it has the same osmolarity as that in the interstitial spaces that surround the colon; therefore, it will not change the fluid balance in the body. It is the only safe fluid to use for cleansing enemas for infants and children because they can tolerate very little change in fluid and electrolyte balance. This solution is also used for elderly patients for the same reason.

Hypertonic saline solution can be administered quickly and easily and is effective for relieving constipation or for eliminating barium sulfate residue after a barium study. Hypertonic solutions pull fluid from the interstitial spaces around the sigmoid colon and fill the bowel with fluid, thereby initiating peristalsis. Only a small amount of solution is required to do this (120 to 180 mL). Hypertonic saline enemas are often available under the name Fleet enema. Hypertonic enemas should not be administered to dehydrated patients or to infants and children.

Oil-Retention Enemas

The oil-retention enema is given for relief of chronic constipation or fecal impaction. It may also be used to eliminate any barium sulfate remaining after a GI series. A small amount of mineral oil or olive oil (120 to 140 mL) is instilled into the rectum and the patient is requested to retain the oil for as long a time as possible, preferably up to 1 hour, and then expel it. The oil lubricates the rectum and colon and softens the fecal material, thereby making it easier to expel.

Tap Water Enemas

Tap water may be used to cleanse the bowel preceding diagnostic imaging procedures; however, the radiographer must remember that there is a potential for fluid toxicity if this is used. The procedure for administration is the same as the soapsuds enema, which is described in the following section.

Soapsuds (SS) Enemas

Soap may be added to tap water or to normal saline to increase the irritation of the intestine, thereby promoting peristalsis and defecation. The only soap safe to use for this purpose is a pure castile soap. Detergents and strong soaps may result in intestinal inflammation.

The Self-Administered Cleansing Enema

If a patient is coming from home to the radiographic imaging department for a barium study of the lower bowel, he or she must be taught to self-administer an enema effectively. The radiographer must be able to assume this teaching responsibility. Instruct the patient to purchase an enema kit when going to the pharmacy for the laxative medication. The enema prescribed is usually a cleansing enema; the adult patient is required to add 1000 mL water and 20 mL liquid soap. Carefully explain to the patient which type of enema set is needed because there are many to choose from. The patient should know that, even if the laxative has the desired effect, he or she will not be adequately prepared if the enema is not taken as instructed.

LOWER GI TRACT STUDIES

Studies performed to diagnose pathological conditions of the lower GI tract use a combination of barium and

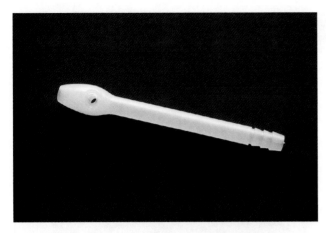

FIGURE 13-1 Plain tip for a barium enema.

air or carbon dioxide (double contrast) or barium alone (single contrast). If there is an indication that the patient has a disease entity or injury that would result in a perforation or tear of the lower GI tract, use a water-soluble iodinated contrast agent rather than barium. This is done to protect against barium peritonitis, a condition that results from barium leakage into the peritoneal cavity.

Much larger tubing is required than is used for a cleansing enema to allow the viscous suspension to be instilled into the lower bowel. The tubing may have a plain tip (Fig. 13-1), a tip with an inflatable cuff attached, or a tip that is used for double-contrast studies. This type of tip has two lumens—one for the inflatable cuff and one for instillation of air into the patient's bowel (Fig. 13-2). If the physician selects a tip with an inflatable cuff, the cuff is inflated after the tip is inserted in the rectum. This holds the enema tip in place and prevents involuntary expulsion of barium. Never inflate the cuff until it is positioned beyond the anal sphincter.

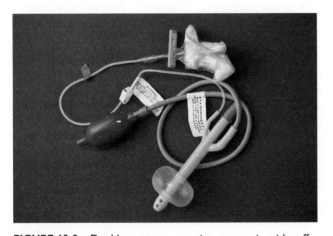

FIGURE 13-2 Double-contrast retention enema tip with cuff inflated.

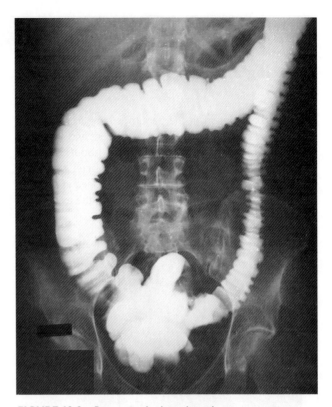

FIGURE 13-3 Barium in the large bowel.

Barium is available in a prepared, prepackaged form. Barium comes as either a liquid suspension or as a powder, which must be mixed with water immediately before the procedure. When adding water to the suspension, remember that the consistency should be dense so that x-rays are absorbed (Fig. 13-3). After it is mixed with water, barium should remain in suspension for some time before resettling; it should also be able to flow freely. Foam is undesirable in the mixture because, if present, the barium suspension will not coat the mucosal walls evenly, which is necessary for diagnostic purposes.

The amount of barium needed for a single-contrast study of an adult is generally 1500 mL, although it may vary. The amount used for infants or children is much less and depends on their age and size. The correct amount is instilled in the patient by the radiologist in charge of the procedure. A normal saline solution may be mixed with the barium instead of water to prevent electrolyte imbalance if the patient is an infant, a child, or a frail elderly person. The barium solution is passed through the tubing in the same manner as the solution for a cleansing enema to displace the air in the tubing before insertion of the tip. Premixed preparations of barium should be remixed so that the suspension is uniform, and they should be administered at room temperature.

Placing an Enema Tip

The bag containing the barium is hung from a metal standard. A clamp on the tubing opens and closes the tubing easily (Fig. 13-4). Place the bag about 30 inches higher than the table. The tip is usually placed in the rectum prior to the radiologist being summoned in order to allow the radiologist to immediately begin the exam upon entering the room.

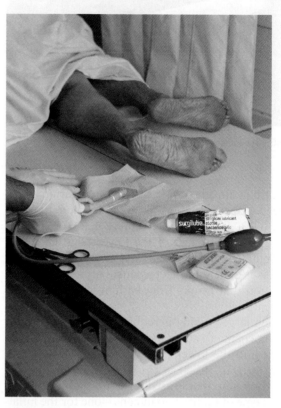

FIGURE 13-5   Be sure the enema tip is well lubricated.

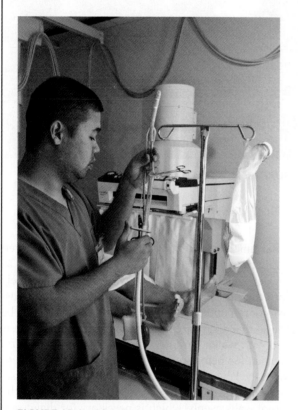

FIGURE 13-4   After hanging the enema bag, clear the tubing of air by releasing the lower clamp.

The procedure for the placing the enema tip in an adult is as follows:

1. Place the patient in the Sims position and drape him or her to provide privacy yet expose the anal area.

2. Put on clean gloves and heavily lubricate the enema tip (Fig. 13-5).

3. Instruct the patient to exhale slowly as the tip is inserted 3 to 4 inches or until it passes the anal sphincter. Do not use force to insert the tip because of the potential for laceration of the mucous membranes. If

the tip cannot be easily inserted, the radiologist may have to perform this under fluoroscopy.

4. Once the tip is in place, return the patient to the supine position.

When a retention-type tip with an inflatable cuff is used to administer barium, the cuff is inflated with a hand inflation pump. The cuff must be inserted beyond the rectal sphincter before it is inflated. Inflation of the cuff may tear the patient's rectal tissues if it is not properly placed. Initially, inflate the cuff with no more than 10 mL of air for an adult patient. If more air is desired, the radiologist may add more under fluoroscopy.

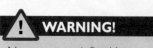

WARNING!

Never use an inflatable enema tip in an infant or child who is undergoing a barium enema.

(continued)

Occasionally, a patient has an allergy to items made of latex (including barium enema tips with inflatable cuffs). Asking the patient if he or she is allergic to latex and assuring that the barium enema tip being used does not contain latex will prevent an allergic reaction from occurring. Most inflatable cuff enema tips are now manufactured without the use of latex.

Pediatric patients undergoing a barium enema require special consideration. The barium mixture may need to be more diluted than for an adult. Certainly the amount of barium that will be required to perform the procedure will be less. Do not use an inflatable cuff for an infant or a child. There are a variety of commercially available pediatric enema tips that can be used. For infants a 10F catheter is used or even a 12 Foley urinary catheter. Never inflate the balloon on a catheter in the rectum of an infant. Sometimes, the barium enema will be performed in a therapeutic manner rather than as a diagnostic procedure. As illustrated in Figure 13-6, intussusception is a situation in which the bowel telescopes into itself. If this is the case, barium may be forced under pressure into the bowel to try to push the telescoped section back down into place.

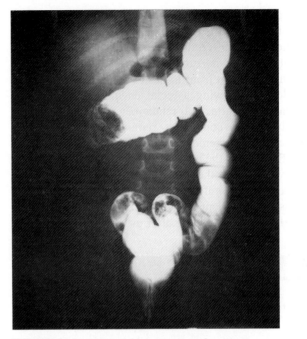

FIGURE 13-6 Pediatric barium enema showing intussusception on the ascending colon.

PATIENT CARE CONSIDERATIONS DURING LOWER GI TRACT STUDIES

Remember that patients are extremely uncomfortable during this type of procedure and usually highly anxious. They are forfeiting their dignity and comfort to discover the cause of their illness. The radiographer must be aware of this and do what is necessary to alleviate the patient's discomfort and anxiety.

Some patients may not feel that they are able to hold the enema in due to spasms and abdominal cramping. Instruct the patient to alert the radiologist of cramps so that the flow of barium may be turned off to allow the spasm to subside. An anticholinergic drug or glucagon is often prescribed and administered intravenously before or during the examination to reduce gastric motility, which may help decrease the cramping. If the patient is an insulin-dependent diabetic, glucagon is contraindicated. If the patient receives an anticholinergic drug or glucagon, observe him or her for adverse reactions through the examination and for 30 minutes after the examination. Possible adverse reactions from glucagon include nausea, vomiting, hives, and flushing. Possible adverse reactions from anticholinergic drugs include dry mouth, thirst, tachycardia, urinary retention, and blurred vision. If the patient is to receive these medications, he or she should have another person available to drive him or her home.

CALL OUT!

Determine if the patient is an insulin-dependent diabetic prior to giving glucagon.

Inform the patient that he or she will be moved into several positions to afford maximum visualization while the examination is in progress. Explain that the radiologist will be giving instructions that the patient may mistakenly think are being addressed to him or her. Tell a patient that commands such as "open" or "close" are not intended for them. Also inform the patient that the urge to defecate will be relieved as soon as the procedure is over and he or she is taken to the lavatory.

Air is often placed into the bowel during this examination. When a double-contrast study is to be performed, the radiologist will limit the amount of barium that is instilled into the patient. The barium is then turned off, and air is instilled into the patient's bowel through a second lumen of the enema tip. The instillation of air provides for high contrast between the air and the barium and is an excellent method in diagnosing polyps and diverticula of the bowel.

The patient will be extremely uncomfortable during this study. Remind the patient that cramping and the urge to defecate are both normal sensations. By staying close to reassure the patient, the radiographer is able to facilitate a smoother procedure.

The patient is often requested to move about on the table during the examination, and the table may be positioned at different angles. Assist the patient by keeping the enema tubing from being tangled as the patient rolls from front to back or side to side.

Before removing a rectal enema tip that has an inflatable cuff attached, remember to deflate the cuff. The barium is sometimes removed by gravity flow before the tip is removed. Place the barium bag lower than the level of the patient's hips and allow the barium to flow back into the bag. The air is then permitted to escape from the cuff. After this, gently remove the tip and assist the patient to the lavatory. Instruct the patient what he or she should do after evacuating the bowels.

> ⚠️ **WARNING!**
>
> Remember to deflate the retention cuff before removing the enema tip.

Patient Care Instructions after Studies of the Lower GI Tract

A patient must never be dismissed from the radiographic imaging department after a procedure without instruction in post-examination care. This is particularly true for the patient who has received barium because, without adequate care, the barium may be retained, which can cause fecal impaction or intestinal obstruction. The patient may also suffer from extreme dehydration as a result of preparation for the study.

Explain to the patient that his or her stools will be white or very light colored until all the barium is expelled. Some physicians regularly prescribe a laxative medication or an enema following barium studies. If the physician in charge of the patient does not do this, tell the patient that if he has not had a bowel movement within 24 hours after the procedure, he or she should contact the physician. Stress the importance of eliminating the barium.

It is also extremely important for the patient to increase fluid intake and fiber in the diet for several days if this is not medically contraindicated. The patient should be instructed to rest after the examination. If the patient feels weak or faint; has abdominal pain, constipation, or rectal bleeding; is not passing **flatus;** or has polyuria, nocturia, or abdominal distention, the patient must contact his or her physician.

> 📢 **CALL OUT!**
>
> Constipation is a common side effect of barium enemas. Instruct the patient to increase fluid intake to prevent this.

THE PATIENT WITH AN INTESTINAL STOMA

Several conditions of the lower GI tract require the creation of a **stoma** through which the contents of the bowel can be eliminated. A stoma is created by bringing a loop of bowel to the skin surface of the abdomen. Some diseases that are treated in this manner are cancer, **diverticulitis,** and ulcerative colitis. Traumatic injuries of the bowel may also require this type of treatment.

The surgical procedure to repair the bowel and create the **ostomy** is named by the area of bowel on which the operation is done. For instance, if the opening is from the colon, it is called a **colostomy;** if it is from the ileum, it is known as an **ileostomy** (Fig. 13-7). The stoma may be temporary, performed to rest and heal a diseased portion of the bowel; or, it may be permanent, done to remove a diseased or traumatized portion of the bowel.

The stoma may have either one or two openings, depending on the type of surgery that was performed. When two openings are surgically created, one opening is located toward the rectum and the other toward the small bowel. One opening, called the proximal stoma, emits fecal material. The other opening, the distal stoma, is relatively nonfunctioning and emits only mucus. Some stoma patients (also called ostomy patients) have had their rectum and lower bowel removed; others have not. A patient who has an ostomy may require barium studies for further diagnosis or further study of the progression of the disease.

Ostomy causes a major change in a patient's body image and many persons with a new colostomy or ileostomy stoma are going through a grieving process. This is particularly true of younger patients. They may be angry, depressed, in a stage of denial, or just beginning to accept the fact that they must learn to live with this physical change.

Caring for the patient with a new ostomy requires sensitivity and a matter-of-fact attitude. It is suggested that the radiography student who has never seen an ostomy should observe the diagnostic studies being performed for these patients until he or she can care for them easily.

The ostomy patient will have a dressing or drainage pouch in place over the area of the stoma (Fig. 13-8). The dressing is removed while wearing clean gloves. The procedure for dressing change is discussed in Chapter 5. Remove the drainage pouch, and put it aside in a safe place to be reused. The patient may want to do this him or herself. The pouch must be kept dry in order for it to be reused.

A patient who has a colostomy or ileostomy and is going to have a barium study of the lower GI tract

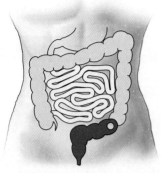
Sigmoid Colostomy

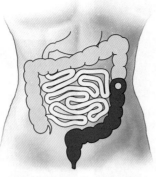
Descending Colostomy

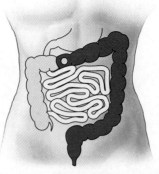
Transverse (Single B) Colostomy

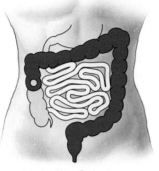
Ascending Colostomy

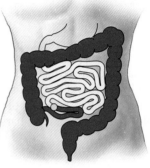
Ileostomy

FIGURE 13-7   Locations of various colostomies and the location of an ileostomy.

needs special instructions to be adequately prepared. If the hospital has an enterostomal therapist, the patient may have been instructed through this person. If not, the radiologist and the patient's physician should give the instruction before and after the procedure. All ostomy patients should be instructed to bring an extra pouch with them if they are coming from outside the hospital. Dietary, laxative, and cleansing preparations vary depending on the type and location of the ostomy.

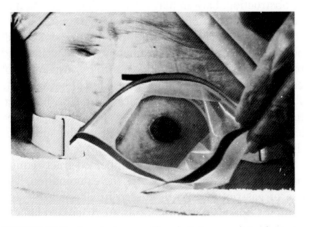

FIGURE 13-8   A colostomy with a drainage pouch in place.

Administering a Barium Enema to an Ostomy Patient

Ostomy patients have barium studies for diagnostic purposes, and the procedure is somewhat different from that performed on a person with normally functioning bowels. The radiographer must plan the procedure with the radiologist before beginning in order to ensure the patient's comfort and safety. A cone-shaped tip with a long drainage bag that attaches to it after the procedure is frequently the instillation instrument of choice (Fig. 13-9A and B). Occasionally, a small catheter with an inflatable cuff is used. Other ostomy tips may be used, depending on the patient's situation and the preference of the physician. Examples are the nipple tip and the double-barrel tip. The patient who has had the ostomy for some time may prefer to insert the tip him- or herself.

After lubricating the tip of the cone, hand it to the patient for insertion. Be aware that some radiologists prefer to insert the tip and tape it in place. After the cone has been inserted, the procedure is the same as for other patients. The patient may be placed in various positions; however, do not place the patient in a prone position because this may cause injury at the stoma site. Don't begin to instill the barium until the physician who is conducting the examination is present to supervise

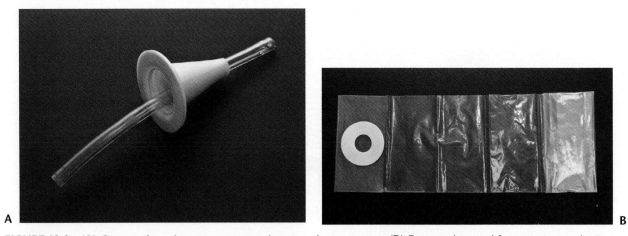

A   B

FIGURE 13-9   (A) Cone tip for colostomy patients undergoing a barium enema. (B) Drainage bag used for emptying out barium from a stoma after a barium enema procedure.

the procedure. If the patient's rectum and lower bowel are present, barium may be instilled into the ostomy and also into the lower bowel through the rectum. Because these patients have lost portions of their intestines, a considerably smaller amount of barium suspension is needed.

 WARNING!

Never place a stoma patient in the prone position as this may cause damage to the patient's ostomy site.

When the examination is complete, attach the drainage bag to the cone and drain the barium into it. When the drainage is complete, the patient whose physical condition permits may be taken to the lavatory with the drainage bag sill in place; there the drainage bag may be cleaned and the ostomy pouch replaced. Give the patient as much assistance as needed and offer towels, washcloths, and any other articles he or she may need. Allow the patient privacy if he or she is able to be independent in his or her care.

STUDIES OF THE UPPER GI TRACT AND SMALL BOWEL

Barium examinations of the upper GI tract and small intestine are called an upper GI series and small bowel follow through (SBFT), respectively. They are performed to diagnose pathological conditions of the pharynx, esophagus, stomach, duodenum, and small intestine. The patient is usually instructed to remain on a low-residue diet for 2 to 3 days before the examination and to go on a food fast for 8 hours before the examination.

The patient must be instructed not to smoke or chew gum before the examination because this increases gastric secretions, which may cause dilution of the contrast agent. In most instances, medications that the patient routinely takes are restricted for 8 hours before the examination. Enemas are usually not required. The patient must be informed that the examination may take several hours when having a SBFT study; he or she should be encouraged to bring reading material to pass the time.

Adverse reactions from glucagon may be nausea, vomiting, hives, and flushing. Adverse reactions from anticholinergic drugs may be dry mouth, thirst, tachycardia, urinary retention, and blurred vision. If the patient is to receive these medications, another person should be available to drive the patient home. Adverse reactions to barium are not common.

The physician will order a water-soluble iodinated contrast agent if the patient has a possible pathological perforation or obstruction of the upper GI tract and if barium is contraindicated. In the event of a perforation or obstruction, barium may intensify the obstruction or pass into the abdominal cavity.

The patient should be informed that he or she will be expected to drink approximately 12 oz of flavored barium. For some examinations, a thick suspension of barium is followed by a thin suspension of barium. The solution does not have an unpleasant flavor; however, the chalkiness may be difficult to tolerate. It may be less distasteful for the patient to drink the substance through a straw.

Some examinations of the upper GI tract require passage of a gastric tube before the examination. The use of gastric tubes is discussed in Chapter 14, and complex upper GI examinations are discussed later in this text.

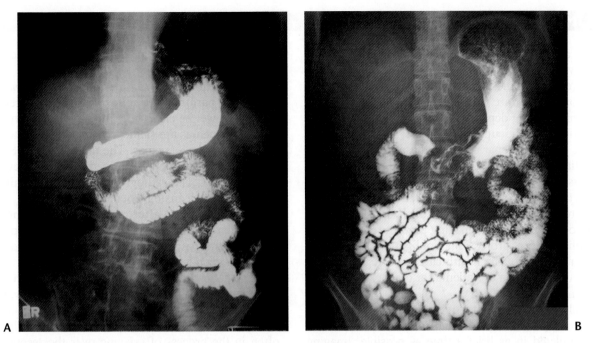

FIGURE 13-10   (**A**) A stomach filled with barium. (**B**) Barium filled stomach and small bowel.

After the barium is swallowed and passes through the digestive tract, fluoroscopic examination outlines peristalsis and the contours of the upper GI tract (Fig. 13-10A). Spot films are taken as directed by the radiologist. Double contrast with air is often used; when this is done, the patient should be informed of this and warned that he or she will have a feeling of fullness. It is important that the patient be told not to burp or allow the gas from the stomach to come out. As in the lower GI examination, the air provides contrast with the barium to outline the stomach for better visualization of the mucosal lining.

The patient must also be informed that during the examination, he or she will be positioned in upright, supine, and side-lying position while the passage of barium is viewed fluoroscopically. If the passage of barium is delayed or if a SBFT examination is also ordered (Fig. 13-10B), the examination will take much longer, with intervals during which the patient simply waits, lying on the table. Occasionally, changing the patient's position or allowing the patient to move about may assist the contrast agent to pass through the upper GI tract.

Infants and children require minimal preparation for upper GI procedures. Nothing to eat or drink is the main requirement with the length of time being determined by the age of the patient. Babies need only be NPO for about 3 to 4 hours prior to an exam-ination, while the 1-year-old child should not have anything to eat for 4 to 6 hours. The older the child, the longer it takes his or her stomach to empty. Hungry babies will drink from a bottle of barium despite the taste. It may be a challenge to get an older child to drink the "special milkshake." Allowing the child to sip from a straw may make it more attractive for them. Some children who have already developed a dislike for certain foods may present more of a challenge to the radiographer. Finding creative ways to introduce the barium will alleviate the need to use a **nasogastric tube**.

Instructions after Barium Studies of the Upper GI Tract

If there are no contraindications, the patient must receive instructions to increase fluid and fiber intake for several days after the upper GI series using barium. He or she may resume eating immediately after the examination unless another examination is to follow. Also inform the patient that the stools will be light in color and that, if no bowel movement occurs within 24 hours, he or she must notify the requesting physician, who may wish to prescribe a laxative. The patient must be instructed not to allow constipation, because fecal impaction or bowel obstruction may result. If rectal or gastric bleeding occurs, the patient must seek medical treatment immediately.

SUMMARY

There are two types of contrast agents: positive and negative. The most commonly used contrasts are the positive type. Studies using barium and barium in combination with air are frequently conducted in the radiographic imaging department to diagnose pathological conditions of the upper and lower gastrointestinal tracts. Correct preparation for these examinations is essential for a successful outcome. The radiographer's professional responsibility is to teach the patient the correct methods of preparing for barium studies and the care and precautions that he or she must take after these or any diagnostic imaging procedures. The radiographer has a professional obligation to instruct other members of the health care team regarding the correct preparation of patients for diagnostic imaging examinations.

Scheduling for a series of diagnostic imaging examinations requires careful planning so that the studies can be completed in as brief a time as possible. Imaging examinations must also be scheduled so that they will not conflict with other diagnostic procedures that may be prescribed. Knowledge concerning which diagnostic imaging examinations will interfere with other tests will expedite the process for the patient by allowing the schedule to move forward smoothly. The very young, the elderly, and the patient with diabetes mellitus must be scheduled to accommodate their dietary restrictions and frailties.

Preparation for examinations of the lower GI tract using barium as a contrast agent usually requires that the bowel be cleansed with enemas. The types of cleansing enemas are saline, hypertonic, oil-retention, tap water, and SS enemas. The tap water and SS enemas are the most often prescribed to precede lower GI examinations. The radiographer may be required to perform the cleansing enema if the patient is not properly prepared after arriving in the imaging department. Proper care must be taken to prevent injury to the patient during the administration of a cleansing enema.

The patient with an ostomy may also require a barium enema. The procedure and the tip used vary for these patients. The radiographer must be sensitive in his or her care of ostomy patients because they are often in the process of grieving over the recent alteration in body image. Recent ostomy patients must be related to in a therapeutic manner.

Barium studies of the upper GI tract are frequently done to diagnose pathological conditions of the pharynx, esophagus, stomach, duodenum, and jejunum. The preparation before and after these studies varies somewhat from that of the lower GI series.

CHAPTER 13 TEST

1. Before removing the retention-style enema tip, what is the most important thing to remember?
2. Barium is a relatively nontoxic contrast agent.
   a. True
   b. False
3. Mr. and Mrs. Ob Noxious bring their 3-year-son into the department for an upper GI examination. They have been concerned because he has been spitting out all of his food saying that he is not hungry. They suspect that he has a tumor in his stomach. The child immediately begins screaming that he will not drink any of "that stuff." What is your best response in this situation?
   a. Ask the parents to wait outside while you do the examination
   b. Try to calm the child down
   c. Tell the family to leave and return when the child is under control
   d. Ask for sedation for the child
4. What would be the worst response in the above scenario?

5. A double-contrast study of the gastrointestinal tract includes which of the following. Circle all that apply.
   a. Use of room air
   b. Use of barium
   c. Use of nitrogen
   d. Use of carbon dioxide
   e. Use of a water-soluble contrast agent
6. If the patient has the large bowel removed at the sigmoid area and the opening is made on the anterior surface of the abdomen, the patient is said to have a:
   a. Colostomy
   b. Ileostomy
   c. Sigmoidostomy
   d. Colonostomy
7. After a barium study, the patient must receive the following after-care instructions. Circle all that apply.
   a. Increase fluid intake for the next 24-48 hours
   b. Call the physician if no bowel movement has occurred within the next hour

c. Expect to see light-colored stools for a few days
d. If constipation seems to be a problem, take a laxative
e. Increase fiber intake for 24-48 hours
f. Call the physician if blood is noticed in the stool

8. Place the following examinations in order for scheduling. Use the same number for those that can be scheduled together as one examination.
   a. _____ Upper GI
   b. _____ Esophagram
   c. _____ Barium enema
   d. _____ Abdominal radiographs
   e. _____ Small bowel follow through

9. What is the preparation for an infant who is scheduled to have an upper GI done?

10. Robbie Overnight, a 73-year-old male sheduled for a barium enema, comes into the department and is obviously concerned about the study. He says, "My friend told me that the barium will turn hard in my bowel and have to be removed. Is that true?" Place a "B" in front of the best response and a "W" in front of the worst response.
    a. _____ "Yes."
    b. _____ "That is a possibility, but we are going to take every precaution to not allow that to happen."
    c. _____ "Did your doctor tell you anything about this examination?"
    d. _____ "After the examination, I will tell you how to get rid of the barium."
    e. _____ "I see that you have some concerns. Let me explain to you now what will happen after the exam is over so that you will feel comfortable during the procedure."

11. Why is air used in the performance of barium studies of the gastrointestinal tract?

12. Mr. Albert Barium has questions regarding his upcoming lower GI study. From the following list of items, circle all the responses that would be correct to tell him.
    a. Oh, don't worry, the barium won't kill you.
    b. You should drink lots of water after the study is over.
    c. The barium should be eliminated from your system within 24 to 48 hours.
    d. After the examination, your doctor will phone you with the results.
    e. We will make sure that you are the first person we put on the table!

Caring for Patients Needing Alternative Medical Treatments

STUDENT LEARNING OUTCOMES

After studying this chapter, the student will be able to:

1. Explain the reasons for nasogastric and nasoenteric intubation and the radiographer's responsibilities when these tubes are in place.

2. Describe the precautions needed when caring for a patient who has a gastrostomy tube in place.

3. Describe the patient care considerations when working with a patient who requires parenteral nutrition or has a central venous catheter.

4. Describe the symptoms of a patient who needs suctioning, and explain the action the radiographer would take in this situation.

5. Explain the precautions necessary when working with a patient who has a tracheostomy.

6. List the precautions that are required when working with a patient requiring mechanical ventilation.

7. List the patient care precautions taken for the patient who has a chest tube in place with water-sealed drainage.

8. Describe the patient care considerations for the patient who has a tissue drain in place.

KEY TERMS

Asphyxiation: Severe hypoxia leading to hypoxemia, hypercapnea, loss of consciousness, and death

Bolus: A concentrated mass of a pharmaceutical preparation, such as an opaque contrast medium given intravenously or swallowed

Cannula: A tube used to allow fluids, gases, or other substances into or out of the body

Dyspneic: Having shortness of breath or difficulty breathing

Fowler position: Position in which the head of the patient's bed is raised 18 to 20 inches above the level of the heart with the knees also elevated

Gastrostomy: Creation of an opening in the stomach to provide food and liquid administration

Hemostat: A clamp-like instrument used to control flow of fluids or blood

Lavage: The process of washing out an organ, usually the stomach, bladder, or bowel

Nasoenteric tube: A tube made of the same materials and inserted in much the same way as a nasogastric tube; however, a nasoenteric tube is allowed to pass into the duodenum and small intestine by means of peristalsis

Nasogastric tube: A tube of soft rubber or plastic inserted through the nostril and into the stomach

Saline solution: A solution consisting of a percentage of sodium chloride and distilled water that has the same osmolarity as that of body fluids

Nasogastric (NG) and **nasoenteric** (NE) **tubes** are inserted for therapeutic and diagnostic purposes. These tubes have a hollow lumen through which secretions and air may be evacuated or through which medications, nourishment, or diagnostic contrast agents may be instilled. The radiographer must be able to care for and transport patients with these tubes in place. The purposes of gastric suction and the ability to attach or discontinue it when the physician's orders require it must also be understood to prevent any injury to the patient.

Studies are done in diagnostic imaging departments that require the passage of NG or NE tubes before the examination. While radiographers do not insert these tubes, preparation of the patient may be required if the tube is to be inserted in the diagnostic imaging department. What type of equipment to assemble and how to assist with the procedure are requisite knowledge.

Occasionally, a patient requiring a procedure will have a gastrostomy tube in place. These tubes may be required for persons who are gravely debilitated and unable to obtain nutrition in a normal physiological manner. These patients must be cared for in a safe and sensitive manner.

Patients who are unable to take in nutrients though the gastrointestinal (GI) system, either partially or completely, may be nourished intravenously. This can be accomplished in the short term parenterally by peripheral intravenous means and in the long term by reliance on central venous catheters.

Occasionally, it is necessary for the patient who has vomited or who has an accumulation of blood or secretions in the mouth or throat to be suctioned while under the care of the radiographer. The radiographer does not perform these procedures, but quick assessment of the patient is critical so that the procedure can be done quickly to prevent aspiration of the fluid into the lungs or respiratory failure.

Patients with the tracheostomy tubes in place may also need diagnostic imaging examinations. They must receive proper care to prevent injury and to keep them comfortable while the examination is in progress.

Patients who are unable to maintain adequate respiration may require mechanical ventilation to support life. Mobile radiography is a frequent occurrence; therefore, precautions when working on these patients are required.

Chest tubes are inserted after surgical procedures, injury, or diseases of the lungs to permit drainage of fluid or air out of the pleural space. If air and fluid become trapped in the pleural space, pressure builds and creates what is called a tension pneumothorax. If this condition is not relieved, the resulting respiratory distress may produce a life-threatening situation. The precautions needed to care for patients with a chest tube must also be learned.

After surgical procedures, a variety of tissue drains are placed in the areas of the body that poorly tolerate an accumulation of fluid. The radiographer must be able to recognize these drains and direct patient care in a manner that prevents dislodging the drains.

NASOGASTRIC AND NASOENTERIC TUBES

NG tubes are made of polyurethane, silicone, or rubber. They are inserted through the nasopharynx into the stomach, the duodenum, or the jejunum. If a patient has an anatomic or physiologic reason why the nose cannot be used for passage, the tube may be inserted through the mouth over the tongue. NG tubes are also used for diagnostic examinations, for administration of feedings or medications, to treat intestinal obstruction, and to control bleeding (Table 14-1).

NE tubes are made of the same materials as NG tubes and are inserted in much the same way as NG tubes; however, they are allowed to pass into the duodenum and small intestine by means of peristalsis. They are also used for decompression, diagnosis, and treatment purposes (Table 14-2).

Two of the most common NG tubes are the Levin and the sump tube (Fig. 14-1). Other NG tubes often seen are the Nutriflex, the Moss, and the Sengstaken-Blakemore esophageal NG tube. The Levin tube is a single-lumen tube with holes near its tip. The sump tube is a radiopaque, double-lumen tube. The opening of the second lumen is a blue extension off the proximal end of the tube. This is the end that remains outside and is called a "pigtail." This end is always left open to room air for the purpose of maintaining a continuous flow of atmospheric air into the stomach, thereby controlling the amount of suction pressure that may be placed on the gastric mucosa. This is a means of preventing injury and ulceration of these tissues.

The Nutriflex tube is used primarily for feeding. It has a mercury-weighted tip and is coated with a lubricant that becomes activated when moistened by gastric secretions.

The Moss tube is a more complex triple-lumen tube. One lumen has an inflatable balloon to anchor it in the stomach. The second lumen is used for aspiration of fluid, and the third is for duodenal feeding (Fig. 14-2).

The Sengstaken-Blakemore (S-B) tube is also a triple-lumen tube; two of the lumens have balloons. The balloons are inflated to exert pressure on bleeding esophageal varices. The third lumen is used for **lavage** and to monitor for hemorrhage. The balloon pressure must be maintained at all times, but if the patient becomes **dyspneic**, the balloon pressure must be relieved at once by cutting the balloon lumens with

TABLE 14-1   Common Nasogastric Tubes

Names	# of Lumens	Description	Use
Levin	1	Plastic tube that is passed through the nose into the stomach	Gastric decompression
Sump	2	Radiopaque tube with a plug pigtail that lets air flow into the stomach	Drain fluid from the stomach
Nutriflex	1	Mercury-weighted tip; coated with a gastric secretion-activated lubricant	Feedings
Moss	3	Has a balloon to anchor into stomach while 2nd and 3rd lumens are used for aspiration and feeding	Aspiration of fluid; duodenal feeding
Sengstaken-Blakemore	3	Thick catheter with 2 balloons used to exert pressure against walls of esophagus	Control of bleeding from esophageal varices

scissors. The radiographer must not attempt to care for a patient with an S-B tube in place without the patient's nurse on hand. **Asphyxiation** or aspiration of gastric contents into the lungs is possible without keen and continuous monitoring. The patient with an S-B tube in place is usually cared for in the intensive care unit, and portable radiographic images are ordered.

Three of the most commonly used NE tubes are the Cantor, the Harris, and the Miller-Abbott. The Cantor and Harris tubes have a single lumen; the Miller-Abbott tube is a double-lumen tube. One lumen of the Miller-Abbott tube is used for intestinal decompression; the other is for the introduction of mercury after insertion. Some single-lumen tubes are weighted with a metal tip. The progress of the tube may be observed in the diagnostic imaging department fluoroscopically.

Radiographs are taken after passage of these tubes to establish correct placement (Fig. 14-3).

Passage of Nasogastric and Nasoenteric Tubes

Radiographers are not responsible for inserting NG or NE tubes. A registered nurse usually inserts an NG tube; a registered nurse or a physician inserts the NE tube. Insertion of a tube is an uncomfortable and frightening procedure for the patient, who is often very ill. If this procedure is to take place in the radiographic imaging department, explain to the patient what is being done and for what purpose. Assure the patient that if he or she concentrates on swallowing and breathing as the tube is inserted, the procedure will go smoothly and quickly.

TABLE 14-2   Common Nasoenteric Tubes

Names	# of Lumens	Description	Use
Cantor	1	Long tube with a small mercury-filled bag at the end; contains drainage holes for aspiration	Relieves obstructions in the small intestine
Harris	1	Mercury-weighted tube passed through the nose and carried through the digestive tract by gravity	Gastric and intestinal decompression
Miller-Abbott	2	Long small-caliber catheter; one is a perforated metal tip, and the other has a collapsible balloon; radiopaque tube	Decompression

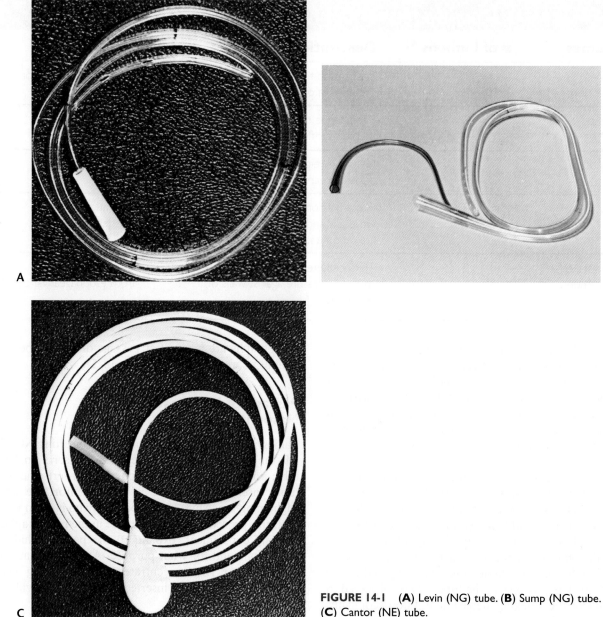

FIGURE 14-1 (**A**) Levin (NG) tube. (**B**) Sump (NG) tube. (**C**) Cantor (NE) tube.

The physician may swab the nasal passages and spray the oropharynx with tetracaine (Pontocaine) to promote the patient's comfort by anesthetizing the area and suppressing the gag reflex. A gargle with a liquid anesthetic may also facilitate the procedure.

The patient is placed in a **Fowler position** with pillows supporting the head and shoulders. When the physician or nurse is ready to insert the tube, the distal end is lubricated with a water-soluble lubricant and the patient is instructed to swallow as it is passed. The tube should go down easily and with little force. When the tube is believed to be in the stomach, as shown in Figure 14-4, an initial radiograph verifies its position. If the tube is to be in place for a considerable length of time, its placement may be verified by attaching the end of the NG tube to a 20- to 30-mL syringe and withdrawing gastric fluid. The fluid is tested with litmus paper, which must test acidic to ensure that the tube is in the correct position. When it is certain that the tube has reached the stomach, reassure the patient and make him or her comfortable. NG tubes are taped in place, but NE tubes are not taped because their position is achieved through peristaltic action. The Levin tube is securely taped so that it is not accidentally withdrawn. It should never be necessary to repeat passage of a gastric tube because of careless handling. There should be no pulling pressure on the tube. Patients with gastric tubes in place are not to eat or drink anything unless

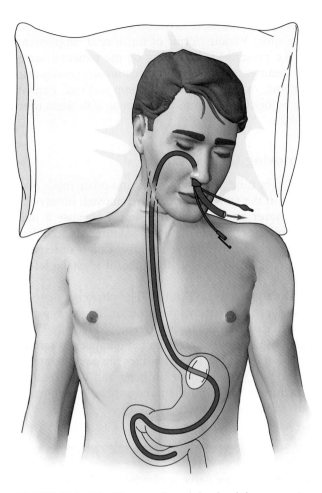

FIGURE 14-2 The Moss esophageal duodenal decompression and feeding tube has three chambers; the first anchors it in the stomach, the second is for aspiration, and the third is for feeding.

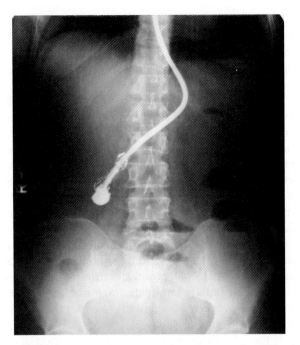

FIGURE 14-4 Radiograph taken after insertion of an NG tube. This is done to verify the tube's position.

the physician specifically orders it. Patients who may accidentally pull their NG tubes out may have immobilizers on their hands. If this is the case, the radiographer must make certain that the hands are tied securely when leaving the bedside after a mobile radiograph. The patient must not be able to reach up and pull the NG tube from its location.

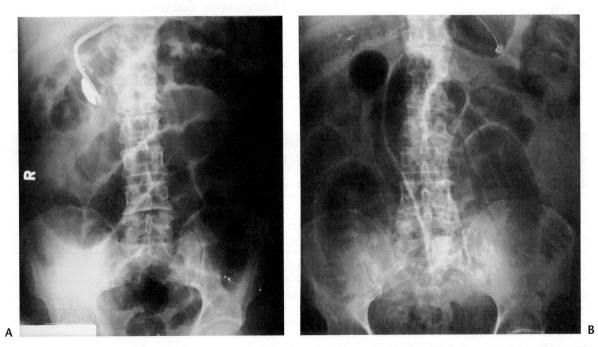

FIGURE 14-3 **(A)** Radiograph of a small bowel obstruction with a nasoenteric tube in place. **(B)** Radiograph of a small bowel ileus with an nasogastric tube in place.

Placement of an NG tube must be ascertained before any medication, food, water, or contrast agent is administered into it. If this is not done, accidental administration of an agent into the pleural cavity may occur with adverse consequences for the patient.

The correct position of an NG or NE tube initially may be determined with a radiographic image or by fluoroscopy. Obviously, a radiograph cannot be used each time it is necessary to know whether the tube is correctly positioned. The other means of determining the correct placement of an NG or NE tube is by aspirating the tube with a syringe. The aspirant is then tested with litmus paper to measure its acidity. Gastric contents are acidic (pH approximately 3). The pH of the intestinal secretions is less acidic (pH approximately 6 to 6.5). The pH of respiratory secretions is not acidic (pH 7 or greater). Note that small bowel and respiration pH levels are similar but are far greater than intestinal secretions. Tubes properly placed in the stomach show a pH in the range from 1 to 4.

If there is any doubt concerning the position of an NG or NE tube, nothing should be administered into it. If instillation of an agent has begun, discontinue it immediately. If the patient seems to have regurgitated gastric contents, the radiographer must summon assistance immediately and prepare to assist with suctioning. To reduce the risk of aspiration, the patient with an NG or NE tube should be placed in a semi-Fowler's position during and for 30 minutes after administration of any agent into the tube.

Nasoenteric Feeding Tubes

These are several narrow-lumen tubes that are inserted for the purpose of feeding patients. They are used for patients who are unable to obtain nourishment or take oral medications in a natural manner and who are expected to obtain nourishment by this method for some time. Various forms of nutritional supplements may be prescribed depending on the patient's needs. The feedings may be given by continuous gravity drip, by **bolus**, or by a controlled pump method. Patients may be discharged from the hospital with these tubes in place.

Removing Gastric Tubes

The Levin tube, the sump tube, and other tubes positioned in the stomach are easily removed; however, it must never be assumed that simply because a radiographic examination that involved its use is complete, it is permissible to remove the tube. Unless ordered by the physician to remove the tube, it must be left in place.

Do not remove NE tubes. The physician or registered nurse may remove the tube, or it may be passed through the intestinal tract and removed rectally. While it is not in the purview of the radiographer to remove the NG tube, Table 14-3 identifies the equipment that will be necessary to have on hand and describes the procedure in the event the radiographer is required to assist in the procedure.

📢 CALL OUT!

Radiographers are never to remove an NE tube.

Transferring Patients with Nasogastric Suction

NG and NE tubes are used before or after surgical procedures that involve the digestive system, for illness of the GI system to keep the stomach and bowel free of

TABLE 14-3	Equipment and Procedure to Remove an NG Tube
Equipment	**Procedure**
Emesis basin	Identify the patient and explain the procedure
Tissues and paper towels	Wash hands and put on the protective apparel
Impermeable waste receptacle	Loosen tape, disconnect suction
Clean disposable gloves	Instruct the patient to take in a deep breath
Face shield	Gently withdraw the tube, wrap in paper toweling, and place in disposal bag
Impermeable gown	Make the patient comfortable and dispose of items correctly

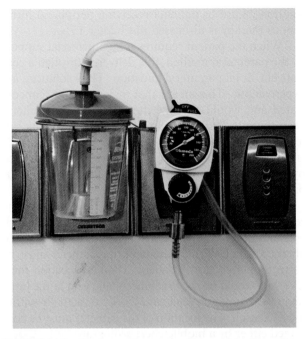

FIGURE 14-5 Suction equipment is often used in diagnostic imaging. It is piped to the department from a central area in the hospital. The vacuum collecting canister is disposable.

gastric contents, and for gastric decompression. The tube may be attached to a suction apparatus that is either portable or piped into the room from a central hospital unit (Fig. 14-5). The suction is maintained either continuously or intermittently, as the patient's needs demand. When the radiographer is responsible for transferring a patient who is having either continuous or intermittent gastric suctioning, the physicians' orders must be verified before making the transfer. If it is permissible to discontinue the suction, the length of time that it can be interrupted safely must be known. If it is for only a short time, be certain that suction can be reestablished in the diagnostic imaging department. This can be accomplished by taking the patient's portable suction machine with him or her or by using the suction available in the department. The amount of suction must also be known so that the pressure can be accurately adjusted. The amount of pressure that is ordered varies, and the correct level can be determined by reading the physician's orders or by asking the nurse in charge of the patient to do this. The maximum amount of suction that can be used is a pressure equal to 25 mm Hg for an adult patient. More than this can damage the gastric mucosa.

If the suction must be disconnected for a period of time, the radiographer is allowed to do this. If the tube is a single-lumen tube, a pair of gloves, a clamp, 2 rubber bands, and a package of sterile gauze sponges will be needed. Follow these procedures to discontinue suction:

1. Explain the procedure to the patient while opening the package of sponges and putting on the gloves.
2. Turn off the suction; clamp the gastric tube with the clamp, and place one gauze pad over the end of the tube, securing it with a rubber band.
3. Cover the connecting end of the suction tubing with the other sponge, and secure it with a rubber band. This gauze covering keeps both ends of the tubing clean while not in use.
4. Secure the suction tubing on the machine so that it will not fall onto the floor, and make certain that the NG or NE tube will not be dislodged during the transfer.
5. Proceed with the transfer by wheelchair or gurney as required.
6. If the suction is to be restarted in the diagnostic imaging department on arrival, set the suction pressure gauge, turn on the suction, and reattach it to the tubing. This procedure is repeated when transferring the patient back to the room.

If the NG tube is a double-lumen tube, never clamp it closed with a **hemostat** or regular clamping device because this may cause the lumens to adhere to each other and destroy the double-lumen effect. To prevent leakage from this type of tube, the barrel of the piston syringe may be inserted into the suction-drainage lumen (the blue pigtail). It is then pinned to the gown with the barrel upward to prevent reflux drainage.

> ### CALL OUT!
> Never clamp a double-lumen NG tube because this may destroy the effect.

THE PATIENT WITH A GASTROSTOMY TUBE

A **gastrostomy** is the surgical creation of an opening into the stomach. Through this opening, a tube is placed from the inside of the stomach to the external abdominal wall for the purpose of feeding a patient who cannot tolerate oral food intake (Fig. 14-6). This can be a temporary or permanent provision. The tube can be sutured in place or may be held in place with a crossbar that holds the tube against the wall of the stomach.

The patient with a newly applied gastrostomy tube has an unhealed surgical incision and will have a dressing in place. An older gastrostomy may or may not have a dressing applied. The tube is closed off after feeding with a clamp or a plug-in adapter to prevent leakage of gastric fluid or food. The tube is then coiled and kept in place with tape or a small dressing.

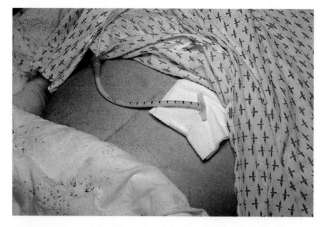

FIGURE 14-6 A PEG tube with the site protected by a dressing that covers the exit site (From *Brunner & Suddarth's Textbook of Medical-Surgical Nursing*, 11th ed. Philadelphia: Lippincott Williams & Wilkins, 2008).

While caring for a person with a gastrostomy tube in place, the radiographer must be aware of the potential for infection. If the operative area around the gastrostomy tube is not healed, sterile gloves must be worn if contact with the open area is possible. This is to prevent introduction of microorganisms that may result in infection. The potential for dislodging the tube is also present. Take care to prevent this. There must not be any tension placed on the tube.

The radiographer must be sensitive to the feelings of the patient with a gastrostomy. The patient may be grieving owing to the change in his or her body image or because of a chronic illness. Sensitive and thoughtful communication is required and the patient who is able to should be allowed to direct the care of the tube.

THE PATIENT WITH A CENTRAL VENOUS CATHETER

Central venous catheters and implanted ports are being used more frequently for patients who must have long-term medication administration, frequent blood transfusion, hyperosmolar solutions, or total parenteral nutrition.

When a patient does not have an adequate nutritional intake and cannot tolerate nourishment by means of the GI tract, he or she may be ordered to receive partial or total nutrition by an intravenous route. Partial parenteral nutrition is used when the patient is able to supply a part of his or her nutritional requirements by natural means. A large-gauge catheter is inserted into a large peripheral vein in the arm, and a parenteral solution containing a combination of lipid emulsion and amino acid/dextrose solution is administered as needed to satisfy the patient's nutritional needs. Vitamins and minerals are often added to these solutions. Care of patients receiving peripheral intravenous therapy is discussed in Chapter 15.

When the patient requires total nutritional support by the parenteral method, it is delivered through a central vein. Total parenteral nutrition (TPN) solutions are hyperosmotic. This means that they are highly concentrated and would damage the intima of a peripheral vein; therefore, a large vein in the central venous system is used. Because fluid imbalance may result if TPN is administered too rapidly, administration is controlled by a pump or an infusion controller. Intravenous pumps are discussed in Chapter 15.

Central venous catheters are used for measuring the central venous pressure (CVP) as well as allowing nutrients and other fluid to be instilled into the patient. To obtain a true CVP measurement, the catheter must be correctly placed in the patient. The best location for a CVP line would be the brachiocephalic vein at the junction of the superior vena cava (SVC) or actually within the SVC itself. The location of the catheter must be confirmed either by a mobile chest radiograph or by C-arm fluoroscopy during the actual insertion of the catheter. The line should be seen just medial to the anterior border of the first rib on the image (Fig. 14-7A).

There are several types of central venous catheters. The tunneled type is inserted into the subclavian or internal jugular vein and then advanced into the SVC or the right atrium. The exit site is on the anterior chest. Most central venous catheters have more than one lumen and several access ports at the exit site (Fig. 14-7B).

The Hickman and Broviac catheters are two commonly used tunnel-type central venous catheters. Two other commonly used central venous catheters are the peripherally inserted central (PIC) and the Groshong. The PIC catheter may be peripherally inserted into the patient's arm and advanced until its tip lies in a central vein. Radiographers are often called on to provide C-arm fluoroscopy in the operating suite during the placement of one of these catheters.

Another alternative central venous catheter is an implanted port. These are meant for patients who have long-term illnesses that require frequent intravenous medications or transfusions. The port is made of plastic, titanium, or stainless steel. It is implanted into the subcutaneous tissue, usually in the chest, and sutured in place. The port is not visible but can be felt as a small, hard surface under the subcutaneous tissue. A catheter from the port is then inserted into the subclavian or internal jugular vein. A needle, called the Huber needle, is inserted to access the central vein through the port.

While caring for a patient with a central venous catheter or port in place, great care must used to prevent infection at the insertion site. If a dressing around the catheter must be removed, a physician's order to do so must be received first. Medical aseptic technique is used to remove the dressing. If the dressing is in the

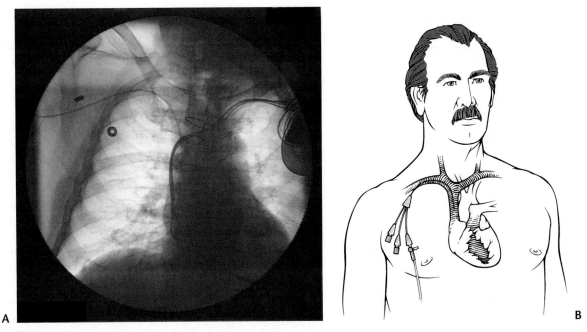

FIGURE 14-7 **(A)** Radiograph showing not only the central venous catheter in place on the patient's right side, but also a pacemaker on the left side. The image is made in the negative mode. **(B)** Subclavian triple-lumen catheter for total parenteral nutrition and other adjunct therapy. The catheter is threaded through the subclavian vein and placed in the vena cava.

upper thoracic region, both the health care worker and the patient should wear a mask to prevent breathing on the area. The dressing must be removed carefully to avoid dislodging or moving the needle.

EMERGENCY SUCTIONING

Occasionally an infant, a child, an unconscious patient, or a very weak and debilitated patient is unable to clear emesis, sputum, or other drainage from the nose, mouth, nasopharynx, or oropharynx by coughing or swallowing. The conscious patient is placed in a semi-Fowler position and is assisted to clear the airway. If the patient has a potential spinal cord injury and is in a back brace and a collar and begins to vomit, log roll the patient to the side with face directed downward. No movement of the patient's head or neck should be allowed. If the airway is not cleared quickly, the patient may need to be suctioned. Signs that indicate that a patient may need to receive nasopharyngeal or oropharyngeal suctioning are:

1. Profuse vomiting in a patient who cannot voluntarily change position
2. Audible rattling or gurgling sounds coming from the patient's throat
3. Signs of respiratory distress

Persons with these symptoms may require mechanical suctioning to remove the secretions to prevent aspiration or respiratory arrest.

Suctioning is an emergency procedure. It is not within the scope of practice for a radiographer to perform suctioning procedures because there are many instances in which suctioning may be contraindicated. The need for suctioning must be determined by a health care professional who has been educated for this and who is familiar with the patient's condition. Some contraindications for suctioning may be head and facial injuries, bleeding esophageal varices, nasal deformities, trauma, cerebral aneurisms, tight wheezing, bronchospasm, and croup.

The radiographer must be able to determine if the patient needs to be suctioned, to call for the physician or the registered nurse to do this if necessary, and to assist with the procedure. The radiographer is responsible for checking the emergency suctioning equipment in the department each day to be certain that it is in good working order and that all necessary items are available.

THE PATIENT WITH A TRACHEOSTOMY

A tracheostomy is an opening into the trachea created surgically either to relieve respiratory distress caused by an obstruction of the upper airway or to improve respiratory function by permitting better access of air to the lower respiratory tract. This may be done as either a temporary or a permanent measure. Patients who require this procedure may have suffered traumatic injury or may be paralyzed, unconscious, or suffering from a disease that interferes with respiration.

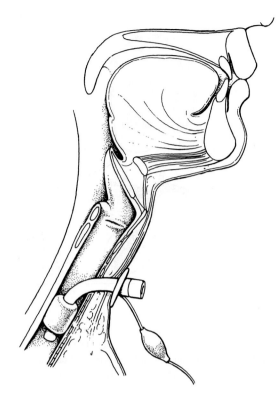

FIGURE 14-8 Tracheostomy tube placement.

After the surgical incision is made and the opening exists, a tracheostomy tube is inserted into the opening (Fig. 14-8). Tracheostomy tubes are equipped with an obturator to ensure safe insertion; the obturator is removed as soon as the tube is in place.

There are several types of tracheostomy tubes. They are usually made of plastic but may be metal. They have a cuff that helps seal the tracheostomy to prevent air leaks and aspiration of gastric contents (Fig. 14-9). Most tracheostomy tubes have an inner **cannula** that is locked into place. The tracheostomy tube is held in place at the back of the neck with ties or tapes. The tubes that are used for infants and small children do not usually have the cuff because they fit tightly enough without one.

Patients with newly inserted tracheostomy tubes are very fearful. They are unable to speak because the opening in the windpipe prevents air from being forced from the lungs past the vocal cords and into the larynx. They are afraid of choking because they are unable to remove secretions that accumulate in the tracheostomy tube. These secretions must be suctioned out by a registered nurse. If a patient with a new tracheostomy is brought to the diagnostic imaging department, a nurse qualified to care for this patient should accompany him or her. Sterile suction catheters, suctioning equipment, and oxygen administration equipment must be prepared before the patient arrives in the department. The semi-Fowler position is usually most comfortable for these patients, and bolsters or pillows should be provided so that the best position for the patient can be maintained.

While caring for the patient with a tracheostomy, plan the care with the patient's nurse and the patient before any diagnostic imaging procedure is begun. The tracheostomy tube must not be removed, and the tapes holding it in place must not be untied for any reason, because the tracheostomy tube may be dislodged and may not be able to be replaced immediately. All procedures must be explained to the patient in order to alleviate anxiety. If the patient appears to be breathing noisily or with difficulty, immediately stop working and allow the nurse to suction the patient or otherwise relieve the discomfort.

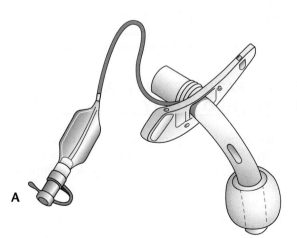

FIGURE 14-9 (**A**) Fenestrated tube. (**B**) Double cuff tube.

THE PATIENT ON A MECHANICAL VENTILATOR

The radiographer will be frequently called to the intensive care unit of the acute care hospital to take radiographs of patients who are being ventilated mechanically. Patients who continue to need mechanical ventilation may be transferred to extended care facilities or to their homes. Because mechanical ventilators support life, it is of great importance that all precautions be understood when taking care of a patient whose breathing is supported by mechanical means.

A patient who cannot breathe spontaneously or whose respiration is inadequate to oxygenate the blood is a candidate for mechanical ventilation. The need for this may be the result of a pathological condition that alters gas exchange, oxygen perfusion, or both. These are called gas exchange disorders. Examples of these might be pulmonary emboli or severe respiratory disease.

The need for mechanical ventilation may be the result of a disease process that affects the mechanics of breathing by interfering with the neurological or neuromuscular functions related to breathing. These are called extrapulmonary disorders. Examples of extrapulmonary disorders that may require mechanical ventilation to support respiration are cerebral vascular accidents and Guillain-Barré syndrome.

There are two general classifications of mechanical ventilators: negative-pressure and positive-pressure ventilators. Negative-pressure ventilators are most likely seen in the home. They exert a negative pressure on the chest wall. When this occurs, air rushes into the negatively pressurized space to refill it and it is again removed. While negative-pressure ventilators are cumbersome, they have the advantage of not requiring an artificial airway for use.

Positive-pressure ventilators are the more commonly used type. There are three general categories of positive-pressure ventilators: pressure-cycled, time-cycled, and volume-cycled. They inflate the lungs by exerting positive pressure on the lungs, stopping inspiration when a preset pressure is attained. The lungs are then allowed to expire passively. All positive-pressure ventilators require an artificial airway, either an endotracheal tube or a tracheostomy. The volume-cycled ventilator is the most often used. The machine stops inspiration when it has delivered a predetermined volume of gas in spite of the amount of pressure needed to deliver it. Expiration is passive (Fig. 14-10).

When radiographing a patient who is on a positive-pressure ventilator, consult the nurse assigned to care for the patient before beginning to work. Take the following precautions for a patient who is being ventilated by positive pressure:

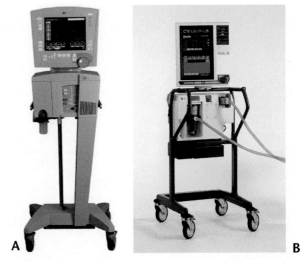

FIGURE 14-10   Positive-pressure ventilators. (**A**) AVA machine. (**B**) Puritan-Bennett 840 Ventilator System.

1. Obtain as much assistance as necessary to move the patient safely.
2. Do not place tension on any intravenous tubing or on the tube to the ventilator.
3. Do not displace the endotracheal tube or tracheostomy tube.
4. Do not disconnect the power to the ventilator.
5. Do not disconnect the spirometer.
6. Have the patient's nurse stand by. Provide the nurse with a radiation protection apron if he or she is to be in the room.
7. If the patient becomes suddenly restless or confused or seems to be fighting the respirator, stop and notify the nurse immediately.
8. Use meticulous medical aseptic technique when working with the patient to prevent infection. Put on gloves if there is any possibility of being in contact with blood or body fluids.

If displacement or malfunction of any part of the equipment occurs, an alarm will sound on the machine. This may indicate a life-threatening problem that must be attended to immediately. The potential complications due to a positive-pressure ventilator equipment displacement or malfunction include cardiovascular compromise related to inadequate oxygenation; pneumothorax resulting from excessive ventilator pressure; or infection resulting from exposure to microorganisms introduced into the pulmonary system.

The patient who is on a positive-pressure ventilator is unable to communicate because of the endotracheal tube or a newly acquired tracheostomy. This is extremely frustrating for the patient. An explanation of what is about to happen goes a long way toward relieving this frustration, as does providing the patient with a means to give written feedback if he or she is able to write.

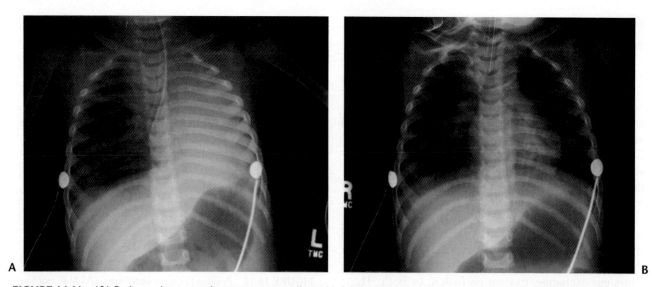

FIGURE 14-11   (A) Radiographic image demonstrating a collapsed left lung due to incorrect endotracheal tube placement. (B) This image shows that the left lung has now reinflated when the ET tube was withdrawn and the tip of the tube is above the carina.

Endotracheal Tubes

Tubes are often inserted through the mouth into the trachea as a means of establishing or opening an airway on patients. After being placed in the trachea, a cuff is inflated, which keeps the airway open. At the same time, the tube prevents aspiration of foreign objects into the bronchus.

Correct placement of the tube is approximately 5 to 7 cm above the tracheal bifurcation (carina). A chest radiograph should always be obtained after intubations to ascertain proper placement of the tube. Up to 20% of all endotracheal tubes require repositioning after initial insertion. Because of the anatomical position of the right main bronchus, tubes that are inserted too far usually enter the right bronchus. This will cause collapse of the left lung (Fig. 14-11A and B). A tube positioned too high in the trachea may cause air to enter the stomach, causing the patient to regurgitate any gastric contents. This regurgitation may lead to aspiration pneumonia.

Radiographs should be taken on a daily basis to ensure that the tube has not accidentally shifted. The tube can be moved by the patient's coughing, the weight of the ventilator tubing, or the movement of the patient by a health care worker.

THE PATIENT WITH A CHEST TUBE AND WATER-SEALED DRAINAGE

The pressure in the pleural cavity is normally lower than atmospheric pressure, but disease or injury can alter this. Air in the pleural cavity known as a pneumothorax causes a collapse of the lung. A condition created by a collection of blood in the pleural cavity that prevents the lungs from expanding normally is called a *hemothorax,* while fluid other than blood that builds up in the pleural cavity is called *pleural effusion.* In any case, the lung is unable to expand and get enough oxygen necessary to fulfill the body's requirements.

A thoracotomy, the surgical creation of an opening into the chest cavity, is performed to diagnose or treat diseases or injury to the lungs or pleura.

Conditions such as these require the placement of one or more chest tubes inserted into the pleural cavity. The chest tube is attached to a water-sealed drainage unit to remove any air or fluid from the pleural cavity (Fig. 14-12). This is done to reestablish the correct intrapleural pressure and to allow the lungs to expand normally.

A water-sealed drainage system is established by connecting the chest tube that originates in the pleural cavity to a clear tube that ends in a chamber containing sterile water or sterile normal **saline solution.** The tube leading from the chest tube remains below water level at all times to maintain the seal. When the patient inhales, air and fluid from the intrapleural spaces are drawn into the drainage tube and emptied into a chamber prepared to receive them. Since the fluid in the drainage chamber is heavier than air, it cannot be drawn back into the tub on inspiration, nor can air from the atmosphere enter because of the water seal.

There are several variations of the water-sealed systems. There may be one, two, or three chambers. Additional chambers, also with water seals, are needed for drainage from the patient's pleural cavity and for suction regulation if suction is also attached to the chest tube. If two chest tubes are coming from the

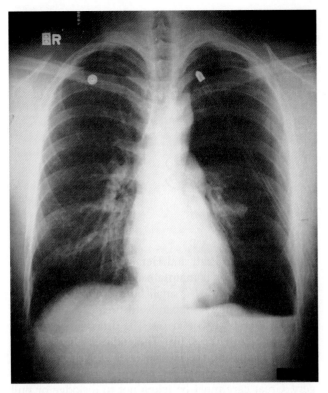

FIGURE 14-12 A chest tube is present in the left lung of this patient with a complete pneumothorax. The opaque tip can be clearly seen above the left clavicle.

pleural cavity, a Y connector joins the two tubes near the patient's body and continues to the water-sealed drainage apparatus. Several commercial water-sealed drainage systems are on the market; most are disposable (Fig. 14-13).

The following items are important to remember when caring for a patient with a chest tube with water-sealed drainage:

1. Keep the tubing from the pleural cavity to the drainage chamber as straight as possible. If it is long, loosely coil it on the patient's bed, and do not allow it to fall below the level of the patient's chest.

2. All connections must be tightly taped to the tubing, and stoppers must fit tightly into receptacles.

3. A heavy sterile dressing and tape are kept at the patient's bedside so that if the tubing is accidentally dislodged from the pleural cavity, the dressing can be taped to the open area immediately.

4. Do not empty water-sealed chambers or raise them. The water seal must remain below the patient's chest at all times.

5. Do not clamp chest tubes.

6. If a water-seal chamber is continuously bubbling, notify the patient's nurse immediately, since this may indicate a leak in the system. There should be a steady rise and fall of the water as the patient breathes.

7. Immediately report to the patient's nurse rapid, shallow breathing, cyanosis, or a complaint from the patient of a feeling of pressure on his chest.

8. The drainage tube from the chest should be long enough to allow free patient movement. If the patient must be moved for radiographic exposures, do not allow tension to be placed on the chest tube or the patient to be positioned in a way that causes the tubing to be kinked or sealed off.

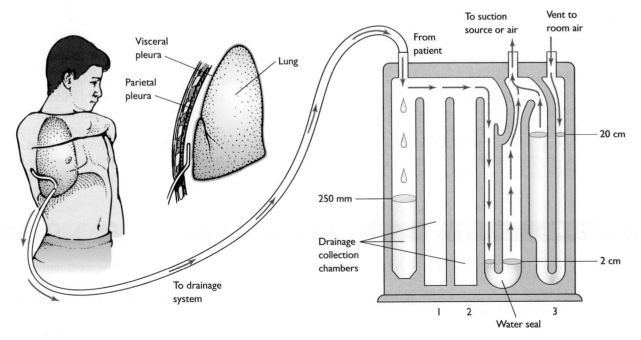

FIGURE 14-13 An example of a disposable chest drainage system.

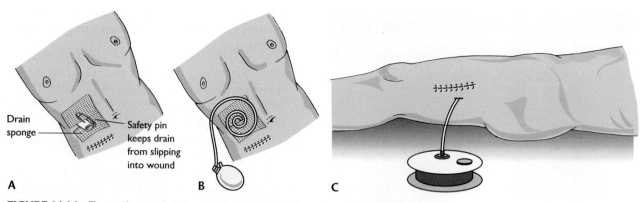

FIGURE 14-14   Types of surgical drains. (**A**) Penrose. (**B**) Jackson-Pratt. (**C**) Hemovac.

> ### 📢 CALL OUT!
>
> Always ascertain whether the patient has a chest tube before moving him or her and placing the image receptor, since these tubes are often hidden under the blankets.

TISSUE DRAINS

Tissue drains are placed at or near wound sites or operative sites when large amounts of drainage are expected. This drainage interferes with the healing process because the body reabsorbs it too slowly. In some circumstances, it may produce infection or result in formation of a fistula.

The Penrose, Jackson-Pratt, and Hemovac drains are three of the most common postoperative tissue drains. They are often placed in areas in which the surgical procedure calls for large amounts of tissue dissection or in areas with an increased blood supply, such as the breast, the neck, and the kidney. They are also placed in the abdominal area. One end of the tube or drain is placed in or near the operative site, and the other end exits through the body wall. The surgeon removes them when the drainage diminishes.

The Penrose drain is a soft rubber tube, which is kept from slipping into the surgical wound or beneath the body wall by a sterile safety pin (Fig. 14-14A). It is allowed to drain into the surgical dressing.

The Jackson-Pratt and Hemovac drains are plastic drainage tubes that maintain constant, low, negative pressure by means of a small bulb, which is squeezed together and slowly expands to create low-pressure suction (Fig. 14-14B and C). The drainage goes from the tubing into the bulb. The radiographer is most likely to encounter the Hemovac drain in the recovery room while radiographing a patient just out of hip surgery. Great care must be taken not to dislodge or pull on this drain while placing the image receptor.

Other types of drains are placed into the hollow organs of the body and may be sutured in place and attached to a collection bag. Some of these are the T tube, which may be placed into the common bile duct; the cecostomy tube, which is placed in the cecum; and the cystostomy tube, which is placed in the kidney.

All these drains must be identified during the assessment of the patient and care must be taken to avoid any tension on these drains, which might dislodge them partially or completely. Infection control must also be a concern. The presence of a tissue drain indicates that the patient has an opening directly into the body where infection may be easily introduced. If radiographing the patient includes touching an area in which a drain is inserted, surgical aseptic technique must be used to prevent introduction of new microorganisms into the wound. This requires hand washing and donning sterile gloves as described in Chapter 5. Always wear gloves and perform a 30-second hand wash when coming into contact with drainage from these areas.

SUMMARY

Nasogastric (NG) and nasoenteric (NE) tubes are inserted into the stomach and small intestine for varying medical purposes. They are used for gastric decompression, for diagnosis of diseases of the GI tract, for treatment of diseases of the GI tract, and for feeding persons who are unable to swallow food in the normal

manner. Mechanical suction often accompanies NG and NE intubation. The radiographer may have to transport patients who have NG or NE tubes in place, including those who need suction.

Before transferring a patient who has a gastric tube in place and is receiving continuous gastric suction, consult the patient's nurse to determine if it is permissible to discontinue the suction and, if so, for how long. The patient should be moved carefully. If the suction is continuous, it must be restarted at the same pressure as in the hospital room as soon as the patient reaches the radiographic imaging department.

The sump gastric tube is a double-lumen tube designed to maintain a continuous flow of atmospheric air into the stomach. This tube must never be clamped with a regular clamp or hemostat, since such clamping may destroy the double-lumen effect of the tube.

The gastric tubes most often used in the diagnostic imaging department are the Levin tube and the Cantor tube. The Levin tube enters the stomach, and the Cantor enters the small intestine. The radiographer may remove Levin tubes if a physician's order to do so is received. Gently withdraw the tube and wrap it in several thicknesses of paper toweling, place it in an impermeable bag, and dispose of it with the contaminated waste. If it cannot be easily removed, call the physician to remove it. The radiographer does not remove NE tubes. Either a registered nurse or the physician removes them, or they are allowed to pass through the intestinal tract to be removed rectally.

Gastrostomy tubes are surgically inserted directly into the stomach for the purpose of providing a means into the stomach for nourishing a person unable to take food or fluids by mouth for an indefinite period of time. When caring for a patient with a gastrostomy tube in place, take precautions not to dislodge the tube or to introduce infection at the insertion site. The radiographer must also understand that that person with a recently inserted gastrostomy tube may be grieving over the alteration in his or her body image and must therefore be treated with sensitivity.

Patients who are unable to receive nutrients through the GI tract may need to be nourished by partial or total parenteral nutrition (TPN). Partial parenteral nutrition is delivered by the peripheral intravenous route. The central venous route delivers TPN. This is because the nutrients in the TPN formula may injure the intima of small blood vessels. There are many other reasons for the use of central venous catheters; therefore, the radiographer must be able to recognize their presence and take the necessary precautions if they are in place.

While the radiographer will not perform nasopharyngeal or oropharyngeal suctioning procedures, he or she is responsible for having equipment prepared and for assisting with the procedure. When it is required, it is usually an emergency procedure done to prevent aspiration of secretions into the lungs or respiratory arrest.

The patient with a tracheostomy may require radiographic imaging. These patients may be extremely apprehensive. They are unable to speak and unable to clear their tracheostomy tube of secretions that accumulate. A nurse who is able to suction a tracheostomy should accompany the patient who has a new tracheostomy to the diagnostic imaging department. If the patient needs to be suctioned, the radiographer must stop whatever is being done to allow the nurse to perform this procedure.

Mechanical ventilators are used to support respiratory function when a disease process or an obstruction prevents normal respiration. Mechanical ventilators support life when no other means is available; therefore, the radiographer must understand the precautions necessary when caring for a patient who is ventilator dependent. Most patients are on positive-pressure ventilators, which require an artificial airway for their use. This may be either a tracheostomy or an endotracheal tube. Never disconnect the ventilator from its power source and obtain adequate assistance when radiographing a ventilator patient to prevent other life-threatening problems.

Patients who have chest tubes connected to water-sealed drainage systems are often radiographed on a daily basis with the mobile unit. Remember to keep the tubing coiled at the patient's chest level, to keep all connections tightly sealed to maintain the water seal at all times, not to lift the water-sealed bottle higher than the patient's chest level, not to clamp or kink the drainage tube, and to notify the patient's nurse immediately if the patient is in respiratory distress or if there is a continuous bubbling in the water-sealed chamber.

There are various tissue drains used for the purpose of removing excessive fluid from an operative site to hasten the healing process and prevent infection. If a tissue drain is present, do not allow tension to be placed on the drain that might dislodge it. Take appropriate infection control precautions when caring for the patient who has a drain in place.

CHAPTER 14 TEST

1. While caring for a patient, who has an NG tube in place, what needs to be done? Circle all that apply.
   a. Find out if the tube is to be reconnected to suction and if so what is the amount of pressure.
   b. Take care not to dislodge the tube.
   c. Remove the tube before the patient leaves the department.
2. An alert patient whose swallowing reflex is intact is placed into what position in preparation for suctioning?

a. Prone
b. Sims
c. Semi-Fowler
d. Lateral

3. What are two points to remember when caring for a patient with a new tracheostomy in place?
   a. He or she may be talkative and may need to be suctioned.
   b. He or she will be anxious and unable to speak.
   c. He or she will be in the stage of denial and will express anger.
   d. He or she will be unconscious and will be accompanied by a nurse.

4. When caring for a patient who has a chest tube with water-sealed drainage, what must be remembered? Circle all that apply.
   a. The water seal must be maintained at all times.
   b. Continuous bubbling into the water-sealed chamber is an indication that all is well.
   c. The tubing may be clamped if necessary.
   d. Most patients with chest tubes complain of respiratory distress.
   e. Never lift the drainage system above the patient's chest.

5. Signs and symptoms that indicate a patient needs to be suctioned are (circle all that apply):
   a. Audible rattling and gurgling sounds from the patient's throat
   b. Gagging
   c. Breathing with difficulty
   d. Profuse vomiting in a patient who cannot voluntarily change positions

6. When caring for a patient who has a tissue drain in place:
   a. Disregard these drains because they are not the radiographer's concern.
   b. Prevent tension on the drain and use surgical aseptic technique if in direct contact with the drain.
   c. Measure intake and output from the drain.
   d. Remove the drain because it will impede the success of the radiograph.

7. When disconnecting a sump gastric tube (a tube with a double lumen):
   a. Clamp the tube with a regular clamp and then place sterile gauze over each end.
   b. Clamp the tube closed with a hemostat.
   c. Increase the amount of suction pressure.
   d. Place a piston syringe in the open end of the gastric tube or place the "pig tail" over it.
   e. Decrease the amount of suction pressure.

8. List 2 types of NG tubes that will be commonly seen in the radiography department.

9. Name three types of tissue drains. Which one is more commonly seen in the recovery room while radiographing a hip surgery patient?

10. Name two types of mechanical ventilators and state which type is most commonly used.

11. List the precautions taken when radiographing a patient who has a central venous catheter in place.

12. Describe why a chest radiograph is taken when a patient has been intubated.

CHAPTER 15

Pharmacology for the Radiographer

STUDENT LEARNING OUTCOMES

After completing the chapter, the student will be able to:

1. Explain the legal accountability of all health care professionals who administer drugs and list the precautions and restrictions necessary when drugs are administered.

2. Discuss drug standards and methods of control of drugs with potential for abuse.

3. Explain methods of naming drugs and the sources of drugs.

4. Define "over-the-counter" drugs and explain use of herbal and dietary supplements.

5. Describe pharmacokinetic and pharmacodynamic principles pertaining to drugs.

6. Describe the physiologic processes involved in drug absorption, distribution, metabolism, and excretion, and differentiate between the side effects and adverse effects of drugs used in imaging.

7. Identify and describe routes of drug administration.

8. Describe the methods and techniques for administering various types of contrast agents.

9. Delineate areas appropriate for venipuncture sites and describe potential complications associated with intravenous drug administration and action that must be taken to alleviate or prevent complications.

10. Differentiate and document dose calculations for adult and pediatric patients receiving contrast agents.

KEY TERMS

Addiction: A dependence on a drug beyond voluntary control

Adverse effects: Undesirable and often dangerous effects of drugs

Affinity: The chemical force that impels particular atoms or molecules to unite

Agranulocytosis: An acute disease condition that presents with an extremely low number of polymorphonuclear leukocytes

Alternative therapies: Natural plant extracts, herbs, vitamins, minerals, and therapeutic techniques such as massage and acupuncture

Angina: A severe constricting pain or sensation in the chest that may radiate to shoulder or arm; related to coronary artery disease

Aqueous: Watery

Blood-brain barrier: Anatomic structure that prevents certain substances from accessing the brain

Blood dyscrasias: Pathologic conditions of the cellular elements of the blood

Broad spectrum: (Antibiotics) effective against a wide variety of microorganisms

Buccal: In the mouth adjacent to the cheek

Contraindication: Any symptom or circumstance that renders use of a drug inadvisable

Cutaneous: Relating to the skin

Dependence: Reliance on a drug that may be physiologic or psychologic in nature

Drug-drug interaction: One drug interacting or interfering with the action of another drug

Enteral: Within the gastrointestinal tract

Extended spectrum: (Antibiotics) effective against more microbes than broad spectrum penicillin

Extravasation: Fluid passing out of a blood vessel into surrounding tissues

First trimester of pregnancy: The first 3 months of pregnancy

STUDENT LEARNING OUTCOMES

(Continued)

11. List precautions to be taken during drug administration and the radiographer's accountability to correctly assess the patient prior to administering a drug.

12. State components of a patient's drug history and explain the procedure to be followed if a medication error is made.

13. List symptoms that indicate infiltration or extravasation of a drug into surrounding tissues and explain the radiographer's action and responsibility if an adverse drug reaction occurs.

14. Demonstrate preparation of sites for intravenous drug administration and the correct method of administering intravenous contrast agents.

15. Demonstrate radiographer's patient care responsibilities before, during, and after an infiltration of any contrast agent and the method of discontinuing an intravenous injection.

16. Identify and define common medical abbreviations pertaining to drug administration.

KEY TERMS *(Continued)*

Hypnotic: A drug that causes sleep

Hypokalemia: An abnormally low concentration of potassium ions in the bloodstream

Hypothyroidism: Reduced amount of thyroid hormone leading to a disease process

Indication: The basis for initiation of treatment or use of a particular drug

Intra-arterial: Within the artery

Intra-articular: Into the cavity of the joint

Intracardiac: Into the chambers of the heart

Intralesional: Applied directly into a lesion or wound

Lipoid: Pertaining to fat

Macromolecular: A molecule in a finely divided state dispersed in liquid or solid media

Narcotic: Any drug synthetic or naturally occurring that induces a state of stuporous analgesia

Neurologic: Related to the nervous system

Oral: By mouth

Parenteral or parenterally: Refers to administration of a drug by penetrating the skin

Rectal: Inserted into the rectum

Retrograde procedure: Instillation of contrast in opposite direction of physiologic flow of fluids in the body

Side effects: Mild, common reactions to drugs

Sublingual: Under the tongue

Thrombocytopenia: An abnormally small number of platelets in the circulating blood

Thrombosis: Clotting within a blood vessel

Thyrotoxicosis: A disease state related to excess amounts of thyroid hormone

Tinnitus: Sound in the ears that can be ringing, whistling, hissing, roaring, or booming in the absence of acoustic stimuli

Topical: Designed for or involving local application and action (the skin)

Toxic level: A drug given in a strength that is physiologically harmful

Toxic reaction: A life-threatening effect of a drug that may occur immediately or over a long period of the particular drug's administration

Urticaria: An eruption of itchy wheels, hives

Vaginal: Drug administration into the vagina

Vasodilatation: A widening of the lumen of blood vessels

Vasovagal response: Related to action of the vagus nerve upon blood vessels resulting in rapid pulse, cold sweats, bradycardia, hypotension, and syncope

Pharmacology is the study of drug actions and drug interactions with living organisms. Drugs are chemical substances that are not required for normal maintenance of body function and produce a biological effect in an organism. The word *pharmacology* comes from the Greek words *pharmakon,* meaning drug or poison, and *logos,* meaning study; therefore, pharmacology is a study of drugs. All drugs are, or can be if misused, poisons (Aigins, 1995). If used correctly, they are meant to relieve human diseases and suffering.

The position of the American Society of Radiologic Technologists is that "venipuncture falls within the profession's Scope of Practice and Practice Standards and that it shall be included in the didactic and clinical curriculum with demonstrated competencies of all appropriate disciplines regardless of the state or institution where such curriculum is taught." For this reason, pharmacology and the clinical component of venipuncture are included in this chapter.

There are three categories assigned to substances applied or administered for therapeutic purposes. They are drugs or medications, biologics, and **alternative therapies.**

A *drug* is a chemical agent capable of producing biologic responses in the body. These responses may be desirable (therapeutic) or undesirable (adverse). After a drug is administered, it is called a *medication.* A *biologic* is an agent naturally produced in animal cells, microorganisms, or by the body itself such as hormones, natural blood products, or vaccines. *Alternative therapies* include natural plant extracts, herbs, vitamins, minerals, dietary supplemental, and therapeutic techniques that may be considered unconventional such as acupuncture (Adams, Josephson, and Holland, 2005).

The professional radiographer who administers drugs is expected to know the safe dosage, the safe route of administration, limitations of the drug he administers, the **side effects,** the potential **adverse** and **toxic reactions,** the **indications** and **contraindications** for its use. He must also know the potential hazards of any drug that is incorrectly or unsafely administered. If drug administration errors are made due to lack of knowledge, the person who administers the drug is legally liable. Radiologic technology students who are permitted to administer drugs must adhere to the specific ethical and legal guidelines established for drug administration. The student must be supervised by a licensed professional; professional liability coverage must be adequate and the student must also demonstrate competency before performing drug administration without supervision.

> **📣 CALL OUT!**
>
> Any radiographer or radiographic technology student who administers drugs must demonstrate competency before administering drugs without supervision.

Pharmacology and its clinical application is a scientific discipline unto itself and cannot be covered adequately without combining theoretical knowledge and clinical coursework. Drug therapy is a complex and ever-changing aspect of patient care. The radiographer is not licensed to dispense drugs. He cannot enter a hospital pharmacy and select a drug. He is legally liable if any drug taken from a dispensary results in adverse effects. If a drug error is made by the radiographer, he must document the incident completely and fill out an institutional incident report according to the policy of the facility in which he is employed.

DRUG STANDARDS AND CONTROL

The federal government of the United States has strict standards for control of drug safety that are strictly enforced. In the early 1900s drug enforcement laws were established to ensure the safety of drugs sold for public use. Through the years these laws have been amended to ascertain that drugs are thoroughly tested and proven safe before marketing. Table 15-1 lists the most recent laws that regulate drug production and sale.

There are a list of drugs that must bear the legend "caution: federal law prohibits dispensing without prescription." They are as follows:

Drugs that must be administered **parenterally**
Drugs that are **hypnotic** or **narcotic**
Drugs that may cause **dependence**
Drugs that contain derivatives of habit-forming substances
Drugs that may be toxic if not administered under the supervision of a physician, dentist, or nurse practitioner
Drugs that are new and limited to investigational use and are not safe if indiscriminately used

Drugs that are considered safe for self-administration are called over-the-counter drugs (OTC drugs). Some drugs that must be prescribed may also be purchased as OTC drugs because they are marketed in a lesser potency when sold in this manner. OTC drugs must also be reviewed by a panel of reviewers appointed by the FDA and deemed safe for self-administration. When taking a patient's drug history as part of an initial interview, note that the patient's use of OTC drugs and alternative medications is important information because these agents may affect treatment.

The use of alternative therapies by the general public has increased tremendously in the past 5 years. In 2004 sales of herbal and dietary supplements has grown into an over $4.4 billion dollar business. This amount does not include massage therapy, yoga, and

TABLE 15-1   Laws That Regulate Drug Production and Sale

1906: **Food and Drug Administration (FDA):** established as an agency of the Department of Health and Human Services. Branches of the FDA include the Center for Drug Evaluation and Research, which controls whether prescription drugs and over-the-counter drugs may be used for therapy, and the Center for Biologics Evaluation and Research, which regulates use of serums, vaccines, and blood products.

1938: **Food, Drug and Cosmetic Act:** prevents marketing of drugs not thoroughly tested. Provides the requirement that drug companies must apply to the Food and Drug Administration before marketing any new drug.

1986: **Childhood Vaccine Act:** regulates safety of biologics.

1992: **Prescription Drug User Fee Act:** requires nongeneric drug and biologic manufacturers to pay fees to be used for improvements in drug review.

1994: **Dietary Supplement Health and Education Act:** requires clear labeling of dietary supplements and allows the FDA to remove those that are a risk to the public.

1997: **FDA Modernization Act:** reauthorizes the Prescription Drug User Fee Act and reforms the drug review process.

other healing methods that do not involve the ingestion of a substance.

Alternative dietary and herbal supplements are not regulated by the FDA. They are regulated and classified as foods, not drugs. There is no requirement to prove the efficacy, quality, or safety of these substances. The Dietary Supplement Health and Education Act enacted in 1994 forbids the producers of these drugs from making claims that discuss disease or the cure of an ailment; however, they may claim effectiveness on body structure and/or function. This act deemed these products independent of FDA rules.

Supplements in this classification are too numerous to include in this text, but the radiographer taking a health and medication history must include questions concerning the patient's use of these substances as many may react in an adverse manner with other drugs.

Since 1980 the only official books or publications of drug standards in the United States are the *United States Pharmacopeia* (USP) and the *National Formulary* (NF). The drugs listed in these books meet the high standards of quality, purity, and strength. There are several other good references for drugs that one may consult in the clinical area; however, drugs that meet the criteria of the United States Pharmacopeia can be identified by the letters USP after the drug's official name.

Great Britain and Canada also have strict drug legislation programs. The United Nations, through the World Health Organization, provides technical assistance with drug research and use. Drug enforcement agencies throughout the world cooperate to control the use and problems associated with habit-forming drugs internationally.

DRUG CONTROL

Drug abuse continues to increase in the United States and throughout the world with each passing year. The words *addiction* and *dependence* are often used interchangeably. **Addiction** refers to an overwhelming feeling of physical need for a particular drug that must be met at all costs. Dependence may be a physical or psychological need for a particular drug. If the need is physical, when the drug is no longer available, the body develops physical signs of discomfort that are called *withdrawal.* If the need is psychological, the dependent person has no physical signs of discomfort, but continues to need the feeling that the drug produces. These abnormal needs create addiction and potential for abuse of a drug.

In an effort to restrict drug abuse, the United States enacted the Controlled Substances Act in 1971. This law was also meant to increase research and to assist persons dependent on drugs with rehabilitation. In 1973, the Drug Enforcement Administration (DEA) in the Department of Justice became the nation's only legal drug enforcement agency.

Drugs labeled as controlled substances have been categorized by the Controlled Substances Act into schedules according to numbers related to their potential for abuse. The drug schedules are listed in Table 15-2.

DRUG SOURCES, NAMES, AND ACTIONS

Drugs come from many natural and synthetic sources. Some are produced from animal sources such as hormonal drugs. Many come from plant sources such as

TABLE 15-2   Drug Schedules

Schedule	Characteristics	Dispensing Restrictions	Examples
I	High abuse potential; not recognized for medical use; may lead to severe dependence	Limited or no therapeutic use	Heroin, LSD, marijuana, cocaine, and others
II	High abuse potential; accepted for medical use; may lead to severe dependence	Hand-written prescription by a licensed person; no refills; container must have warning label	Opioids, methadone, morphine, and others
III	Less abuse potential; accepted for medical use; may lead to dependence	Written or oral prescription required; container must have warning label	Codeine, hydrocodeine with aspirin or Tylenol, nonamphetamine stimulants
IV	Lower abuse potential; may lead to limited dependence	Written or oral prescription that expires in 6 months	Benzodiazepines, nonnarcotic analgesics
V	Low level of dependence	May or may not require prescription	Antidiarrheals, cough medicines with codeine

digitalis and atropine. Others are produced from microorganisms as are many antibiotics. Minerals are the source of calcium, iron, and other dietary supplements and herbal remedies. Drugs from synthetic materials are made in laboratories. Some drugs are genetically engineered and used to treat specific diseases. Epoetin alfa (Epogen), used to treat some anemias, is an example of such a drug.

Learning drug names is complicated because most drugs have several names. The same drug may be sold under many different *proprietary* or *trade* names. The trade or proprietary name is assigned to a drug by a particular manufacturer of the drug. In the United States, the initial developer of a drug has an exclusive right to name and market a drug for 17 years. Because it often takes several years for that drug to be approved for general use, some of those 17 years may be lost before it is marketed. No other company is allowed to produce this drug until the 17 years has expired.

The *chemical name* of a drug presents its exact chemical formula of a drug and always remains the same. The chemical name is often cumbersome, and one is seldom required to remember it as it is rarely used in daily clinical practice.

The *generic name* of a drug is the name given to the drug before its official approval for use. It is assigned by the United States Adopted Name Council. Usually the generic name is less complicated and easier to remember than the chemical name. This is the name

used by the FDA, the U.S. Pharmacopoeia, and the World Health Organization to describe the drug. There is one generic name for each drug and, because it is often used, it must be learned by all persons who administer drugs. For instance, a drug frequently administered prior to imaging procedures is **parenteral** diazepam. Diazepam is the generic name for Valium, and its chemical formula is 7-chloro-1,3-dihydro-1-methl-5-phenyl-2H-1,4-benzodiazepin-2-one. The radiographer must be able to identify drugs by their trade name and their generic name. It is not essential to learn the chemical formula of each drug.

A drug does not have the capacity to change cellular structure, but acts to either increase or decrease the rate and range of a normal or abnormal physiologic process going on within the cells of the body. Drugs are administered for a number of reasons. They are as follows: to relieve undesired symptoms; to prevent disease; to cure disease; and to diagnose disease or pathological conditions. The radiographer administers drugs primarily to diagnose disease or pathological conditions. On occasion, he may administer a drug to relieve anxiety or pain prior to a diagnostic procedure.

Drugs are absorbed, distributed, metabolized, and then excreted from the body. As this process takes place, the drug reaches a point at which it has its *intended effect.* This is called the *onset of action.* As it continues to be absorbed, the drug reaches its *peak concentration level.*

This is the time during which the drug attains its *maximum therapeutic response.* This means that the drug is able to produce its most desired curative or remedial effect. The time during which the drug is in the body in an amount large enough to be therapeutic is called its *duration of action.* As the drug is excreted from the body, the concentration level subsides to a point at which there is little or no intended effect.

It is seldom possible for a health care practitioner to keep up with all new drugs that are marketed. Anyone who administers drugs must be able to obtain information concerning any drug he administers from reliable sources before he administers a drug with which he is not familiar. Some reliable references are as follows: *The American Hospital Formulary Service Drug Information, Drug Facts and Comparisons, Handbook of Nonprescription Drugs, Physician's Desk Reference (PDR),and United States Pharmacopeia.* All of these references are updated yearly. The radiographer must learn where a reliable drug reference is available in his workplace and consult it as necessary. A current pharmacology textbook should be a part of the library of any person who administers drugs.

THE ACTION OF DRUGS WITHIN THE BODY

Depending on their physical makeup, drugs taken into the body act in different ways. All drugs must be in liquid form to be absorbed. For this reason, drugs that are administered in solid or tablet form must go through a phase called the *pharmaceutic phase* before they can be absorbed. This means that the solid form of the drug must be broken down into tiny particles to be dissolved into the body fluids of the gastrointestinal tract. Enteric-coated tablets do not go through the pharmaceutic phase of absorption until they reach the small intestine where they are dissolved in an alkaline media. Drugs that are administered orally in liquid form or drugs that are administered parenterally do not go through this phase.

PHARMACOKINETICS

The processes that control absorption, distribution, metabolism, and excretion of drugs by the body are called *pharmacokinetics.* All persons process drugs differently depending on their age, nutritional status, ethnicity, existing physical condition, immune status, state of mind, sex, weight, environmental factors, and time of day.

A drug must advance from its dosage form into a form that makes it biologically available for passage into the systemic circulation. In other words, a drug must be absorbed and taken through the bloodstream

to its intended site in order to act. The amount of drug that actually reaches the systemic circulation becomes *bioavailable* or reaches a state of bioavailability. Drug absorption varies from person to person and depends on the absorptive surface available. A damaged or absent intended drug surface alters the length of time it takes a drug to reach its intended site. Drugs may be absorbed by either passive or active transport or by *pinocytosis,* a form of active transport.

Drugs move to their site of absorption and then must penetrate the cell membrane at that site. This is accomplished by varying methods. One method is *passive diffusion,* which requires no cellular energy. The drug simply moves across a cell membrane from another area of lower concentration to one of higher concentration. When the concentration equalizes on both sides of the cell membrane, the transport is complete. *Lipid solubility* is the most important determinant in deciding whether a drug will cross cell membranes, although water solubility is also of importance. Most drugs cross cell membranes by passive diffusion.

Active transport is another method of drug absorption. This method requires energy from the cell and a carrier molecule such as an enzyme or protein that forms complexes with drug molecules on the membrane surface to carry them through the membrane and then leave them by disassociation. Active transport is necessary to move some drugs and electrolytes such as sodium and potassium from outside to inside a cell. *Pinocytosis* is a type of active transport in which a cell engulfs a drug particle, forms a protective coat around it, and transports it across the cell membrane. Fat-soluble vitamins are transported in this manner.

Drugs taken orally are usually absorbed in the small intestine, which has a large surface for absorption. If a portion of the small intestine has been removed or is scarred, the ability to absorb a drug is reduced.

The quantity of blood flow to absorption surfaces affects the rate at which a drug is absorbed. For instance, a drug is absorbed much more rapidly when it is administered intramuscularly in the deltoid muscle than in the gluteal muscle because the blood flow is greater in the deltoid. A person who is in severe pain or in a state of acute stress may have decreased ability to absorb a drug.

First-Pass Effect

When a drug is taken by mouth and swallowed into the stomach, it goes from the small intestine to the mesenteric vascular system, and then to the portal vein, and from there into the liver before it is transported into the systemic circulation. Because of this travel through the gastric and hepatic circulation, a portion of the drug is metabolized en route and becomes inactive. This partial metabolism of a drug before it reaches the systemic circulation is called a *first-pass effect.* In the cases of many drugs taken orally, this effect requires that a larger dose of a drug be administered so that a portion of the drug remains to perform its intended effect. Drugs that can be administered by **sublingual, vaginal,** or parenteral route avoid the first-pass effect by going directly into the systemic circulation; however, these routes of administration may be contraindicated for other reasons.

Some drugs, after absorption, are moved from the bloodstream into the liver and then through the biliary tract, where they are excreted in bile or return to the small intestine and back into the bloodstream. This action, called *enterohepatic recycling,* allows the drug to persist in the body for long periods of time.

> **⚠ WARNING!**
> The dosages of most drugs given by mouth are generally much larger than those given by parenteral routes because they are susceptible to the first-pass effect!

Distribution

After a drug is absorbed into the body, it is distributed to its intended target site. The rate and extent of distribution depends on adequate blood circulation, protein binding, and the drug's affinity for **lipoid** or **aqueous** tissues. Drugs move quickly to body organs that have a rich supply of blood, such as the heart, liver, and kidneys. They reach muscles and fatty tissues more slowly.

As a drug travels through the circulatory system, it may come into contact with plasma proteins and bind to them or remain free. If bound to plasma protein, the drug becomes inactive. Only free drugs are able to act on cells. As the free drug acts, there is a decrease in plasma drug levels, which allows a portion of the bound drug to be released and become active. The slow release of the drug allows blood levels of a drug to remain somewhat constant. The health status of the person receiving the drug and the drug itself affects drug distribution.

If two or more drugs compete for a plasma-binding site, the drug with the strongest **affinity** for the site acquires it. This allows a greater amount of the other drug free to act and may result in a **toxic level** of that drug or result in a **drug-drug interaction.**

Lipid-soluble drugs are stored in lipoid tissues. Highly lipid-soluble drugs remain stored in fatty tissues and are released very slowly. Drugs that are intended to penetrate the **blood-brain barrier** must be highly lipid soluble and bind minimally with plasma proteins to achieve their intended effect.

Because of the nonselective nature of the placenta, most drugs are able to pass that barrier and affect the developing fetus. The toxicity of drugs to the fetus during the **first trimester of pregnancy** makes it mandatory that the pregnant mother receive no medication without the explicit orders of her physician. Only drugs that are absolutely necessary to maintain the optimum health of the mother should be given. This is important for the radiographer to remember as he cares for female patients of childbearing age.

> **⚠ WARNING!**
> All female patients of childbearing age must be screened before receiving any drug to ascertain whether they are pregnant!

Metabolism

The process by which the body alters the chemical structure of a drug or other foreign substance is called *metabolism* or *biotransformation.* These terms are interchangeable. Generally, this process reduces lipid solubility to render the drug ready for excretion.

Most drugs are metabolized in the liver by means of a complex chemical action involving enzymes. These enzymes act on a wide variety of compounds. In certain drugs, tissues from plasma, kidneys, lungs, and the intestinal mucosa may be involved.

Age, health status, time of day, emotional status, the presence of other drugs in the body, genetic variations, and disease states may alter the rate of drug metabolism. An altered metabolic state may allow a drug to accumulate in the body and produce an adverse reaction. Conversely, rapid metabolism of a drug may interfere with the intended effect. Drugs administered orally are significantly metabolized by the first-pass effect through the liver, which also alters their metabolism.

Excretion

Excretion of drugs from the body takes place chiefly in the kidneys. Some drugs are excreted virtually unchanged through the kidneys whereas others are extensively metabolized with only a small amount of the original drug remaining.

Other sites of drug excretion are through the biliary tract and into the feces or through the enterohepatic cycle and later into the kidneys. Gases and volatile liquids used for anesthesia are excreted by the lungs. Sweat and saliva are of minimal importance in drug excretion.

Some drugs or drug metabolites may cross the epithelium of the mammary glands and be excreted in breast milk. This is important if the mother is breastfeeding an infant and a drug, particularly a narcotic drug, is transferred in high concentrations to the infant.

Half-life

The time it takes for a 50% decrease in a drug's presence in the body is called its *half-life*. It is important for a prescribing health care worker to understand a drug's half-life in order to attain a steady-state concentration in the body. To attain this steady-state, the same amount of a drug must be taken in, as is eliminated in, each 24-hour period. Drugs with a short half-life need to be administered more frequently than a drug with a prolonged half-life in order to be at maximum therapeutic level at all times.

A drug's removal from the body is called its *clearance rate.* The clearance rate of a drug is an important consideration, because a drug with a slow clearance rate that is given too often may accumulate in the body and reach a toxic level.

◼ PHARMACODYNAMICS

Pharmacodynamics is the study of the method or mechanism of drug action on living tissues or the response of tissues to chemical agents at various sites in the body. Drugs may alter physiologic effects in the body in the following ways:

1. By altering blood pressure
2. By altering heart rate
3. By altering urinary output
4. By altering function of the central or peripheral nervous system
5. By altering changes in all other body systems

Drugs do not produce new functions on tissues or organs of the body. Usually, a primary site of drug action is targeted by a drug that is administered systemically; nevertheless, all body tissues are affected in some way by every drug administered.

The intent of drug therapy is to produce a therapeutic effect that may be to control pain, cure a particular disease, alleviate symptoms of a disease, or diagnose a disease. The radiographer will be involved most of the time with drugs used to diagnose disease.

The particular area for which a drug is intended and that receives a maximum effect of a drug is called the *drug receptor.* The function of a cell is altered but not completely changed by a drug. A drug receptor is a **macromolecular** component of body tissue.

Drug receptors have an *affinity* for a particular drug. This means that there is an attraction between the drug and the receptor. Affinity is the factor that determines the concentration of drug necessary to accomplish its intended effect. If there is a strong affinity at the receptor site, the concentration of drug necessary to accomplish its effect is low. This is referred to as the *efficacy* of the drug.

There are both drug *agonists* and *antagonists.* Agonists are drugs that are able to bind with receptors to produce a therapeutic response. Partial binding at the receptor site is also possible and this produces only partial therapeutic response. These are called *partial agonists.* A drug antagonist joins with a receptor and prevents the agonist from performing its intended effect.

The molecular structure of each drug determines the affinity for a receptor. A very small change in a drug molecule can leave the drug's affinity to a receptor unchanged but drastically change the pharmacological action of a drug.

Many drugs exert more than one effect on the body. For instance, a drug given at the recommended dosage will have the intended effect; however, if given in a larger dose, it may have an undesirable effect. The relation between the dosage at which the intended effect of a drug is obtained and the amount that produces an unwanted effect is called the *therapeutic index.* The greater the therapeutic index, the safer the drug is since more can be tolerated without *adverse effect.*

◼ ADVERSE DRUG REACTIONS

Any person who participates in drug administration must be aware of the potential harm that may result from drugs. They may produce many unintended effects. When a drug produces an effect that is mild, common, unintended, and nontoxic, this text will refer to the effect as a *side effect.* When a drug produces an effect that is more severe or life-threatening, it will be referred to as an *adverse effect.* Some adverse effects occur almost immediately after the drug is administered, and some take weeks or months of administration before an untoward reaction is produced.

A *toxic reaction* is an unwanted effect that is an extension of the therapeutic effect, such as an extension of the therapeutic effect. A drug that, when given in the prescribed amount, is therapeutic may become toxic when given in an increased amount; this is considered as overdose. A toxic reaction does not include an allergic reaction or anaphylactic shock, which is classified as an adverse reaction.

Immediate adverse reactions to drugs can include gastric distress and allergic or hypertensive reactions that may range from mild **urticaria** to severe anaphylactic shock. Some drugs are disease-producing themselves and may produce **blood dyscrasias**, hepatic disease, gastric ulcerations, or thrombosis.

Since drugs are tested extensively before they are permitted to be marketed, most adverse reactions have been documented, and it is known that these reactions may occur. The therapeutic or diagnostic purpose of a drug is weighed against the risk factors prior to administration. If the need outweighs the risk, it is prescribed by the physician with caution.

The patient must be educated regarding the potential adverse effects of a drug before it is administered. He must be instructed to notify his physician if adverse reactions occur. Particular care must be given to pregnant women and nursing mothers. All health care workers who administer drugs have the responsibility to understand and educate their patients about any drug that they administer.

> ### (((CALL OUT!
>
> It is the responsibility of all health care workers who administer drugs to understand and educate their patients about any drug they administer!

An unexpected or exacerbated effect from a drug is called a *drug idiosyncrasy*. For example, a drug given to produce sleep instead produces a hyperactive reaction. The cause of this reaction is not clear, but may be due to a genetic deficiency that creates an inability to tolerate certain chemicals.

Drug tolerance occurs when a drug received continually for a length of time creates a change in the response to that drug. Usually, the drug is needed in increasingly larger doses to create the desired effect. Drug tolerance is a sign of drug dependence, and the drugs that are related to this problem are narcotics and tranquilizers. *Tachyphylaxis* is a rapid development of tolerance to a drug.

DRUG INTERACTIONS

The radiographer must learn to consult a *drug compatibility* chart before attempting to mix two drugs into the same syringe. Many drugs, combined with another drug, can become inactivated or form a toxic compound. At times, when two drugs are combined, they increase the effect of each drug when given alone. An example of this is a dose of heparin when given with alcohol increases bleeding. This can equate to one plus one equaling two and is called an *additive reaction. A synergistic drug reaction* may occur when two drugs interact to equal an effect greater than the sum of their separate dosage.

Some drugs are *antagonistic* to other drugs or interfere with the action of another drug. When this occurs the intended drug effect is either neutralized or decreased.

> ### ⚠ WARNING!
>
> Always check a drug compatibility chart or consult the pharmacist before mixing two drugs for administration! Never assume that related drugs can be combined. This may not be the case!

Drugs may also be affected by food if given orally. Directions for drug administration list whether the drug should be taken on an empty stomach or taken with food. These directions must be taken seriously as some drugs may be absorbed into the bloodstream more quickly with food and others may need to be taken on an empty stomach to enhance absorption.

Drugs must be stored according to manufacturer's directions. Drugs that are incorrectly stored may loose their effect quickly.

> ### ⚠ WARNING!
>
> If a drug has a sediment or is discolored, it must not be used. This includes intravenous fluids!

EMERGENCY DRUG USE

Medical personnel who use drugs and equipment from an emergency cart in departments where medical care is rendered must have special education in emergency drug use. These drugs, if used incorrectly, can have lethal effects. Although some emergency drugs are listed in this text, the explanations given here are not adequate to qualify the radiographer to administer them. Health care institutions must have staff members specifically trained in emergency drug procedures and equipment use.

The radiographer has an obligation to know the location of the emergency cart, how to gain access to it when it is needed, and how to summon the emergency team in a timely manner. In a department with limited staff, he may be responsible for maintaining the completeness and currency of the drugs and equipment on the emergency cart. If this is the case, the radiographer must be educated to do this, and maintenance must be done on a daily basis and after each use.

> ### ⚠ WARNING!
>
> During an emergency is not the time to update emergency drugs and equipment. Every minute lost in this pursuit is life-threatening for the patient!

FACTORS ALTERING DRUG RESPONSE

The age of a patient; his weight, gender, and health status; and the route of administration must be considered prior to administering a drug. The number of drugs the patient takes on a regular basis must be considered. Each patient must be assessed before any drug is given. It is not possible in this text to list all of the drugs that may result in adverse effects; however, the radiographer must be aware of all special problems the patient may have. Table 15-3 lists special considerations for patients receiving drugs.

DRUG CLASSIFICATION

Drugs may be classified in several ways. They can be grouped according to their physiologic effects on receptors, their physiologic effects on specific body systems, or their overall physiologic effects. This chapter provides only a brief overview of the physiologic effects of certain drugs on body systems. Contrast agents are discussed, as are some drugs used in imaging and those found on the emergency drug cart.

> ### 📢 CALL OUT!
>
> The drug descriptions in Table 15-4 do not adequately explain the nature of these drugs to anyone who plans to participate in drug administration!

Drugs used in imaging and elsewhere in the practice of medicine are constantly changing. New and better preparations are appearing on the market monthly, and the personnel administering them must be educated in their use before using them.

Table 15-4 lists drugs that are currently in use that the radiographer may encounter in his practice and drugs found on the emergency cart.

CLASSIFICATION OF CONTRAST AGENTS

Approximately 30% of all imaging examinations involve the use of a form of contrast media to aid in the visualization of a body part or body system. The radiographer must have a fundamental understanding of these agents. Contrast agents are categorized as drugs because they can be absorbed into the systemic circulation and may produce a physiologic response on the body. The radiographer must use extreme caution when preparing a contrast agent for injection or ingestion.

Contrast agents are required to visualize areas of the body when the organ or system of interest is too similar to the surrounding area. When an anatomical area is filled or outlined by a positive contrast agent, the organ appears to be *radiopaque* meaning white or light on the image. Negative contrast agents make the organ appear darker on the image. This is known as being *radiolucent.* Negative contrast agents are rarely used in the imaging department because computerized tomography (CT) and magnetic resonance imaging (MRI) have replaced procedures that were once performed with these gaseous materials. Radiopaque contrast media (ROCM) are what the radiographer will be working with most frequently.

Barium is the most common type of contrast used in imaging of the gastrointestinal system (GI). Barium is a metal and does not dissolve; therefore, it is suspended in solution. The metallic component of barium makes it an ideal substance for use as a contrast agent. Gastrografin is another type of contrast used for GI imaging and was discussed in a previous chapter.

All positive contrast agents, except barium, used in diagnostic imaging contain iodine. The high atomic number of iodine, barium, and bromine gives them the ability to decrease radiographic density on the image receptor. Iodine, with an atomic number of 53, is able to absorb the x-ray photons, thus allowing the area of interest to be seen on the radiographic image as a white area (Fig. 15-1). Barium has the atomic number of the metal, barium (56), and is able to accomplish the same absorption of x-ray photons and the same radiopaque image.

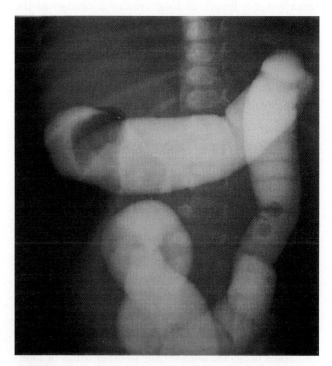

FIGURE 15-1 White area of interest created by use of barium.

TABLE 15-3   Special Considerations When Administering Drugs

Age Group	Physiologic Changes	Precautions
Pregnant women	Many drugs cross the placental barrier. Drug effects depend on fetal age and can result in harm to the fetus.	Drugs during pregnancy must be avoided or administered only to women who absolutely require treatment. If in doubt, inform patient's physician of possible pregnancy before administering any drug.
Infants	Lack well-developed muscle mass; lack the protective mechanisms of older children and adults. Skin is thin and permeable; stomachs lack mucous barrier; temperature control is poor; they become dehydrated easily and have immature liver and kidneys that cannot manage foreign chemicals.	Only persons educated in drug administration to infants must administer medications to them.
Breastfed infants	May have all drugs in maternal circulation transferred to colostrum and breast milk.	Mothers who are breastfeeding may be advised by the physician to cease breastfeeding for a prescribed time if they are to receive radioisotopes or radiation. All other drug therapies must be evaluated as they may harm the infant. A detailed history must be taken, and no drugs should be administered without establishing that they will not harm the infant.
Pediatric patients	At 1 year of age, liver metabolizes more rapidly than in adults; renal function may be more rapid than adults. Standard dosage for children depends on child's weight or body surface. Topical drugs are more easily absorbable through the skin.	Children are not small adults! Physiologic differences vary, and only those experienced in medicating children must administer drugs to them! Topical drugs and solutions, including antiseptics, can cause poisoning in children. Cleanse only with soap and water.
Elderly patients	Blood-brain barrier is more easily penetrated, with increaseing rate of dizziness and confusion. Reduced baroreceptor response increases hypotensive effects of some drugs. Liver size, blood flow, and enzyme production decrease, increasing the half-life of some drugs and leading to possible toxic reactions. Increased adipose tissue in abdominal area may lead to toxicity from fat-soluble drugs. Decreased renal blood flow and filtration decrease elimination of drugs from the body. Slower gastric emptying time and increase in pH of gastric juices increase risk of gastric irritation.	Drugs affecting the central nervous system and cardiovascular system must be given with extreme caution. Patients must be monitored closely and assisted with ambulation to prevent falls. Do not allow elderly patients who have been given drugs to leave the area unattended.

TABLE 15-4   Classification of Drugs

Trade name	Generic name	Uses	Adverse effects
Adrenergic drugs: Constrict blood vessels and stimulate the heart. Many in this category are used in cardiovascular, respiratory, and allergic emergencies.			
Intropin (found on emergency drug cart)	dopamine	shock due to trauma, myocardial infarct, renal failure, chronic cardiac decompensation	hypotension, dyspnea, anginal pain, nausea
Adrenalin chloride (found on emergency cart)	epinephrine	cardiac arrest, acute asthma, hay fever	anxiety, insomnia, restlessness, nausea
Levophed	norepinephrine	shock, hypotension, cardiac arrest	restlessness, hypertension
Isuprel (found on emergency cart)	isoproterenol	shock, acute renal failure	tachycardia, tremors, bronchial edema
Adrenergic blocking agents: Cause increased peripheral circulation and decreased blood pressure.			
Tenormin	atenolol	hypertension, angina	bradycardia, weakness, hypotension
Inderal (found on emergency drug cart)	propranolol	cardiac arrhythmias, myocardial infarct, hypertension	bradycardia, hypotension, hyperglycemia
Antimuscarinic drugs: Increase cardiac output, constrict blood vessels, decrease saliva and bronchial secretions.			
Atropine (found on emergency drug carts)	atropine sulfate	bradycardia, bradyarrhythmia, preoperatively to prevent salivary and bronchial secretions	dry mouth; bradycardia, tachycardia, urine retention
Scopolamine hydrobromide	hyoscine butylbromide	used to treat motion sickness, gastric disturbance, as a preliminary to anesthesia	tachycardia, dry mouth, delirium
Calcium channel blockers: Reduce calcium flow to heart and thereby relax smooth muscle tone and reduce muscle spasm.			
Cardizem (found on emergency drug cart)	diltiazem	used to treat angina and hypertension	peripheral edema, bradycardia
Calan (found on emergency drug carts)	verapamil hydrochloride	used to treat angina, cardiac arrhythmias, hypertension	peripheral edema, bradycardia
Cardiotonics: Increase force of contractions of the heart to reverse cardiac symptoms.			
Lanoxin	digoxin	used to treat congestive heart failure and cardiac arrhythmias	cardiac toxicity, hypertension, cardiac arrest
Dobutrex	dobutamine	short-term treatment of shock related to heart failure	increased heart rate, headache

(continued)

TABLE 15-4   (Continued)

Trade name	Generic name	Uses	Adverse effects
Direct-acting vasodilators: Used for severe hypertension by directly affecting arteriolar smooth muscle. Produce too many adverse effects to be drugs of choice.			
Hyperstat IV	diazoxide	used for hypertensive crisis	headache, seizures, cerebral ischemia
Apresoline	hydralazine	used for severe essential hypertension	tachycardia, lupus-like syndrome
Antiarrhythmics: Used to correct arrhythmias of the heart due to electrical abnormalities in formation or conduction that may be life-threatening.			
Quinaglute (found on emergency drug cart)	quinidine	used to maintain normal cardiac rhythm	hypotension, heart block, liver toxicity
Xylocaine (found on emergency drug cart)	lidocaine hydrochloride	used to treat serious ventricular arrhythmias, also used as local anesthetic	cardiac arrest, respiratory depression, convulsions
Cordarone (found on emergency drug cart)	amiodarone hydro-chloride	used to treat life-threatening ventricular fibrillation	pulmonary toxicity, ataxia, hypothyroidism
Organic nitrates: Used to relax smooth muscles of both arteries and veins; may be short-acting or long-acting.			
Nitrostat	nitroglycerin	short-acting, used to treat sudden onset of **angina** pain	headache, fainting, nausea
Transderm-nitro	nitroglycerine	long-acting patch used to prevent or minimize angina	**cutaneous vasodilatation**, dermatitis
Diuretics: Reduce blood volume through urinary excretion of water to treat hypertension.			
Lasix (found on emergency drug carts)	furosemide	used to treat hypertension, acute pulmonary edema, and congestive heart failure	**hypokalemia**, muscle cramps, nausea
Hydrazide	hydrochlorothiazide	used to treat hypertension	dizziness, weakness, pancreatitis
Analgesics, Antipyretics, and anti-inflammatory drugs: Used to reduce pain, reduce fever, and reduce inflammation in tissues.			
Motrin, Advil, etc.	ibuprofen analgesic drugs (NSAID)	used to treat moderate pain usually related to muscle or **neurologic** origins	gastric distress, renal failure, prolonged bleed time
Aspirin	acetylsalicylic acid	used to treat mild pain or fever, arthritic conditions and inflammatory conditions, to prevent **thrombosis**	**tinnitus**, nausea, gastro-intestinal bleeding
Tylenol	acetaminophen	used to treat moderate pain without anti-inflammatory effects	liver toxicity, hemolytic anemia, skin rash
Opioid analgesics (narcotic): Used to control intense pain and the anxiety that results.			
Morphine	morphine sulfate	all are used to control severe pain; all may create dependence; all are kept in locked cupboards	nausea, restlessness, respiratory depression, shock, death
Demerol	meperidine hydrochloride		
Duragesic	fentanyl citrate		

(continued)

TABLE 15-4 (Continued)

Trade name	Generic name	Uses	Adverse effects
Opioid analgesics with mild to moderate efficacy: Used for less severe pain.			
Codeine Percocet Darvon	codeine sulfate oxycodone hydrochloride propoxyphene napsylate	all used alone and in various combinations with milder analgesics to control less severe pain	sedation, clouded sensorium, dizziness, nausea, constipation, dependence
Antianxiety drugs: Benzodiazepines are used for treatment of anxiety and, in some cases, to treat behavior disorders.			

Xanax
Ativan
Valium (found on
  emergency drug
  carts)
	alprazolam
	lorazepam
	diazepam
		all used to reduce anxiety;
		  at higher doses, produce hypnosis,
		  relax muscles, and may reduce
		  seizure activity
			bradycardia,
			drowsiness,
			severe withdrawal reaction
			  with prolonged use;
			dependence

Drugs affecting the blood: Are used to prevent thrombus formations prior to surgical and imaging procedures. They are also used to prevent extension of thrombi after myocardial infarction, strokes, and pulmonary embolism and venous thrombosis.			

Heparin
 	
Coumadin
	heparin sodium
	
	warfarin sodium
		inhibits formation or fibrin
		  clots; used to maintain
		  potency of venous catheters
		prevention of emboli in
		  chronic atrial fibrillation, deep
		  vein thrombosis, heart
		  valve damage
			hemorrhage,
			  thrombocytopenia,
			  allergic reactions
			hemorrhage, hematuria,
			  hepatitis

Antihyperlipidemic drugs: All are used to prevent formation of atherosclerotic plaques in the blood; thereby preventing strokes and myocardial infarction.			

Lipitor
Mevacor
Zocor
	atorvastatin
	lovastatin
	simvastatin
		lowers LDL cholesterol
		  and total cholesterol in
		  the blood
			headache, nausea,
			arthralgia, liver
			toxicity

Drugs affecting the respiratory system: Used to treat a wide range of respiratory problems; however, those named in this text are used to treat severe disorders seen by the radiographer in his practice.			

Adrenalin
  (listed with adrenergic
  drugs found on
  emergency drug cart)
Proventil
Aminophylline
  seizures
	epinephrine
	
	albuterol sulfate
	theophylline
		all used to treat bronchospasm,
		  asthmatic attacks and
		  anaphylaxis
		
		used to treat chronic
		obstructive pulmonary disease
			shock, loss
			  of appetite,
			  respiratory arrest,
			  dyspnea tremor, muscle
			  cramps, cardiac
			  arrhythmias

Antihistamines: Used to treat anaphylactic shock, upper respiratory disorders, acute urticaria, edema, hypersensitivity reactions, motion sickness, and nausea. Some are used OTC as sleep medications.			

Benadryl (found
  on emergency
  drug carts)
Chlor-trimeton
 	
Phenergan
	diphenhydramine
	
	chlorpheniramine
	
	promethazine
		used to prevent anaphylaxis
		
		used to treat symptoms
		  of colds and allergies
		used often for sedative effects;
		  for motion sickness
			drowsiness, dizziness,
			  dry mouth,

⚠️ **WARNING!**

Do not administer antihistamines to patients with asthma or to patients who are to operate motor vehicles!

(continued)

TABLE 15-4   (Continued)

Trade name	Generic name	Uses	Adverse effects
Antiemetic drugs: Used to treat motion sickness, nausea and vomiting. All are used for similar purposes but belong to various drug categories and have various adverse effects.			
Compazine	prochlorperazine	the radiographer administering	
Transderm-Scop	scopolamine	these drugs must familiarize himself	
Dramamine	dimenhydrinate	with the potential adverse effects of	
Vistaril	hydroxyzine	these drugs individually	
Drugs that act on the gastrointestinal (GI) system: Drugs in this category are used to treat gastric ulcers, esophageal reflux, constipation, and diarrhea.			
Tagamet	cimetidine	all used for short-term palliative	diarrhea,
Zantac	ranitidine	treatment of peptic ulcers, gastro-	confusion,
Pepcid	famotidine	esophageal reflux, heartburn	anxiety,
Prilosec	omeprazole		headache
Protonix	pantoprazole		
Antacids: Used to treat heartburn and indigestion by neutralizing gastric acidity and decreasing the rate of gastric emptying time.			
Amphogel	aluminum hydroxide		diarrhea,
Maalox	magnesium hydroxide and		intestinal
Sodium bicarbonate	aluminum hydroxide also		impaction,
(found on emergency	used in cardiac arrest to		alkalosis
drug cart)	reduce acidosis		
Drugs used to treat constipation: Drugs used to treat constipation are classified as either *cathartics or laxatives.* Cathartics cause bowel evacuation by increasing peristalsis, and laxatives promote bowel evacuation by increasing the bulk of the feces, by softening the stool, or by lubricating the intestinal wall. Laxatives are generally less harsh than cathartics.			
Some examples of each follow:			
Milk of Magnesia	magnesium hydroxide	a saline cathartic	hypokalemia,
Cascara sagrada		an irritant cathartic	abdominal
			cramping, nausea
Colace	docusate sodium	a stool softener	all drugs used to
Metamucil	psyllium	a bulk-forming	treat constipa-
		laxative	tion may result
			in dependence
Drugs used to treat diarrhea: All may result in fecal impaction and abdominal cramping.			
Pepto-Bismol	bismuth subsalicylate		
Imodium	loperamide		
Lomotil	diphenoxylate hydrochloride and atropine		
Drugs used to treat endocrine disorders: Drugs in this medical specialty area are used for treatment of a wide range of diseases that include diabetes mellitus, diabetes insipidus, thyroid dysfunction, sexual dysfunction, and autoimmune diseases. The endocrine system is composed of the hypothalamus; the pituitary, thyroid, parathyroid, and adrenal glands; and the pancreas, ovaries, and testes. To list drugs in each of these categories is beyond the scope of this text; therefore, only those used most commonly will be mentioned.			
Drugs that affect the thyroid gland:			
Levoxyl	levothyroxine sodium	used to treat **hypothyroidism** and **thyrotoxicosis**	nervousness, weight loss, tremor,
Cytomel	liothyronine sodium		cardiac arrest

(continued)

TABLE 15-4 (Continued)

Trade name	Generic name	Uses	Adverse effects
Tapazole	methimazole	used to treat hyperthyroidism	**agranulocytosis**
PTU	propylthiouracil		hepatitis, loss of hair, jaundice

Glucocorticoids: Used as replacement therapy in diseases of the adrenal glands; for relief of inflammatory symptoms; for severe allergic reactions; and for relief of stress caused by trauma or other stress reactions resulting in physical insults to the body. Some of the most widely prescribed are as follows:

Cortef (found on emergency drug carts)	hydrocortisone	short acting	hyperglycemia, moon face, peptic ulcers,
Cortone	cortisone	short acting	behavioral
Medrol	methylprednisolone	intermediate acting	disturbances,
Decadron	dexamethasone	long acting	edema, infection

⚠ **WARNING!**

Do not stop glucocorticoid drugs abruptly after long-term therapy. To do so may be fatal. They must be administered by a health care professional who is knowledgeable. Great caution must be exercised if given intravenously or intramuscularly. They may not be given intrathecally!

Insulin and oral hypoglycemic drugs: Patients are treated with either insulin (for insulin-dependent diabetes) or oral hypoglycemic agents (for non-insulin-dependent diabetes).

Insulin preparations used at present are human insulins, synthetic insulins, and insulin analogs. They range from rapid-acting to long-acting types and are too numerous and complex to be discussed in this text.

The adverse effects of insulin are hypoglycemia that ranges from mild to severe and can lead very quickly, if not treated, to coma and death.

Oral hypoglycemic drugs: Used to treat type 2 diabetes mellitus. Some frequently prescribed are:

Glugophage	metformin	renal and hepatic impairment,
Glucotrol	glipizide	weight loss, diarrhea,
DiaBeta	glyburide	hypoglycemia

Drugs used to treat osteoporosis: Used to aid in prevention and/or treatment of loss of bone mass related to postmenopausal women, sedentary or immobilized persons, and persons on long-term steroid therapy.

Premarin	estrogen replacement therapy	nausea, headaches, fluid retention, endometrial cancer if not used in conjunction with progesterone
Fosamax	alendronate sodium	headache, bone pain, nausea, diarrhea,
Actonel	risedronate sodium	headache, abdominal pain, arthralgia, bone pain

Anti-infective: This drug classification has grown so large that this text will only list the classes of each drug with one or two randomly chosen prototypes in each category. Those chosen do not reflect author's preference.

Drugs used for bacterial infections:
Penicillins:

Augmentin	amoxicillin-clavulanate	**broad spectrum**	nausea, diarrhea,
Geopen	carbenicillin	**extended spectrum**	anaphylaxis

Sulfonamides: Used to treat urinary tract infections and some topical infections.

Gantanol	sulfamethoxazole	used in combination with trimethoprim to treat *shigella*, and *Pneumocystis carinii* pneumonia	blood dyscrasias, hypersensitivity reaction

(continued)

TABLE 15-4   (Continued)

Trade name	Generic name	Uses	Adverse effects

> ⚠ **WARNING!**
> Sulfonamides are contraindicated during pregnancy and lactation and for children less than 2 years old!

Cephalosporins: Divided into four groups called *generations* based on their activity against particular bacteria.

Keflex	cephalexin	first generation	all are subject to hypersensitivity
Ceclor	cefaclor	second generation	reactions, gastric disturbances
Rocephin	ceftriaxone	third generation	ranging from mild to severe.

Tetracyclines, macrolides, and lincosamides: All are broad-spectrum antibiotics used to treat susceptible microorganisms.

Vibramycin	doxycycline	a tetracycline	all are subject to hyper-
Zithromax	azithromycin	a macrolide	sensitivity reactions,
Cleocin	clindamycin	a lincosamide	nausea, hematologic and gastric disturbances

Fluoroquinolones and aminoglycosides: More powerful drugs used to treat resistant microorganisms.

Cipro	ciprofloxacin	a fluoroquinolone	both drug may result in
Garamycin	gentamicin	an aminoglycoside	hypersensitivity reactions, superinfections, and pseudomembranous colitis; ototoxicity and nephrotoxicity may result with aminoglycosides

Antiviral drugs: Have relatively limited use but general uses are as follows: treatment of herpes simplex and herpes zoster infections; AIDS-related infections, cytomegalovirus, genital herpes, influenza A, and respiratory syncytial virus.

Zovirax	acyclovir	to treat herpes simplex and herpes zoster	headache, nausea, diarrhea, many
Symmetrel	amantadine	to prevent influenza A	other adverse
Sustiva	efavirenz	to treat HIV infection	effects
Amphocin	amphotericin B	to treat systemic fungal infections	intravenous use headache, fever
Lotrimin	clotrimazole	to treat topical fungal infections	skin irritation, burning

Antiparasitic drugs: Used to kill invasive parasites and to prevent or treat malaria.

Vermox	mebendazole	to treat pinworm, roundworm, American	abdominal pain, diarrhea
Aralen	chloroquine	hookworm, whipworm to prevent or treat malaria	hypotension, ECG changes, nausea, diarrhea

Fluids, electrolytes and nutrients

Intravenous replacement of fluid, electrolytes, and nutrients is part of the medical care of most patients treated in acute care hospitals. Intravenous (IV) fluids are frequently administered in imaging as part of the diagnostic plan of care. It is not within the radiographer's scope of practice to select the intravenous solution to be administered; however, he must recognize the reasons for their use and the potential hazards of these preparations.

Depletion of or an excess of one electrolyte affects the concentration of all others. For the body to function in a state of health, the correct balance of fluids, electrolytes, and nutrients must be maintained. When a person is acutely ill, this balance is maintained by intravenous therapy.

There are many prepared combinations of fluid and electrolyte solutions for IV use. Vitamins, minerals, and medications may be added to these solutions or given separately as prescribed. Parenteral solutions for IV nutrition are also available.

(continued)

TABLE 15-4   (Continued)

Parenteral Solutions: Used as replacement agents or as simple solutions containing dextrose in various concentrations and normal saline. The radiographer will work with this type of solution when the patient needs an IV line available but does not require electrolytes or nutrients. Some are as follows:

5% dextrose in water	all are isotonic solutions
0.9% NaCl (normal saline)	

Lactated Ringer's solution	
0.33% NaCl	are hypotonic solutions
0.45% NaCl	

5% dextrose in 0.45% NaCl	are hypertonic solutions
10% dextrose in water	
5% destrose in 0>9% NaCl	

Electrolytes: Replacement of electrolytes may be prescribed by intravenous (IV), intramuscular (IM), or oral route. Those widely used are listed:

Sodium (Na+)	controls and regulates volume of body fluids
Potassium (K+)	chief regulator of cellular enzyme activity and cellular water content
Calcium (Ca^{2+})	necessary for nerve impulse transmission and blood clotting
Magnesuim (Mg^{2+})	important for the metabolism of carbohydrates and proteins
Chloride (Cl)	acts with sodium to maintain osmotic pressure of Blood
Bicarbonate (HCO_3)	essential for acid-base balance
(found on emergency	
drug carts)	
Phosphate (PO_4)	helps maintain the body's acid-base balance

Adverse reactions to any one of the electrolytes may lead to nausea, anxiety, and hypotension or even to coma and death.

Vitamins: maintenance of good health requires an adequate daily intake of vitamins and minerals. The precursors of vitamins called *provitamins* may only be supplied through dietary intake. An indequate amount of most vitamins in the diet will lead to disease. The vitamin are: A, B complex, B_{12}, folate, niacin (B_3), pantothenic acid, pyridoxine (B_6), riboflavin (B_2), thiamine (B_1), C, D, E, and K. The sources and functions of the vitamins are not within the scope of this text.

Minerals: Minerals are inorganic substances needed to maintain health. They are needed only in minute amounts and are available in a nutritious diet. The primary minerals are: calcium, chloride, magnesium, phosphorus, iodine, zinc, copper, potassium, sodium sulfur, manganese, and selenium.

Iodinated contrast agents are used in the examination of the GI tract, kidneys, gallbladder, pancreas, heart, brain, uterus, spinal column, arteries, veins, and joints. Contrast agents are used to increase the visibility of body cavities, organs, and the vascular system in diagnostic imaging, fluoroscopy, and other imaging modalities such as CT and MRI. Special imaging procedures are discussed in Chapter 16.

Selecting a Contrast Agent

Variables the physician considers when selecting a contrast agent are the following:

1. Its ability to mix with body fluids
2. The viscosity
3. The ionic strength
4. Its persistence in the body
5. The osmolality
6. The iodine content
7. The potential for toxicity

Most contrast agents are water-based and the body will absorb water-based contrasts in time. A limited number of procedures require an oil-based contrast agent. These may be excreted from the body in a natural manner or may be removed at the end of the procedure.

Iodinated contrast agents are administered by oral, vaginal, intravenous, and intra-arterial routes. They may also be directly instilled into the organ through a **retrograde procedure** or directly into the joints or body cavities. Contrast agents are distributed easily to areas where visualization is required for diagnosis and then excreted from the body in a relatively safe manner.

Drugs used to treat most illnesses are administered in small dosages at selected intervals, whereas contrast agents are often administered in a large dose at one time called a *bolus*. Most drugs used for treating illness that are administered intravascularly are *isotonic*. That is, they have the same concentration of solute as other body fluids; therefore, they exert the same amount of osmotic pressure as the body fluid with which they are combining. Contrast agents have osmolalities much higher than the body fluid with which they are combining. They are highly viscous, and when administered intravascularly, they prompt a sudden shift in body fluid from the interstitial spaces and cells into the systemic circulation. The radiographer must be aware that the physiologic effect of this change may produce an adverse effect on the patient.

Ionic and Nonionic Contrast Agents

Radiodensity in body tissues of the contrast agent is related to the percentage of iodine in the contrast medium. Two commonly used iodinated substances are iothalamate and diatrizoate. Each of these contain methylglucamine (meglumine) salts or sodium salts or a combination of the two. Meglumine compounds are less toxic but more viscous than sodium compounds. All positive contrast media are made up of a cation (a positive charge) and an anion (a negative charge). The cation is either the sodium or the meglumine compound. The anion is basically the same in all media, with the exception of one side chain, and this determines the remainder of the makeup of the contrast agent.

The chemical structures of the nonionic and ionic contrast media are significantly different. Ionic contrast media are salts of iodinated benzoic acid derivatives that were depended upon for radiographic and CT imaging in the past. As salts, the ionic contrast media consist of a positively charged cation and a negatively charged anion. They are also strong acids and are completely dissociated (ionized) in solution. For every three iodine atoms in a contrast solution, there are two particles for osmolality, one anion, and one cation.

It is the iodine in contrast agents that provides the contrast (density difference) between the organ and the surrounding tissues. Advances in iodinated radiopaque contrast agents resulted when research was focused on the ratio between the number of iodine atoms present and the number of particles in solution. The chemical makeup of ionic and nonionic contrast differs in the number of particles in solution and not the number of iodine compounds. It was discovered that if the cation was removed there was no diagnostic information lost since the cation did not contain any of the image-producing iodine. The cation was replaced with a compound such as glucose that does not disassociate in solution. The result was a contrast agent that still contained the three iodine atoms for contrast and only one

particle for osmolality. The lower osmolality factor defines the group of contrasts known as nonionic contrasts, or low osmolar contrast media (LOCM).

With the salt compound removed, the patient was less likely to suffer adverse reactions and was more comfortable during the procedure. When possible, these LOCMs are chosen by the physician as they have a wider margin of safety.

The osmolality (the weight of the ion) of a contrast agent is a significant factor considered when side effects may cause severe complications for the patient. Conventional ionic agents are significantly hyperosmotic to body fluids such as blood because they dissociate into separate ions in solution. This can cause adverse effects that vary from cardiac events, vein cramping, and pain to abnormal fluid retention. The osmolality of nonionic contrast agents is closer to that of human plasma than ionic agents at a similar iodine concentration. Imaging departments differ in choice of LOCM for all patients versus selective use of LOCM only on patients at increased risk for adverse reactions. Patients of choice for LOCM include the following:

1. Patients with a history of previous adverse reaction to contrast agents
2. Patients with asthmatic conditions
3. Patients with known cardiac conditions
4. Patients who are severely debilitated
5. Patients at high risk for contrast **extravasation**
6. Patients for whom the physician feels there is an indication for its use

Table 15-5 lists the contrast agents.

Patient Reactions to Contrast Agents and Radiographer's Response

Reactions to contrast media occur most often when the agent is administered intravenously or intra-arterially. Expected side effects must be explained to the patient before the procedure begins to alleviate anxiety. These include a feeling of warmth and flushing and a metallic taste in the mouth. Adverse reactions are not predictable and may be life-threatening.

Ionic, high-osmolality iodinated contrast agents are most frequently associated with adverse events. These reactions range from mild to severe. Skill in detecting and dealing with potential adverse symptoms makes the difference in patient outcomes. The radiographer is the health care worker who is usually present to observe these symptoms. His skill in assessing problems quickly and initiating emergency action is essential.

The American College of Radiology has identified classifications for adverse reactions as mild (or minor), moderate, and severe. A fourth reaction has been identified as being a reaction to the procedure itself rather than to the contrast agent. This is called a **vasovagal response**

TABLE 15-5   Contrast Agents

Nonionic Intravascular Contrast Agents

Product	Chemical Structure	% Salt Concentration	% Iodine Concentrnation
Omnipaque 140	Iohexol	0	14
Omnipaque 180	Iohexol	0	18
Omnipaque 240	Iohexol 51.8%	0	24
Omnipaque 300	Iohexol 64.7%	0	30
Omnipaque 350	Iohexol 75.5%	0	35
Ultravist 150	Iopromide	15	150
Ultravist 240	Iopromide	24	240
Ultravist 300	Iopromide	30	300
Ultravist 370	Iopromide	37	370
Optiray 160	Ioversol 34%	16	160
Optiray 240	Ioversol 51%	24	240
Optiray 300	Ioversol 64%	30	300
Optiray 320	Ioversol 68%	32	320
Optiray 350	Ioversol 74%	35	350
Isovue 200	Iopamidol 40.8%	20	200
Isovue 250	Iopamidol 51%	25	250
Isovue 300	Iopamidol 61.2%	30	300
Isovue 370	Iopamidol 75.5%	37	370
Visipaque 270	Iodixanol	27	270
Visipaque 320	Iodixanol	32	320

Ionic Intravascular Contrast Agents

Product	Chemical Structure	% Salt Concentration	% Iodine Concentration
Conray	Iothalamate/Meglumine	60	28.2
Conray 30	Iothalamate/Meglumine	30	14.1
Conray 43	Iothalamate/Meglumine	43	20.2
Contay 400	Iothalamate/Sodium	66.9	40
Reno-DIP	Diatriozoate/Meglumine	30	14.1
Reno-60	Diatriozoate/Meglumine	60	28.2
Renografin 60	Diatrizoate/Combo	52 Meg, 8 Sodium	29.25
RenoCal-76	Diatrizoate/Combo	66 Meg, 10 Sodium	37
Hypaque-Meglumine 60%	Diatrizoate/Meglumine	60	28.2
Hypaque-Sodium 50%	Diatrizoate/Sodium	50	30
Hypaque 76	Diatrizoate/Combo	Meg 66, 19.6 Sodium	37
Hexabrix 32	Ioxaglate/Combo	Meg 39.3, 19.6 Sodium	19.6

Ionic Gastrointestinal Agents

Gastrografin	Diatrizoate/Combo	Meglumine	37

Ionic Uroradiological Agents

Hypaque-Cysto	Diatrizoate/Meglumine	30	14.1
Cysto Conray	Iothalamate/Meglumine	17.2	8.1
Conray	Iothalamate/Meglumine	43	20.2

and occurs when the patient experiences high anxiety concerning the procedure and its result.

Invasive radiographic procedures are frequently stressful. The patient's mental status before and during a procedure requiring administration of a contrast agent is significant. The radiographer must be able to identify the highly anxious patient during the initial assessment interview. Critical thinking skills and use of therapeutic communication techniques must be used to alleviate patient anxiety. The radiographer may assist in reducing anxiety in the following ways:

1. Assessment of the patient's understanding of the procedure
2. Informing the patient in detail concerning how the examination will proceed
3. Explanation of the expected side effects and assurance that these are not unusual
4. Allowing the patient to express feelings of anxiety and obtaining patient feedback to ascertain his complete understanding of the procedure

Thoughtful care by the radiographer will aid in establishing a feeling of trust in the patient and will assist in avoiding adverse reactions.

Patient Assessment prior to Administration of Contrast Medium

Before administration of a contrast agent, it is the obligation of the radiographer to obtain a detailed assessment of those aspects of the patient's medical history that might portend an allergic reaction. Prevention of serious adverse effects is the goal of this assessment; however, the radiographer must also be prepared to initiate correct medical treatment should a reaction occur. This includes adequate patient preparation for any procedure and ensuring that all equipment and personnel are available to treat any reaction. Most imaging departments have a standard form that includes the following:

1. Patient's age
2. History of impaired hepatic function (liver disease)
3. History of impaired renal function (kidney disease)
4. History of allergic or anaphylactic reactions
5. History of thyroid disease
6. Last menstrual period and possible pregnancy
7. Nursing mother
8. Sensitivity to aspirin
9. History of diabetes mellitus
10. History of sickle cell disease
11. History of hypertension
12. History of pheochromocytoma
13. History of seizures
14. Medication history
15. History of previous reactions to medications or contrast agents
16. Allergy to seafood

The patient's emotional status should be noted on the form and signed by the radiographer.

During any injection of contrast medium, the patient must be monitored for abnormal responses or reactions. The emergency cart, equipment, and medical response personnel must be immediately available. The radiographer must be alert for extravasation of the contrast agent. If it should occur, he must immediately stop the IV and apply warm compresses to the area to reduce pain and tissue damage.

Potential side effects of contrast are as follows.

Clinical Manifestations of Expected Side Effects
- A feeling of flushing or warmth
- Nausea and/or vomiting
- Headache
- Pain at the injection site
- Altered taste, may be metallic

Radiographer's Response
1. Slow the rate of the contrast infusion.
2. Observe the patient closely and offer reassurance.

Clinical Manifestations of a Vasovagal Reaction
- Pallor
- Cold sweats
- Rapid pulse
- Syncope or complaint of feeling faint
- Bradycardia
- Hypotension

Radiographer's Response
1. Stop the infusion of contrast medium.
2. Place the patient in flat or Trendelenburg position.
3. Notify the radiologist.
4. Remain with the patient and offer reassurance.

Clinical Manifestations of Mild Adverse Reaction
- Nausea, vomiting
- Cough
- Feeling of warmth
- Headache
- Dizziness
- Shaking
- Itching
- Pallor

Radiographer's Response
1. Stop the infusion and notify the radiologist or radiology nurse.
2. Remain with the patient and offer reassurance.

3. Prepare to assist in the administration of an anti-histamine or subcutaneous epinephrine.

Clinical Manifestations of a Moderate Adverse Reaction
- Tachycardia or bradycardia
- Hypertension or hypotension
- Dyspnea
- Bronchospasm or wheezing
- Patient complains of feeling of throat closing (laryngeal edema)

Radiographer's Response
1. Stop the infusion.
2. Notify the radiologist and the radiology nurse.
3. Call for the emergency team if symptoms progress rapidly.
4. Remain with the patient and offer reassurance.
5. Prepare to administer oxygen and intravenous medications.
6. If the patient is in respiratory distress, place him in semi-Fowler's position.
7. Position patient who is vomiting in a position to prevent aspiration.

Clinical Manifestations of a Severe Anaphylactic Reaction
- Dyspnea related to laryngeal edema
- Hypotension
- Seizures
- Cardiac arrhythmia
- Lack of patient response
- Cardiac arrest

Radiographer's Response
1. Call for emergency response team (Code Blue).
2. Notify the radiologist and radiology nurse.
3. Prepare to use AED (automated external defibrillator).
4. Prepare to administer oxygen and intravenous medications.

> ⚠ **WARNING!**
>
> Patients who are receiving iodinated contrast agents must not be left unattended. An anaphylactic reaction may occur quickly and without warning!

For most imaging procedures that require use of a contrast agent, a peripheral intravenous infusion is started to maintain hydration and to permit emergency administration of medications if the situation requires. This ensures that there will be quick intravenous access in an emergency.

Although most reactions to contrast media occur within the first several minutes after administration, a delayed reaction is possible. The patient may have left the department before the reaction occurs; therefore, he must be instructed to return immediately to the emergency department if he has the following symptoms: fever, joint pain, malaise, skin rash, difficult breathing, or swollen lymph nodes.

▮ UNIVERSAL PRECAUTIONS IN DRUG ADMINISTRATION

All drugs (medications) are potentially harmful. The radiographer must never become casual or careless when administering drugs or assisting with drug administration. One must never administer a drug that has not been specifically ordered by a physician. All health care workers who administer drugs must understand the intended action, contraindications, side effects, and potential adverse effects of any drug they administer.

If a radiographer is not familiar with a drug being administered, he should consult the pharmacist or an available literary source prior to administering the drug. If the radiographer does not know or cannot find information about a drug, it must not be administered!

> ⚠ **WARNING!**
>
> The radiographer must remember that contrast agents are drugs and the precautions listed in this chapter pertain to these agents as well!

The radiographer must adhere to the five rights of drug administration at all times. They are as follows:

1. The right patient
2. The right drug
3. The right amount or dose
4. The right route
5. The right time

Other precautions that must be taken before administration of any drug are as follows:

1. Read all drug labels carefully before drawing up or pouring a drug. Check the name, strength, and dosage of the drug.
2. If a drug contains a sediment or appears to be cloudy, do not use until the pharmacist approves the drug.
3. Check the expiration date of the drug on the label. If that date has passed, do not use.

4. Do not use drugs from unmarked, or poorly marked containers. Discard them.

5. Measure exact amounts of every drug used. If medication is left over, do not replace it in the container; discard it according to institutional policy.

6. Drugs must be stored in accordance with the manufacturer's specifications. No drug should be stored in an area where temperature and humidity vary greatly or are extreme. Low room temperature is advised.

7. If a medication is a liquid to be poured, pour away from the label.

8. Do not combine two drugs in a syringe without verifying their compatibility with the pharmacist. If in doubt, do not combine!

9. Before selecting a medication, check the label of the container three times: before taking it from storage, before pouring it or drawing it up, and after it has been prepared for administration.

10. Take only one drug to one patient at one time and remain with the patient until it has been taken. Do not leave the patient to take the drug later.

11. When approaching a patient who is to receive a drug, ask the patient to state his or her name. Do not accept the fact that a patient answers to what is thought to be the correct name. An anxious patient may respond incorrectly. Read the name label on the patient's wrist.

12. After identifying the patient, explain to him how the drug is to be taken.

13. A drug history of allergies must be taken before any drug is administered. See patient interview.

14. The radiographer must not administer a drug that he has not prepared.

15. Report and document any drug that the patient refuses to take.

16. Document any drug administered immediately according to department procedure.

17. Do not leave a patient unattended who may be having a drug reaction!

18. A patient who has received a sedative, hypnotic, antianxiety, or narcotic analgesic drug must not be allowed to drive himself or herself home.

19. A child who has received a medication and is sleeping may not leave the department until fully awake.

20. Patients must be observed for 1 hour before leaving the department alone after receiving any drug.

 WARNING!

Patients who receive narcotic analgesics or hypnotics may suffer respiratory depression and shock and must not be left unattended.

TABLE 15-6   Common Standard Medical Abbreviations

PO = by mouth	ac = before meals
IM = intramuscular	pc = after meals
IV = intravenous	hs = at bedtime
STAT = at once	PRN = as necessary
VO = verbal order	q = every
SC or SQ = subcutaneous	qd = every day
ID = intradermal	tid = three times a day
bid = twice a day	q2hrs = every 2 hours
gtt = drop	mL = milliliter
cc = cubic centimeter	

ABBREVIATIONS RELATED TO DRUG ADMINISTRATION

There are standard medical abbreviations with which the radiographer must familiarize himself prior to working with drug administration. Table 15-6 lists those most commonly used.

THE MEDICATION ORDER AND DOCUMENTATION

Licensed physicians, dentists, podiatrists, and, in some states, optometrists can prescribe, dispense, and administer drugs. Under specific circumstances that vary from state to state, nurse practitioners, physician assistants, and pharmacists may order and dispense drugs.

No health care worker may prescribe or administer drugs that are not ordered by a person licensed to do so. In health care settings, an order must be dated, written, and signed by the physician. If the patient is to be cared for in a medical facility, as in a diagnostic imaging department, the order is written on an order sheet or on a computerized order sheet (Fig. 15-2). The written request for an examination using IV contrast medium should include the medical necessity for the examination, the type of contrast to be used, and the manner in which the procedure will be performed. Medical necessity for the procedure is demonstrated by including the signs and symptoms of the patient's problem, a relevant history, the current diagnoses, and a specific reason for the procedure requested. This request must come from the patient's physician.

When a radiographer, acting under the supervision of a radiologist, administers a medication to a patient, it must be recorded in the patient's chart. The time of day, the drug name, the dose, and route of administration must be included in the documentation.

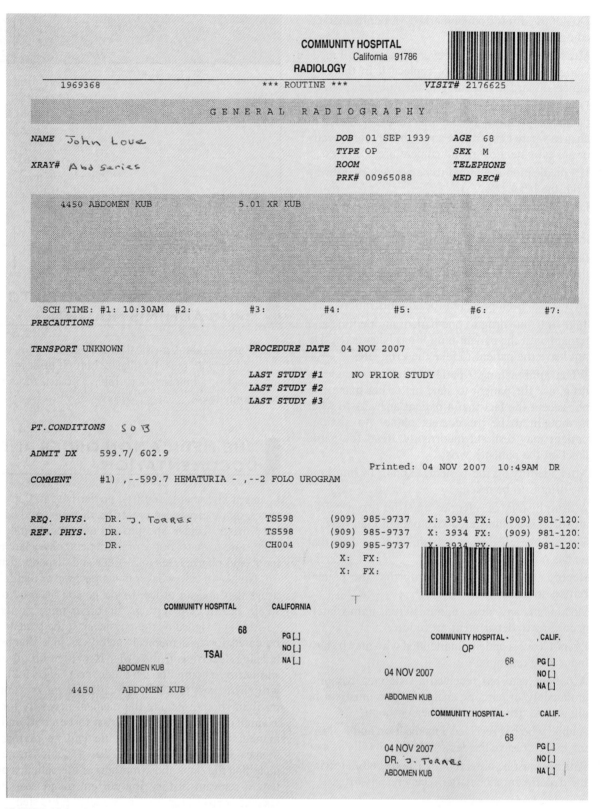

FIGURE 15-2 A computerized order sheet.

The radiographer, or whoever administers the medication, must also sign the chart for identification purposes. The supervising physician then countersigns the entry. The documentation of administration of contrast agents will vary according to institutional protocol. In most cases, the use of contrast media is stated in the radiologist's report following the procedure.

If a patient is to be discharged with a prescription, it will be written on the physician's personal order form. The order will include the following:

The patient's full name, the date, and the time the order is written

The date and time or times that the drug is to be taken

The generic or the trade name of the drug

The dosage and the route of administration

The physician's signature

An example of a physician's order for a hospitalized patient might be as follows:

7 A.M. June 3, 2007
Give Valium, 5 mg PO at 8 A.M.
J. Glucose, Md

MEDICATION ERRORS

All professional health care workers are responsible for their actions. It is the legal and ethical obligation of the radiographer to be knowledgeable about any drug that he administers. If a drug is incorrectly administered or an order is misinterpreted, the radiographer is legally liable. All federal regulations pertaining to controlled substances must be fully understood. The Controlled Substances Act of the federal government restricts personnel who are legally permitted to administer narcotic and hypnotic drugs or any drug that may cause dependence. It also restricts access to these drugs, which are always kept in a locked area. Documentation and accounting for these drugs is also carefully controlled.

Medication errors are an area of frequent litigation in diagnostic imaging. The radiographer who is administering or assisting with administration of drugs is frequently implicated in this type of litigation. If an error in medication administration is made or if the patient has an adverse reaction to a contrast agent, the radiographer involved must assess the patient's condition and notify the prescribing physician immediately.

The error or adverse reaction must be included in the patient's chart. An incident report (sometimes called an unusual occurrence report) will also be required by the facility. A "misadventure" form or a "misadministration" form will also be required. A "misadventure" is one in which the wrong dose or wrong contrast agent brought about the same outcome as that expected by the correct drug or correct dosage.

Every detail of the incident must be included in the report, which becomes the property of the department and is not a part of the patient's chart. Items to include in the report are as follows:

1. The dosage of the drug administered
2. The name of the incorrect drug
3. Why it was administered
4. The patient's reaction
5. How the error was remedied

An example of documentation of the wrong contrast administered follows:

07-07-2007: 0820 hrs Iopamidol 30 mL administered IV. Administered in error instead of Omnipaque.

0830 hrs Dr. Glucophage (radiologist) notified of the error. Initialed by the radiographer.

0840 hrs Dr. Glucophage assessed patient's condition.

0845 hrs B/P 124/70; P 72; R 16 Patient reports no complaints.

The patient must be observed for an appropriate amount of time, and periodic reports on his or her condition are documented until the patient is discharged from the department. If a drug is administered to the wrong patient, the same procedure is followed. Accurate documentation is the best defense if litigation follows.

METHODS OF DRUG ADMINISTRATION

There are basically three routes by which drugs may be administered. They are follows: **enteral, parenteral,** and **topical.** Each will be described below with particular emphasis on the parenteral route.

Enteral Routes

The enteral routes are broken down into **oral, sublingual, buccal,** and **rectal.**

Drugs taken by mouth and swallowed into the stomach are said to be given *orally*. The medical term for this route of administration is PO. It is often the most efficient and most cost-effective method of drug administration. This route is used if the drug will not be destroyed by gastric secretions and when slower absorption and longer duration of drug activity are desired. If the radiographer is to give a drug orally, he will proceed as follows:

1. Place the patient in an upright position.
2. Make sure a glass of water is available.
3. Assess the patient's need for assistance in removing the tablet or capsule from the container.
4. Ask the patient to moisten his mouth with a few sips of water.

5. Observe the patient placing the drug into his mouth. Assist if necessary. If the radiographer must place the drug into the patient's mouth, don gloves to do this. Remove the gloves and wash your hands as directed.

6. Assist the patient to drink water following the drug placement at the back of his mouth.

Do not leave a drug at the patient's bedside to be taken. Make certain the drug is consumed before leaving the patient.

> ###))) CALL OUT!
> Do not break or crush enteric-coated tablets because they may act as gastric irritants or become less effective!

A sublingual drug is placed under the tongue and remains there until it is dissolved completely. The patient must not eat or drink until the drug dissolves. It is not to be swallowed or chewed.

A drug administered by buccal route must be placed against the mucous membranes of the cheek in either the upper or lower jaw. It must remain there until it dissolves. Drugs given by this route are used for local effect and are drugs such as lozenges.

Drugs may be administered by rectum if a patient is nauseated and unable to retain oral drugs. It is difficult to determine correct dosage by this route as absorption may be erratic. Lack of fluid in the rectum also makes absorbability questionable. The radiographer will have little or no reason to administer drugs by rectum.

Topical Routes

Topical drug administration includes the following:

> Drugs administered to the skin for local treatment of lesions or skin conditions.
> Drugs administered to the eyes, nose, and throat.
> Drugs administered to the respiratory mucosa by inhalation.
> Drugs administered to the vagina and, in some cases, to the rectum
> Drugs applied to the skin for intended systemic effect; called *transdermal application.*

It is believed that drugs administered transdermally are absorbed slowly, and a constant blood level of the drug is achieved. The radiographer may care for patients with transdermal patches applied at various areas of the body, generally, the upper thoracic area. This route is used most often for relief of chronic pain and for cardiac therapy.

> ### ⚠ WARNING!
> Children absorb topical drugs more quickly, and they may be highly toxic!

Parenteral Drug Administration

There are several methods of administering drugs by parenteral routes, and they vary depending upon the drug to be administered and the route ordered by the physician. The routes that the radiographer must familiarize himself with are the subcutaneous, intramuscular, intradermal, and intravenous routes. Other routes of parenteral administration are the **intralesional, intra-arterial, intracardiac,** and **intra-articular.** These routes are used only by the physician or specialty nurses.

Equipment used for parenteral injections is dependent upon the route. Any health care worker who plans to administer parenteral medications to children requires special education beyond the scope of this textbook. All parenteral drug administration requires laboratory instruction and practice before administering drugs to actual patients. The procedures described in the following paragraphs pertain to the average adult patient. There are some rules that apply to all parenteral drug administration. They are as follows:

1. All equipment that penetrates the skin including needles, syringes, and the drug itself must be sterile.

2. The patient must be correctly identified.

3. The procedure is explained to the patient and the medication (including contrast media) to be administered is identified.

4. If the patient refuses the drug, document the refusal. Do not insist that the patient accept the drug.

5. The skin at the injection site is cleansed with an antiseptic solution until it is as free of microorganisms as possible.

6. The antiseptic chosen will be dictated by the institution in which you are employed. Alcohol-based preparations are commonly used as many people are allergic to povidone-iodine preparations.

7. All persons administering parenteral drugs must wear gloves during the procedure to prevent exposure to blood.

8. There must be a physician's order for all drugs to be administered. This includes contrast media.

9. The five rights of drug administration must be followed.

10. The drug administered must be documented according to the policy of the department.

11. The patient must be observed closely for 1 hour following drug administration for adverse or allergic reactions.

12. A patient who has had a sedative, tranquilizing, or hypnotic drug may NOT drive him or herself home.

EQUIPMENT FOR DRUG ADMINISTRATION

Needles for parenteral drug administration range in length from 3/8 to 2 inches for average use. Longer needles are used for special procedures. Needles may come attached to a syringe of appropriate size or may come in various sizes packaged separately. Needles are made of stainless steel and consist of the following parts:

- The hub (the part that attaches to the syringe)
- The shaft (the elongated part of the needle)
- The lumen (the hollow tube that runs the length of the shaft)
- The bevel (the sharp angulated tip of the needle)

Selection of the correct size of needle with which to administer a drug is essential. The size of the lumen of the needle can vary from very large to very small. The smaller the lumen, the larger the gauge of the needle (e.g., a 30-gauge needle is much smaller than a 12-gauge needle). The viscosity of the fluid to be injected determines the gauge selected. The area for injection and the condition of the patient determine the length of the needle chosen.

Syringes also vary in size depending on the amount of fluid to be injected. They generally range in capacity from 1 to 50 mL. The parts of the syringe are as follows:

- The tip (the end of the syringe to which the needle is fastened)
- The barrel (the body of the syringe)
- The plunger (the part that fits into the barrel)

Syringes are calibrated in milliliters and minims. One milliliter equals 15 or 16 minims. Syringes are packaged in treated paper or plastic wrappers to maintain sterility, and needles are often attached in the package. The size of the syringe and the size of the needle are printed on the package (Figs. 15-3 and 15-4).

Needle-stick injuries are a serious consequence of incorrect handling of injection supplies. The current types of syringes and needles assist in avoidance of this risk. The rules for working with syringes and needles are as follows:

1. Syringes and needles are disposable and are to be discarded after one use.
2. Syringes and needles are to be discarded in puncture-proof containers labeled *sharps container* that are required to be provided in all areas where drugs are administered even if they contain safety features (Fig. 15-5).

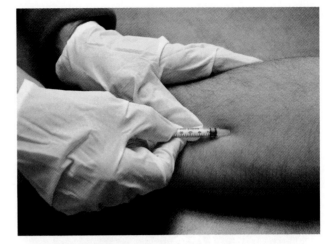

FIGURE 15-3 Photo of syringe.

3. Needles that have been used for an injection must not be recapped. If it has aprotective mechanism, it must be engaged after use (Fig. 15-6).
4. The used syringe must be held by the barrel and carried immediately to the sharps container.
5. Never place a used syringe and needle back onto a tray to be disposed of at a later time.
6. If a needle does not have a protective mechanism in place, a "needle scoop" method may be used to prevent injury (Fig. 15-7).
7. If a needle-stick injury should occur, it must be reported as a "critical incident" as soon as possible following the event.

Packaging of Parenteral Medications

Drugs intended for parenteral administration are packaged to maintain sterility. If they are intended for intramuscular, subcutaneous, or intradermal injection, they are either in an ampule or a vial. Drugs to be administered intravenously may be contained in an ampule or a vial if the amount to be administered is small. If a large amount of fluid or drug is to be administered, it

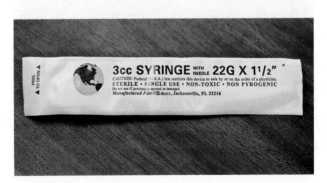

FIGURE 15-4 Photo of packaging for syringes and needles.

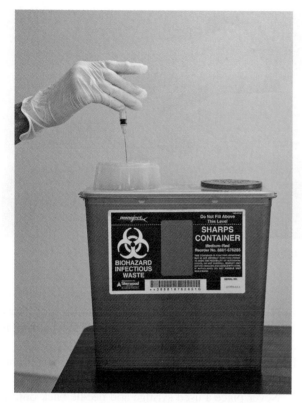

FIGURE 15-5 Discard used needles and syringes in sharps container.

will be contained in a calibrated glass or plastic container (Figs. 15-8, 15-9, and 15-10).

Vials

A vial is a glass container with a rubber stopper circled by a metal band; the band holds the stopper in place. The rubber stopper is protected from contamination by a plastic cap. Some vials are for multidose use. If this is the case, it is considered contaminated after it has been used for 24 hours and must be discarded. The procedure for obtaining a drug from a vial is as follows:

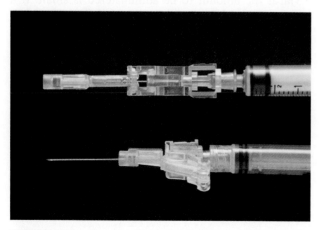

FIGURE 15-6 One type of protective needle device.

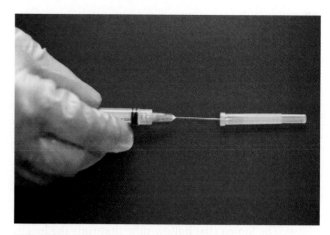

FIGURE 15-7 Needle scoop procedure.

1. Remove the plastic protective cap from the top of the vial.
2. If this a multidose vial and has been opened previously, check the date and time opened and cleanse the rubber top with an alcohol wipe.
3. Determine the dosage desired from the vial and draw up the equivalent amount of air into the syringe.
4. Insert the needle into the vial and inject the air. The fluid will replace the air in the syringe rather quickly.
5. Draw the plunger back until the exact amount of drug is obtained (Fig. 15-11).

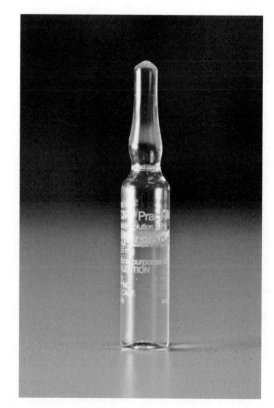

FIGURE 15-8 Ampule.

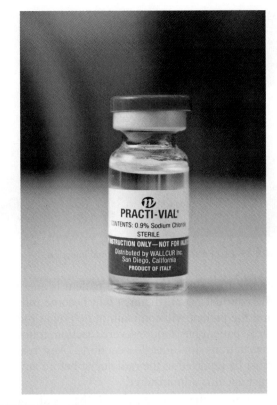

FIGURE 15-9   Vial.

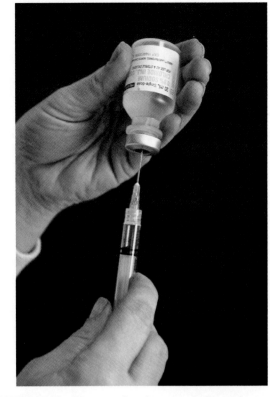

FIGURE 15-11   Preparing drug from a multidose vial.

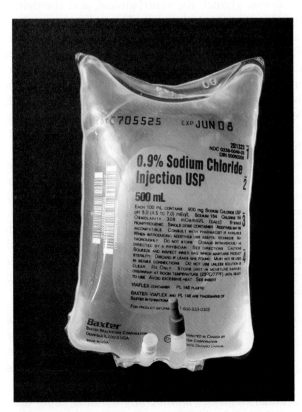

FIGURE 15-10   Intravenous fluid containers.

6. Remove the syringe from the vial, re-read the drug label, and replace it in storage.

Ampules

An ampule is made of glass and contains a single dose of a drug. The ampule is labeled with the name of the drug, the dosage per mL, and the route for administration. Use of the ampule is as follows:

1. The indented area at the neck of the ampule may be opened by filing with a metal file or by simply snapping off the top of the vial.

2. The health care worker must never attempt to snap off the top of an ampule without protecting his hands as the glass may break unevenly and cause a laceration (Fig. 15-12).

3. If a vial shatters when broken open, the medication must be discarded as there may be glass shards in the drug.

4. If all of the drug in an ampule is not used, it must be discarded because it will not remain sterile after the ampule is opened.

Intradermal Administration

Intradermal injections are also called *intracutaneous injections.* For the radiographer's purposes, only the

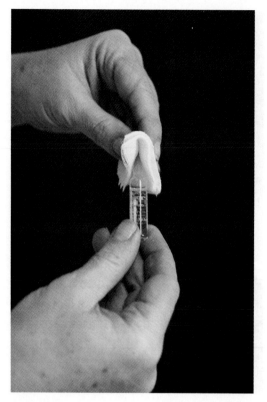

FIGURE 15-12 Do not break top from ampule without protecting hands.

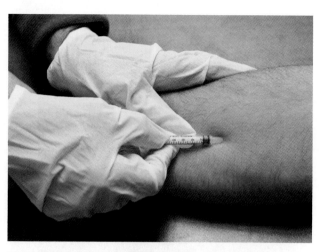

FIGURE 15-13 Performing an intradermal injection.

injection used for testing for sensitivity to a contrast agent will be discussed. The procedure is as follows:

1. Select the agent to be tested. Usually less than 0.5 mL of the agent is used.
2. Select the equipment needed. This includes: a tuberculin syringe, a 25- to 27-gauge needle ½ inch in length, an alcohol wipe, and a pair of clean gloves.
3. Approach the patient and explain the procedure. Select a site for the test: usually administered into the dermis on the inner aspect of the forearm. Areas with excessive hair, scarring, or tattoos must not be used as the results may be difficult to detect.
4. Cleanse the site with an alcohol wipe in a firm, circular motion.
5. Put on gloves.
6. Hold the skin at the area to be injected taut with the nondominant hand.
7. Insert the needle, bevel side up, at a 5- to 15-degree angle. It should be almost flat against the skin.
8. Inject the drug. A small raised area or wheal should be seen at the injection site (Fig. 15-13).
9. Withdraw the needle, and do not massage or cleanse the site. Remove gloves, and dispose of the needle according to rules of standard precautions.
10. Instruct the patient concerning the time to read the results of the test. Usually, the time allowed for

contrast results is brief. If the patient is allergic to the contrast agent, the area will become inflamed and the patient will complain of itching at the site. If the patient has a more severe reaction, follow the instructions for allergic reactions. Any reaction must be reported to the radiologist before any contrast agent is administered.

11. Document the procedure and the result of the injection.

Intramuscular Injections

Intramuscular routes for administration of drugs are the dorsal gluteal, the ventrogluteal, and the deltoid muscles (Fig. 15-14A to C). The radiographer must assess his patient prior to obtaining a site for IM injection. Elderly persons loose muscle mass and may need a shorter needle and a site in which there is an appropriate amount of muscular tissue. The amount of fluid that may be safely administered ranges from 1 to 5 mL. Persons receiving the injection must be relatively large if more than 3 mL of medication is to be injected into the muscle. The radiographer must be educated in a laboratory setting before actually performing this procedure in a clinical setting because incorrect technique may result in harm to the patient. Major blood vessels and nerves traverse muscles used for injection and permanent damage may result. The tissues around the site may also be damaged. Complications that may result from incorrect injection into a muscle are abscesses, necrosis, skin slough, nerve damage, prolonged pain, and periostitis. The procedure is as follows:

1. Assemble equipment needed. This includes the following: a 3- to 5-mL syringe; an 18- to 22- or 23- gauge needle; a 1-inch long needle may be selected for use in the deltoid area or for use on a very thin patient; three alcohol wipes; and a pair of clean gloves.
2. Read the order and identify the drug using the 5 rights of drug administration. Identify the patient.

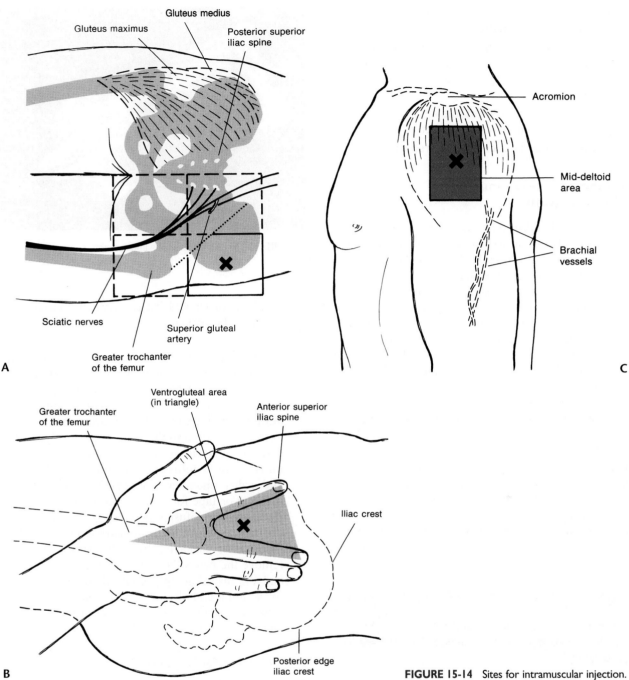

FIGURE 15-14 Sites for intramuscular injection.

Assess the patient to determine the site for injection and any potential allergies to the drug, and explain the procedure to him.

3. Draw up the drug into the syringe. If the medication is an irritating substance such as hydroxyzine, change the needle after it is drawn into the syringe to prevent burning on injection.

4. Position the patient appropriately and cleanse the area with an alcohol wipe. Put on clean gloves and prepare a second alcohol wipe.

5. Place the nondominant hand on the muscle to be injected to support the patient. Quickly insert the needle into the muscle at a 90-degree angle.

6. With the needle inserted, support the needle with the nondominant thumb and index fingers and draw back on the plunger to aspirate, making certain no blood returns into the syringe. If blood appears in the syringe, withdraw the needle and select an alternative site after changing the needle.

7. If no blood appears, inject the drug into the muscle, and quickly withdraw the needle.

8. Wipe the area with the second alcohol wipe. A band aid may be applied if there is a small amount of bleeding following the injection. Remove the gloves.

9. Make the patient comfortable and dispose of the gloves, needle, and syringe correctly.

10. Wash hands and document the procedure.

Peripheral Intravenous Drug Administration

The IV method of drug administration is selected when immediate effect of a drug is desired or when a drug cannot be injected into body tissues without damage. This can be one of the most hazardous routes of drug administration because once a drug is injected directly into the circulatory system, reaction is instantaneous. Any health care worker who administers IV drugs must be aware of the hazards of this route and the life-threatening potential. In many areas of the United States, official authorization is required of all persons administering IV drugs.

Most drugs administered in diagnostic imaging are administered intravenously. A patient receiving an IV drug or contrast agent must not be left alone. Vital signs must be taken before administration and at frequent intervals during IV drug infiltration. Any changes in the patient's vital signs or behavior must be reported immediately to the physician in charge of the patient. The scope of the radiographer's practice has been expanded to include venipuncture; therefore, the radiographer must be able to perform this procedure correctly, safely, and efficiently.

> ### 🔊))) CALL OUT!
>
> The peripheral intravenous route is the only method by which radiographers may administer contrast media parenterally!

Contrast agents may be given by bolus or by infusion. A *bolus* is a designated amount of a drug that is administered at one time, usually over a period of several minutes. An *infusion* usually refers to a larger amount of a drug, fluid, or fluid containing a drug or electrolytes that is administered over a longer period of time ranging from hours to days. Both methods require venipuncture; each requires different equipment.

Supplies Needed for IV Drug Administration

When the radiographer receives a physician's order to administer an intravenous contrast agent, he will proceed as follows:

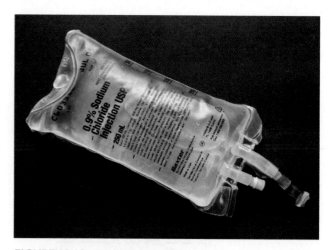

FIGURE 15-15   An intravenous infusion set.

1. Read the order and list the type of contrast, the amount, the patient's name, and the procedure to be performed.

2. Assemble the needed materials: a butterfly needle (also called a scalp vein needle or a winged needle) or an over-the-needle catheter for a prolonged infusion (either of the correct gauge); a tourniquet; antimicrobial swabs; clean gloves; the contrast agent drawn up into the correct size syringe or the contrast in a bag or glass bottle for a continuous infusion; an IV infusion set that includes IV tubing and a drip chamber (Fig. 15-15); clear adhesive dressing or tape for infusion; an IV standard; and if required, an infusion pump (Fig. 15-16). Prepare the contrast agent for administration (Fig. 15-17). Open outer packaging from the infusion set, and remove the protective covering, the drip chamber, and the insertion tip keeping these sterile. Hang the solution and displace all air from the tubing to prevent air emboli. Recap the tip of the tubing to maintain sterility (Fig. 15-18).

Site Selection for Venipuncture

The area selected for venipuncture requires careful assessment before the procedure is begun. The type of contrast, the length of time for the infusion or bolus, and the age and physical condition of the patient are all to be considered when selecting a venipuncture site.

Veins in the hands and arms should be selected rather than those in the lower extremities unless an emergency precludes this. There is a greater hazard of embolus formation in the lower extremities related to IV infusion. Unless a drug is to be injected by bolus, do not select a vein located over a joint, because any movement will dislodge the needle or catheter. If a vein over a joint is selected, the extremity will need to be immobilized. The volar (palm) side of the wrist must

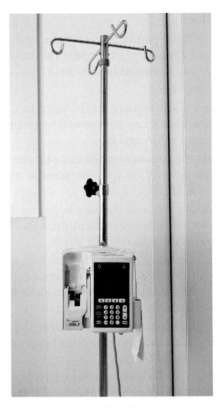

FIGURE 15-16   An intravenous pump.

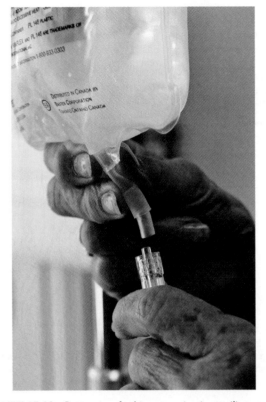

FIGURE 15-18   Recap tip of tubing to maintain sterility.

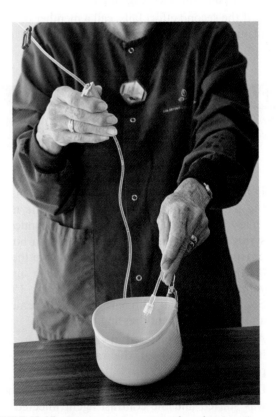

FIGURE 15-17   Prepare contrast agent for administration.

not be used because the radial nerve is in that area and the patient may feel extreme pain. Do not select a very small vein for contrast as there is great danger of leakage into the tissues and pain will result. The basilic or cephalic veins are good choices if available (Fig. 15-19).

Elderly patients must receive special consideration. Their veins are more fragile and have a greater tendency to "roll" as the needle or catheter is inserted. The tissues of the elderly patient are also more fragile, necessitating use of a smaller needle or catheter. The tourniquet is more apt to damage the skin and must be applied with less tension. The elderly patient is also more apt to have an adverse reaction to contrast media. This may be the result of medications the patient has taken prior to their admission to the imaging department, a history of diabetes mellitus, or other medical conditions that result in venous thrombosis.

Contrast media is more likely to dehydrate the elderly patient; therefore, a hydrating intravenous solution is often started prior to the administration of the contrast agent. The elderly patient must be observed closely for any symptom of an adverse reaction as well as **extravasation.**

Pediatric patients are often frightened and have difficulty remaining immobile. Allowing a parent to hold the child's extended arm if possible may be the best way to calm the child and maintain immobility during venipuncture.

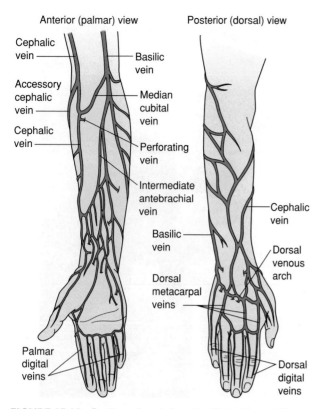

Anterior (palmar) view   Posterior (dorsal) view

Cephalic vein
Accessory cephalic vein
Cephalic vein
Basilic vein
Median cubital vein
Perforating vein
Intermediate antebrachial vein
Basilic vein
Dorsal metacarpal veins
Palmar digital veins
Cephalic vein
Dorsal venous arch
Dorsal digital veins

FIGURE 15-19 Basilic and cephalic veins (From *Brunner & Suddarth's Textbook of Medical-Surgical Nursing*, 11th ed. Baltimore: Lippincott Williams & Wilkins, 2008).

Finding a suitable vein in a small child is often difficult. If the situation permits, a pediatric nurse or pediatric health care specialist should be called upon to perform the venipuncture. Veins on the anterior surface of the forearm are most easily accessible in a child. The size of the butterfly needle or venous catheter must be much smaller than for an adult.

The volume of contrast agent is much lower as is the child's blood volume. The tonicity of the contrast medium must also be considered. Although children do not experience reactions to contrast agents as frequently as adults, anaphylactic reactions and other adverse reactions may occur, and the radiographer must be alert for any adverse or allergic symptom.

The radiographer must recognize that a child or an infant is not able to communicate their feelings; therefore, he must be constantly vigilant if the patient is a child or an infant. The emergency cart and correct sized equipment must be readily available at any time.

> **⚠ WARNING!**
> Oxygen administration equipment, pediatric facemasks, suction, and all other emergency equipment and drugs must be on hand when a child or an infant is the patient!

Venipuncture

1. Approach the patient, identify him, and assess for latex or iodine allergies. Explain the procedure and answer any questions he may have.
2. Wash your hands.
3. Secure the tourniquet over the site selected in such a manner that it can be removed by pulling on one end (Fig. 15-20A and B).
4. Instruct the patient to make two or three tight fists to force more blood into the veins to make them more visible.
5. Put on clean gloves. Gloves need not be sterile; however, all other equipment used that cleans or penetrates the skin must be sterile.
6. Cleanse the area for the venipuncture using firm strokes from center of site to outside. Do this at least three times using a separate swab each time. Allow the area to dry.
7. Hold the skin taut above or below the insertion site. Insert the needle or catheter bevel side up into the vein (Fig. 15-21).
8. When the needle enters the vein, blood returns into the flashback chamber immediately. If no blood returns, the venipuncture was not successful.

    If this is the case, remove the needle and obtain a new needle to start the IV and select a new site. Apply pressure to the failed area with a sterile gauze pad until bleeding stops.

    If the second effort fails, call a member of the IV team or an anesthesiologist to start the IV.

> **⚠ WARNING!**
> Never attempt to reinsert a used needle! Do not subject a patient to multiple punctures!

9. If blood returns, release the tourniquet, instruct the patient to relax his hand, thread the needle ⅛ to ¼ inch further into the vein, and connect the syringe containing the contrast agent if a bolus is ordered. If an infusion is started, remove the needle from the catheter, thread the catheter into the vein, and connect the IV tubing (Fig. 15-22). Secure the catheter with narrow nonallergenic tape and/or a transparent dressing.
10. A bolus is administered at the rate ordered. An infusion is begun at the rate ordered by the physician.
11. Document the procedure including the time the IV was started and the contrast agent injected. The radiographer must sign his documentation.

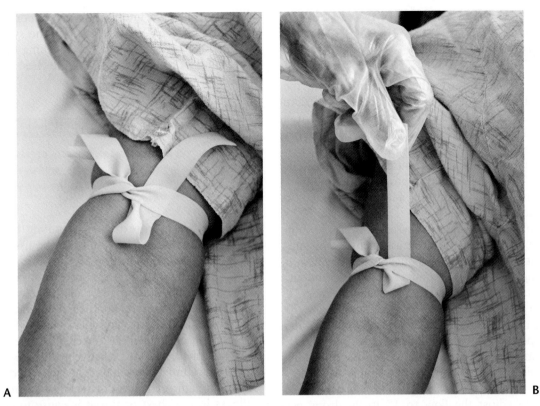

A

B

FIGURE 15-20 (**A**) Secure the tourniquet so that it may be removed by pulling one end. (**B**) Remove the tourniquet by pulling one end.

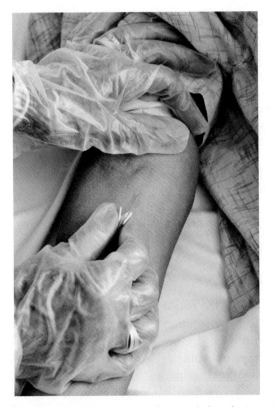

FIGURE 15-21 Hold the skin taut above or below the insertion site.

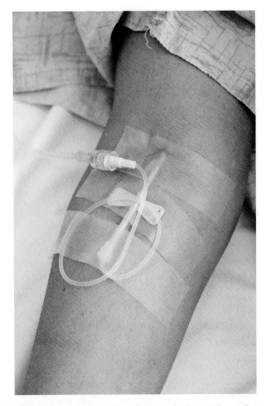

FIGURE 15-22 Connect the tubing and secure the catheter with nonallergenic tape or a transparent dressing.

CARE OF THE PATIENT WITH AN INTRAVENOUS INFUSION IN PLACE

If the IV infusion site is the antecubital vein, the patient's arm must be secured to an arm board to immobilize the elbow joint. The arm may be secured using an elastic bandage applied to avoid circulatory impairment. The arm should be assessed frequently to ensure that there is no discomfort or impaired circulation. The signs and symptoms of circulatory impairment for a patient in a cast, discussed in Chapter 9, may be used.

The infusion site must be assessed every 30 minutes to be certain that the contrast agent is not infiltrating into the surrounding tissues. Ask the patient if he is feeling any pain or discomfort and inspect the surrounding tissues for swelling, coldness, or redness. If this is the case, discontinue the infusion and ask the physician for direction. If the solution is infusing too slowly, reposition the arm and assess the flow. The IV standard must be positioned 18 to 24 inches above the injection site. An infusion pump or a simple clamp may be used to regulate the flow (Fig. 15-23). A safe rule to follow is to adjust the flow to 15 to 20 drops per minute. A large amount of fluid infusing too quickly may result in fluid intoxication or pulmonary edema, both of which are life-threatening. The symptoms of this may be headache, syncope, flushing of the face, complaints of feeling tightness of the chest, shock, and cardiac arrest.

> ⚠️ **WARNING!**
>
> The radiographer must never place pressure on the syringe when administering a bolus of drug or contrast. The fluid must be able to flow into the vein with ease!

Some drugs are extremely irritating to tissues if allowed to infiltrate. The result may be tissue necrosis and subsequent sloughing. At best, it will cause extreme pain. If extravasation occurs, notify the physician immediately, stop the infusion and remove the cannula. Elevate the affected arm and apply either ice packs or warm compresses as ordered. Document the incident naming the location of the area, its appearance, the amount of fluid infiltrated, and the palliative actions taken.

Drugs administered intravenously act very quickly. Any complaint of itching or feeling of congestion or fullness in the chest or throat is cause to cease drug administration. The radiographer must not wait for further evidence of complications. Stop the infusion or bolus and notify the physician.

Discontinuing Intravenous Infusions

An infusion is not discontinued without a physician's order to do so except in situations that call for immediate action. Patients who are receiving IV drugs do not wish to have an IV re-started if it is not necessary as the procedure is uncomfortable. The radiographer must be certain that the IV infusion is to be discontinued and the catheter withdrawn at the termination of a procedure before proceeding.

To discontinue an IV, the following equipment is needed:

Dry sterile 2 by 2 inch gauze sponges
Clean, disposable gloves
Tape

The procedure is as follows:

1. Identify the patient; perform hand hygiene.
2. Stop the solution that may be continuing to be instilled.
3. Prepare a sufficient strip of tape to cover a small pressure dressing.
4. Loosen the tape that holds the needle or catheter in place making certain the hub or the needle or catheter is clearly visible.

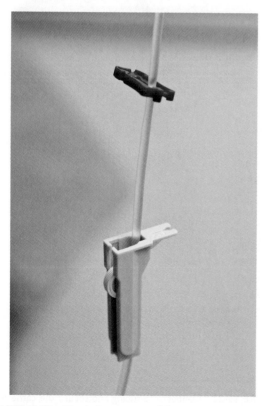

FIGURE 15-23 Simple intravenous clamp.

5. Open the sterile gauze sponge pack using aseptic technique.

6. Put on the clean gloves.

7. Gently withdraw the needle or catheter from the vein completely. Inspect the needle or catheter making sure it has remained intact.

8. Apply pressure to the site with a dry, sterile sponge until bleeding stops—about 2 minutes.

9. When the bleeding stops, use a sterile gauze sponge folded in half, place it over the site of insertion, and tape it in place using some pressure over the sponge. Inform the patient that this dressing may be removed in 1 or 2 hours.

10. Dispose of the materials correctly. Remove gloves and wash hands.

CALL OUT!

The radiographer must not discontinue an IV without orders from the physician!

SUMMARY

All drugs are potentially harmful; therefore, the radiographer must never become casual or careless when administering drugs or assisting with drug administration. The health care worker who participates in drug administration must have both a theoretical and a clinical education in pharmacology. He must also understand the pharmacokinetics and pharmacodynamics of drugs, their intended physiologic actions, and the potential adverse reactions that each can cause.

The radiographer must become familiar with the drugs found on the emergency cart and those frequently used in his department. Contrast media are the drugs the radiographer will use most frequently; therefore, he must be knowledgeable concerning their indications, contraindications, and adverse reactions. Contrast agents are listed in this chapter as either ionic on nonionic agents. The number of iodine particles found in solution of contrast agents influences the possibility and severity of an adverse reaction when administered to the patient. The osmolarity of the agent is also a factor in the severity of an adverse reaction.

The radiographer must carefully assess his patient and compile a history before administering a contrast agent. He must report any negative data gathered from the history to the physician caring for the patient before contrast agent is administered. If the patient has an adverse reaction to a contrast agent, the radiographer must stop the administration of the agent and summon assistance. He must never leave a patient unattended who is receiving a contrast agent or an intravenous infusion.

Any drug administered to a patient must be ordered by a physician or a health care worker who is licensed to do so. There are several methods of obtaining an order for a drug to be administered, including written, verbal, and telephone orders. The radiographer's responsibility is to understand and obtain a legal order before preparing or administering any drug. He must also be able to document the medication administered correctly and learn common medical abbreviations.

It must be remembered that contrast agents are drugs and all precautions pertaining to any other drug also pertains to them. The *five rights of drug administration* are to be followed by the radiographer at all times. Any drug error must be reported and documented correctly. The radiographer must be aware of and follow the federal regulations pertaining to controlled substances.

Each route of drug administration requires its own equipment and procedure. The radiographer must learn the lengths and gauges of needles and venous catheters and the sites for parenteral drug administration. Use of surgical asepsis must be applied for all parenteral drug routes.

The radiographer must be able to prepare the equipment and the site for IV drug administration and take precautions to prevent adverse reactions. This is particularly true for IV drug administration because these drugs travel to the systemic circulation immediately. The radiographer must take special care when the patient is an infant, a child, or an elderly person.

The radiographer must follow the policy concerning administration of IV drugs of the institution in which he is employed. He must also understand the symptoms of early, intermediate, and severe anaphylactic reactions to contrast agents and other drugs and his actions if these occur.

If an IV infusion is to be discontinued, there must be an order by the physician to do so. The correct aseptic procedure must be followed when this procedure is to be completed. Waste materials must be disposed of correctly and standard precautions followed at all times when drugs are administered.

CHAPTER 15 TEST

1. List all aspects of drug administration the radiographer is expected to know.
2. The radiographer who administers a drug incorrectly is not held liable for the error.
   a. True
   b. False
3. Drugs that must bear the legend "caution: federal law prohibits dispensing without prescription" include the following:
   a. Hypnotics and narcotics
   b. Alternative drugs
   c. All diet drugs
   d. All analgesics
4. Alternative dietary and herbal supplements are classified as food, not drugs.
   a. True
   b. False
5. Define *drug dependence* and *drug addiction*.
6. The alternative name for Valium is diazepam. Valium is:
   a. The trade name
   b. The generic name
   c. The chemical name
7. If the radiographer is required to administer a drug with which he is not familiar, he must seek information prior to administering the drug. He would seek such information in which of the following reference books?
   a. The encyclopedia
   b. The radiographer's textbook
   c. *The Physician's Desk Reference*
   d. From his colleague
   e. From the *Los Angeles Times*
8. Drugs given by mouth are generally given in larger doses. This is because:
   a. They absorb more slowly
   b. They absorb more rapidly
   c. They are unreliable
   d. Larger doses ensure that some of the drug will remain to perform the intended effect
9. List the factors that will alter drug absorption in the body.
10. For a drug to reach its therapeutic effect more quickly, a physician might order:
    a. A larger initial dose, and later smaller doses
    b. A smaller initial dose, then a larger dose
    c. A bolus
    d. A maximizing dose
11. Marjorie Merriweather takes oral morphine for chronic pain. After taking the prescribed dosage for 2 weeks, she notices that it no longer seems to be controlling the pain. This reaction is called:
    a. Addiction
    b. Dependency

c. Tolerance
d. An adverse reaction
12. Two drugs must never be mixed in the same syringe for administration before checking their:
    a. Effectiveness
    b. Correct dosage
    c. Compatibility
    d. Expiration dates
13. Drug absorption varies from person to person. The efficiency of drug absorption is largely dependent on:
    a. The time of day
    b. The sex of the individual
    c. The absorptive surface available
    d. The type of drug
14. Drugs given orally are not affected by the first-pass effect.
    a. True
    b. False
15. Factors that may influence the effect of a drug are:
    a. Age and weight
    b. Sex and time of day
    c. Medication history and the patient's temperament
    d. a and b are correct
    e. a, b, and c are correct
16. Match the following terms pertaining to drugs with the correct definition:
    a. The method of drug   (1) half-life
       action on living tissues   (2) metabolism
    b. The effect of a drug that (3) clearance rate
       may be life-threatening   (4) pharmacody-
    c. The process by which   namics
       the body alters the   (5) side effect
       chemical structure   (6) adverse effect
       of a drug
    d. The time it takes for a
       50% decrease of a drug's
       presence in the body
    e. The removal from the body
    f. Unintended but nontoxic effect of a drug
17. Factors the radiographer must consider before administering a drug to a patient include:
    a. The age of the patient
    b. The gender of the patient
    c. The patient's health status
    d. a and b are correct
    e. a, b, and c are correct
18. Contrast agents are categorized as drugs. This is because they are absorbed into the systemic circulation and may produce a physiologic response on the body.
    a. True
    b. False

19. List the variables the physician considers when selecting a contrast agent for use.
20. The physiologic effect of a contrast agent on the patient's body that may create an adverse reaction when administered is due to:
    a. Its low viscosity as compared to other drugs
    b. The fact that it is isotonic
    c. Its high viscosity, which prompts a sudden shift in body fluid from the interstitial spaces and cells into the systemic circulation
    d. Its shift of fluid into the interstitial spaces and cells related to its high viscosity
21. Expected side effects of contrast agents administered by intravascular route are:
    a. Feeling of warmth and flushing
    b. Feeling of being short of breath
    c. Metallic taste in mouth
    d. Complaints of itching
    e. a and c are correct
22. List obligations of the radiographer before he begins administering a contrast agent.
23. A patient is receiving an intravenous contrast agent by bolus intravenous injection. The patient begins to complain of nausea, itching around his eyes, feeling dizzy, and a headache. The radiographer decides the patient is having:
    a. Side effects from the injection
    b. A vasovagal reaction
    c. A mild adverse reaction
    d. A severe adverse reaction
    e. A moderate adverse reaction

24. If coldness and swelling at the site of an intravenous infusion are observed, the radiographer must:
    a. Call a code
    b. Stop the infusion and apply cold or warm compresses
    c. Inform the patient that this is a normal occurrence
    d. Attempt to restart the IV
25. List the five rights of drug administration.
26. Match the following medical abbreviations with the correct term:
    (1) PO   a. milliliter
    (2) IV   b. at once
    (3) STAT   c. every day
    (4) PRN   d. intravenous
    (5) qd   e. by mouth
    (6) mL   f. as necessary
27. List the required items in the radiographer's charting if he administers a drug.
28. All drugs given by parenteral routes are given using:
    a. Medical aseptic technique
    b. Surgical aseptic technique
29. List the items that must be included in the incident report if a drug is administered in error.
30. Discuss the precautions that must be taken when administering a drug to an elderly person.
31. Discuss the precautions that must be taken when administering a drug to a child.

Care of Patients during Special Procedures

STUDENT LEARNING OUTCOMES

After studying this chapter, you will be able to:

1. Describe the potential medical complications, emotional implications, and the patient care and teaching needs for the patient undergoing cardiac catheterization, angiography, and percutaneous transluminal angioplasty.
2. Describe the patient care and teaching needs of the patient for computed tomography.
3. Describe the patient care and teaching needs of the patient before and during ultrasonography.
4. Describe the patient care and teaching needs of the patient before and during magnetic resonance imaging.
5. Explain your responsibilities as the radiographer to the patient for positron emission tomography.
6. List the patient care considerations and teaching responsibilities for the patient receiving nuclear medicine imaging.
7. Explain the teaching and care needs of the patient receiving proton therapy.
8. List the potential side effects, emotional implications, and care and teaching needs of the patient receiving radiation therapy.
9. Describe the patient care considerations and teaching needs before and during mammography.
10. Describe the patient care considerations and teaching needs of the patient having arthrography.
11. Explain the radiographer's role in patient care during lithotripsy.

KEY TERMS

Claustrophobic: Suffering from claustrophobia, which is the fear of being in a confined place

Dehydration: Deprivation of water

Dorsiflex: To move the toes and forefoot upward

Hypoglycemic: Pertaining to an abnormally small concentration of glucose in the circulating blood

Hypotension: An abnormal condition in which the blood pressure is not adequate for normal perfusion and oxygenation of the tissues.

Radioisotope: Radioactive atoms having the same number of protons

Restenosis: Recurrence of stenosis after corrective surgery on the heart valve; narrowing of a structure

Sonographer: Ultrasonographer

Toxicity: State of being poisonous

Transducer: A hand-held device, used in sonography that sends and receives sound wave signals

Patients undergoing special radiographic imaging procedures require special consideration. Many of these patients have been informed that they may have life-threatening illnesses and that the procedure that they are about to undergo will either confirm or rule out this threat. Special imaging procedures are not without pain and risk, and most patients find them anxiety provoking. Even something as innocuous as the diagnostic setting can cause the patient distress.

The atmosphere into which the patient is received is often intimidating for the patients. The imaging room resembles an operating room, and the health care team is either masked and gowned or is hidden behind protective screens, which may require that they address the patient by microphone. This, combined with the prospect of a shortened life span, often elicits from the patient feelings of helplessness, vulnerability, and fear.

Patients receiving radiation or proton therapy may be in various stages of the grieving process. They know that they have a potentially terminal illness and that the prescribed treatment is being administered in an attempt to prolong their lives or provide them some relief from pain during their final days. Working in these diagnostic and treatment areas, one must have exceptional technical skills and superior communication and patient-teaching skills. In these areas of patient care, the physician, the registered nurse, the radiographer, and other health care specialists work together as an interdependent team. Each depends on the other for safe and successful diagnostic and treatment outcomes. All patient care skills presented in the previous chapters of this text need to be applied in these areas.

The intent of this text is to give the radiologic technology student an overview of patient care in these areas so that he or she may benefit from observational experiences and preview potential areas of specialization, which involve additional training and or education. Detailed technical discussion of these procedures is beyond the scope of this text and is mentioned only when relevant to patient care instruction.

CARDIAC CATHETERIZATION AND CORONARY ANGIOGRAPHY, ARTERIOGRAPHY, AND NONSURGICAL INTERVENTIONS

Cardiac catheterization and coronary angiography (Fig. 16-1) are performed by a cardiologist to diagnose coronary artery patency and, if indicated, treat atherosclerosis of the coronary arteries by nonsurgical means. These procedures are performed in a cardiac catheterization laboratory.

The role of a member of this highly technical team is to participate in the patient's education, assessment, and general care. One member of the team, either a radiographer or a nurse, performs a surgical scrub, dons gown and gloves, and prepares the sterile instruments. Another

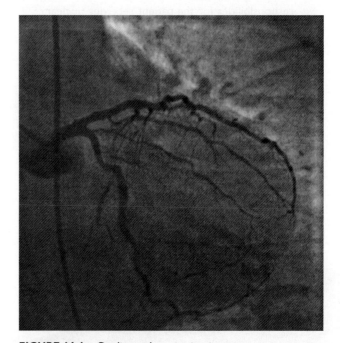

FIGURE 16-1 Cardiac catheterization image.

member of the team performs a sterile skin prep and drapes the patient for the procedure. All members of the team must be alert to any symptoms of respiratory or cardiac distress; be able to monitor vital signs accurately; assist with drug and contrast media administration; apply surgical aseptic technique; and communicate with the patient in a therapeutic manner. Each member of the team must have special education in the problems and potential complications that may result from the procedure. The patient and the medical team must wear shields to protect themselves from unnecessary exposure to radiation during these lengthy procedures, which involve use of fluoroscopy and digital imaging.

The most common sites for insertion of the arterial catheter are the right and left brachial and femoral arteries. The area surrounding the site of catheter insertion is surgically prepared, usually with an iodophor antiseptic as described in Chapter 5. This area is injected with a local anesthetic, and the artery is accessed with a large-bore needle containing a stylet to prevent return blood flow. When the artery has been accessed, the stylet is removed. A guidewire is then inserted through the needle into the artery, and the needle is removed. A catheter is passed over the guidewire into the artery with fluoroscopic guidance. The guidewire is removed, and the catheter is left in place and manipulated to visualize all vessels desired to diagnose potential areas of cardiac pathology.

A low-osmolar contrast media is injected through the catheter, and the cardiac vessels are observed to assess cardiac output; locate and assess the severity of occlusive coronary artery disease; and diagnose congenital heart abnormalities, aneurysms, or other cardiac abnormalities. Treatment of diseased arteries may be performed at the time of the cardiac catheterization. If the coronary arteries are occluded and would benefit from percutaneous transluminal coronary angioplasty, or if the patient has an evolving myocardial infarct, a balloon-tipped catheter is introduced through a guidewire. After the site of occlusion is reached, the balloon is inflated to compress the plaque that is causing the occlusion.

If there is reason to believe that vessel **restenosis** will occur, a stent may be used to maintain patency of the vessel. A stent is an object that provides support and structure to a vessel. It is introduced in the same way that the balloon is introduced and is left in place when the catheter is removed. Some of the potential complications from these procedures are cardiac arrhythmias, embolic stroke, allergic reactions to the contrast media, and infection or hemorrhage at the catheter insertion site.

Arteriography

Arteriography uses the same technology and the same surgical aseptic technique as cardiac angiography to

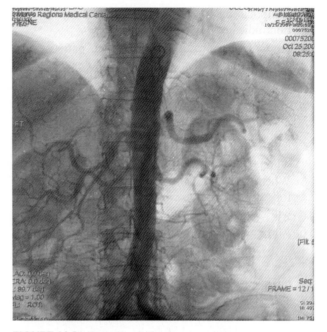

FIGURE 16-2   Arteriogram image.

observe major blood vessels throughout the body. The kidneys (Fig. 16-2), adrenal glands, brain, and abdominal aorta are the most common organs to be assessed by this method. The aorta is the typical route to access the vessels of the lower extremities for diagnosis of circulatory impairment of the lower extremities. Potential complications from arteriography are much the same as with coronary angiography. If the kidneys are the focus of the procedure, renal failure is an added potential problem. If the adrenal glands are the focus, fatal hypertensive crisis may occur if the patient has the disease pheochromocytoma. Medication to prevent this is administered several days before the procedure.

Patient Care before and during Cardiac Catheterization, Angiography, or Arteriography

Nurses in a preoperative area perform most patient care in the hours before these procedures; however, the radiographer must carry out patient teaching and assessment immediately before the procedure. The process varies somewhat depending on the body organ to be assessed, but the process is largely similar, as follows:

1. An informed consent is signed after the patient receives instruction from the physician about all that is involved in the procedure, including all potential adverse effects.

2. Inform the patient before cardiac catheterization of the possible immediate need for coronary surgery if

complications or outcomes from the catheterization indicate.

3. For angiography of the heart, the patient must abstain from food and fluids for 4 to 8 hours before the procedure; however, for angiography in areas other than the heart, the patient is often asked to be well hydrated before the examination.

4. Instruct the patient to empty the bladder; to remove dentures, jewelry, and clothing; and to put on a patient gown.

5. When the patient enters the catheterization laboratory, explain all that will transpire so that he or she will be prepared for the procedure.

6. Allow the patient to express any anxieties or concerns about what is to occur.

7. Assess the patient for allergies to iodine or any medications to be administered.

8. The peripheral pulses are often identified and marked with a pen so that they may be quickly assessed during and after the procedure.

9. If ordered, medication is administered to alleviate anxiety.

10. The patient is transferred to the procedure table and placed in a supine position.

11. The area of catheter insertion is shaved and scrubbed with an antiseptic solution.

12. A peripheral IV line is started for access and to facilitate administration of drugs as needed. The leads for monitoring the heart rate are placed and connected to the oscilloscope.

13. It the patient is a child, he or she may be allowed to bring a CD or DVD player to ease feelings of fear and anxiety.

14. Inform the patient that he or she may be asked to cough or take deep breaths during the procedure to ease feelings of nausea or lightheadedness. Coughing may also correct arrhythmias.

15. A local anesthetic may be administered before arterial puncture.

16. The artery is accessed, the guidewire is inserted, and then the catheter is placed over the wire.

17. The patient is informed that the contrast agent is about to be injected and is told that he or she will feel a burning or flushed feeling from this and must not be concerned.

18. If the angiography is of the adrenal glands, blood pressure must be monitored continually to assess for evidence of a malignant hypertensive crisis.

19. Images are taken in a timed sequence to demonstrate the arterial and venous blood flow to the organ being studied.

20. Nitroglycerin to dilate blood vessels and other drugs may be administered during the procedure.

Patient Care and Teaching after Cardiac Catheterization, Angiography, and Arteriography

Patient care after angiography and cardiac catheterization is relatively uniform and must be carried out meticulously to prevent circulatory deficit, thrombus formation, or hemorrhage. In most instances, the patient is transported to the hospital postanesthesia recovery area or to an intensive coronary care area to be monitored after cardiac catheterization or angiography. The radiographer must understand the monitoring and care required after these examinations so the patient can receive instructions and monitoring before he or she leaves the diagnostic imaging area.

The patient may be extremely fatigued, and any movement required after the procedure must be done with adequate assistance so there is little demand on the patient. Monitor the patient's pulse rate on the side of the invasive procedure every 15 minutes for 1 hour and then every hour until an 8- to 12-hour period is complete and no complication has been detected. The blood pressure is monitored on the side opposite the invasive procedure at the same time intervals. The pulses distal to the site of catheter insertion must also be monitored at frequent, regular intervals for 24 hours after the procedure. After femoral catheterization, the patient should be instructed to move the toes and **dorsiflex** the feet frequently. Also instruct the patient to keep the legs straight and still. Assess the extremities for coldness, cyanosis, pallor, numbness, size of one extremity compared with the other extremity, and tingling. Instruct the patient to inform the nurse if he or she has any of the latter symptoms. If a circulatory deficit occurs, surgical intervention may be necessary to correct the problem. The patient should also inform the nurse of any feeling of wetness at the site of the catheter insertion; this may indicate hemorrhaging.

If a femoral artery was used for the catheter insertion, inform the patient that he or she must remain at bedrest for 10 to 12 hours after the procedure to prevent hemorrhage. A weight or sandbag is often placed over the site of catheter insertion to apply pressure. The patient should also be told to apply pressure at the insertion site when coughing or sneezing. Do not raise the patient's head more than 20 degrees during the immediate postcatheterization period.

If the brachial site was used for catheter insertion, the arm on the side of insertion is kept straight with an armboard for several hours, but the patient may be up as soon as the vital signs are stable. Regardless of the site of insertion, the patient must be monitored for 24 hours for external bleeding or for bleeding into the tissues surrounding the catheter insertion site.

Instruct the patient who has received iodinated contrast media to increase fluid intake to prevent

dehydration and **hypotension**. This may be contraindicated in some patients with congestive heart failure. Patients are often given intravenous fluid replacement therapy during these procedures, but they should be made aware of the need for increased fluid intake.

Record the time that the procedure began and ended, any drugs or contrast agents administered, and the patient's tolerance of the procedure on the patient's chart. Also record the instructions given to the patient after the procedure.

COMPUTED TOMOGRAPHY SCAN

Computed tomography (CT) is a diagnostic imaging procedure that can be used to scan body tissues and organs combining x-ray and computer technology. CT (Fig. 16-3) produces multiple cross-sectional images of body organs, which can be reconstructed into 3-dimensional images. It is a highly effective method of diagnosing disease processes of bones, intracranial, soft tissue structures of the chest, abdomen, and pelvis, and organic pathology.

Contrast media may be introduced by injection to increase tissue density for body and brain scans. Barium solutions may be used to increase organ density of the gastrointestinal organs.

Patient Care and Instruction before Computed Tomography

The patient may be receiving contrast media; therefore, all precautions and questioning that precede administration of that drug are included in pre-CT patient care. The radiographer must spend a few moments explaining the procedure to the patient in order to alleviate anxiety. Tell the patient that he or she is expected to lie still to ensure clear images. Allow the patient to inspect the equipment and to express any feelings of claustrophobia or fear of the procedure. The radiographer must inform the patient

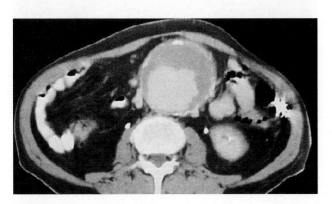

FIGURE 16-3   Abdominal CT.

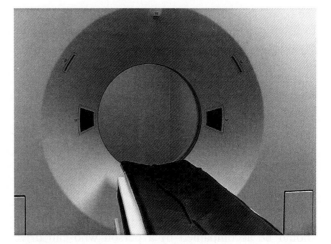

FIGURE 16-4   CT scanner: Gantry.

that he or she may communicate with the radiographer through a microphone in the CT room. The radiographer should show the patient that he will be sitting behind the glass window where he can observe, hear, and communicate with the patient at all times (Fig. 16-4).

The radiographer must establish a feeling of trust in the patient. It is very frightening for patients to feel that they are in a room alone when receiving an intravenous injection, and the radiographer needs to know of the possibility of a reaction. The extremely anxious patient who is in pain and unable to lie quietly may need an analgesic or sedative medication if this can be prescribed.

Inform the patient that he or she may have feelings of nausea, warmth, flushing, and a metallic taste after the contrast media is administered. Place an emesis basin near the patient, where he or she can pick it up easily if need be. Instruct the patient to immediately inform you if he or she has any feelings of pain during the procedure. Inform the patient that the procedure takes 15 minutes to 45 minutes to complete depending on what part of the body is being scanned. The patient must sign an informed consent before receiving a CT scan. The patient's medical history and history of allergies must also be taken before this procedure is begun if contrast is administered.

Computed Tomography of the Body

Patients who are to have CT of the bowel and abdominal organs are allowed nothing to eat or drink 4 to 6 hours prior to the examination. They may receive a barium contrast agent mixed with 8 oz. of orange juice to drink before the scan. A contrast media is also injected intravenously immediately before the CT scan begins.

The radiographer must spend the same amount of time explaining the procedure to the patient before beginning this examination as previously discussed. For the bowel and abdominal CT scan, instruct the patient to listen carefully for instructions to breathe, hold the breath, and release the breath. Tell the patient to expect many of these instructions. If the patient is made to feel like the major focus of the procedure and is kept informed, he or she will be more cooperative and relaxed while the examination is in progress.

Patient Care after Computed Tomography

Patients who have received sedative or antianxiety medication may not drive themselves. Patients who have come from their homes and plan to return home should be accompanied by a person who can drive them or assist them to get there safely.

When contrast media is injected and the procedure is complete, the intravenous line is discontinued by order of the physician, as described in Chapter 13. The patient is then allowed to sit up with assistance. He or she should sit quietly on the table for several minutes before being assisted back to the dressing room, wheelchair, or gurney. If the patient is hospitalized, he or she may be returned to the hospital room with assistance. If going home, assist the patient to the dressing room, and help him or her get dressed, if needed. Observe the patient for at least 1 hour for adverse reaction to drugs and for general instability before discharging the patient from the department.

Instruct the patient who has received a contrast media to increase fluid intake to at least 3000 mL and avoid caffeine for the next 24 hours to aid in excretion of the agent from the body and to prevent dehydration. If the patient has had barium, he or she should follow the instructions in Chapter 13 concerning post-barium administration.

Any adverse reactions that occurred during the CT and any medications that the patient received must be recorded on the patient's chart. Record the time that the procedure began and ended, the patient's tolerance of the procedure, and the instructions that the patient received for post-procedure care.

ULTRASONOGRAPHY

Ultrasound is a method of visualizing the soft tissue structures of the body for diagnosis of diseases without the use of radiation or contrast media. It is a noninvasive, painless procedure that requires the skill of a specially educated technologist, usually a radiographer with additional education. Ultrasound (Fig. 16-5) uses high-frequency sound waves to search for pathological changes in body organs. Images are displayed on a monitor. Permanent copies of the images are also produced (Fig. 16-6).

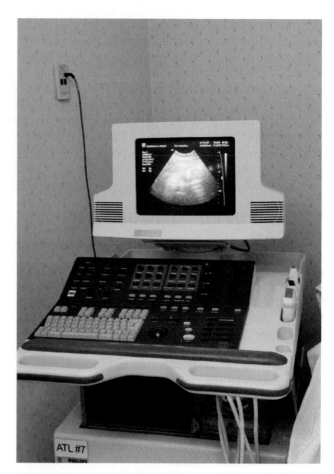

FIGURE 16-5 Ultrasound scanner.

This form of imaging is useful in obstetrics for fetal monitoring, in neurology for diagnosing brain disorders, and in urology for diagnosing urinary bladder, scrotal, prostatic, and renal pathological conditions. It is also used to diagnose vascular aneurysms, as well as pancreatic, gallbladder, thyroid, venous, parathyroid, lymph node, eye, and breast pathological conditions.

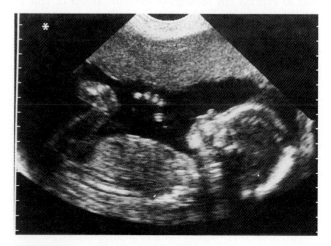

FIGURE 16-6 Ultrasound image: fetus.

This is not an all-inclusive list; new uses for ultrasonography continue to be found. The radiographer who is not trained as an ultrasonographer must have an awareness of the process of ultrasound to correctly schedule imaging procedures to the patient's best advantage.

Patient Care for Ultrasonography

Patient care considerations for ultrasound include instruction in preparation for the procedure, an explanation of the procedure itself, and correct scheduling to prevent unsatisfactory examinations. Little postexamination instruction is needed.

If a patient is to have barium studies as well as an ultrasound examination, the ultrasound examination should be scheduled to precede the barium studies because residual barium in the gastrointestinal tract will interfere with effective ultrasound examinations. If a patient has a tendency to have large amounts of gas in the bowel, the gas will interfere with visualization. A patient with this problem should be instructed to eat low residue foods for 24 to 36 hours before the examination and be scheduled at a time when the bowel will be relatively gas free as is the case in the early morning before breakfast.

CALL OUT!

If a patient is to have barium imaging as well as an ultrasound examination, the ultrasound examination must be scheduled to precede the barium examination because residual barium will interfere with effective ultrasound results!

Active children or patients who are unable to remain quiet because of pain, emotional illness, or anxiety must be scheduled at a time when they can be accompanied by a person who can keep them calm and relaxed. Use of sedative drugs may also be recommended by the physician.

Patients should be informed that this is a painless, noninvasive procedure. A lubricating gel is used as the conductive agent. The **sonographer** will apply the gel. A tap water enema may be required during the procedure for ultrasound of the pelvic area.

A **transducer** is held by the sonographer and is moved over the surface to be examined as the screen is watched and images are produced. The patient must be shown the transducer and reassured that it will cause no pain.

Some examinations require a preparatory cleansing enema and fasting for several hours before the scheduled time. Other ultrasound procedures require the bladder to be filled with fluid. If either of these is

required, the radiographer or the sonographer must explain the preparation to the patient.

Wound dressing, scars, and obesity all are factors to be considered when ultrasound is the imaging technique prescribed. Dressings must be removed, and lubricating gel cannot be applied over an open wound. Scars and obesity prevent good visualization. A clear sterile patch may be worn over wounds if ordered by the physician.

Patient care after sonography is the same as thoughtful patient care after any diagnostic imaging procedure. The lubricating gel must be carefully removed so that the patient's clothing is not soiled by it. If the patient was immersed in water, he or she must be provided with towels and a private area in which to dry and dress. Patients who are in a weakened condition must not be left alone, and any assistance the patient needs must be provided. Patients who have had sedative medication must not be allowed to drive home or return to their hospital room unattended.

MAGNETIC RESONANCE IMAGING

Magnetic resonance imaging (MRI) is a noninvasive procedure used for diagnosing neoplasms as well as vascular, soft tissue, bone and joint, and central nervous system pathological conditions (Fig. 16-7).

MRI is performed by placing the entire body, or a body part, in a magnetic field with radiofrequency waves to produce computerized images of body organs and tissues. These images are replayed on a video screen for diagnosis. MRI has many diagnostic advantages. Among them is the absence of radiation that may harm body cells. It also eliminates the need for iodinated contrast agents and decreases the possibility of anaphylactic reactions.

Patient Care and Education for MRI

Patient education is the key to successful imaging when MRI is the diagnostic procedure selected. Inform the patient that the procedure may take from 30 to 60 minutes to complete. **Claustrophobic** fears are common and emerge when the patient is faced with possibly spending up to 1 hour in a cylinder, in a large room, alone. Accurate information and instruction help to alleviate these fears. Antianxiety medication is often prescribed to assist in relieving the anxiety of the patient. These medications may not be given if blood flow is to be assessed because they may interfere with normal blood flow. Inform the adult patient that he or she will need to lie in a supine position with slight movement between scans. Also inform the patient that

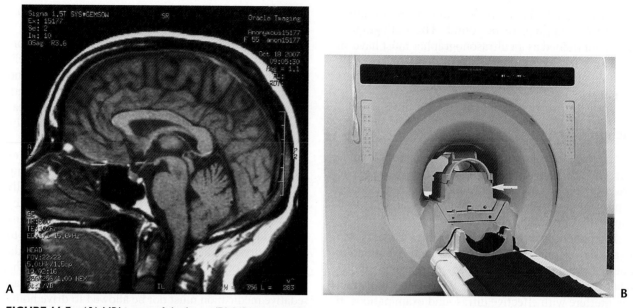

FIGURE 16-7 (**A**) MRI image of the brain. (**B**) MRI scanner: Gantry.

he or she will hear repetitive knocking sounds during the entire examination. The patient may wear earplugs for ear protection due to the knocking sound.

Explain to the patient that, although he or she may feel completely alone, at least two persons will be just on the other side of a glass window. They will be constantly observing the patient, and they can and will be communicating with the patient frequently during the procedure. Show the patient that there is a microphone through which to communicate to the staff. The patient should be allowed to examine the MRI equipment and ask any questions that he or she may have before beginning the procedure. If the patient is a child, a parent may be allowed to sit beside the cylinder and talk to the child during the MRI. Infants should be fed shortly before being placed in the cylinder.

The radiographer can help decrease the patient's anxiety by speaking to him or her frequently and letting the patient know how much time is left before the examination is completed. The radiographer must remember that many patients who are having MRI are anxious and fearful because of possible ominous diagnostic outcomes, as are the parents of children who are having this procedure. Patients may focus on their claustrophobic feelings in an attempt to deny the possibility of a threatening diagnosis. The radiographer must be patient, sensitive, and nonjudgmental when communicating with these patients and their family members. By implying that a patient's feelings are foolish or offering cliché responses, the radiographer may only increase a patient's anxiety. Time must be spent discussing the process and the patient's or the parents' feelings and concerns before beginning MRI. If this is

not done, the patient may be unable to remain as quiet as is necessary for successful imaging.

A medical history, as previously described, must be taken before MRI. History of allergies must be included. If the patient is to receive a contrast agent, the institution may require the patient to sign an informed consent. The patient should be informed that this procedure does not expose him or her to radiation and is relatively painless. The patient who has metal dental work may feel some tingling sensations.

Instruct patients to remove all metal jewelry, dental bridges, clothing with metal closures, belts, metal-containing prostheses, hair clips, and shoes before entering the scanner room. Purses and wallets containing credit cards must be left outside in a secure place because magnetic resonance will deactivate credit cards. You will be responsible for placing the items safely away and for informing patients where their belongings are being kept.

Patients who receive antianxiety or sedative drugs before MRI and those who have a history of asthma and receive a contrast media should be monitored during the procedure. There are pulse oximeters made for use in the MRI chamber.

MRI is contraindicated for people who have internal pacemakers, implanted heart valves, metal orthopedic implants, or surgical clips. It may be contraindicated for pregnant women because the effects of MRI on pregnancy are unknown at present. Patients on life-support equipment or infusion pumps or who are critically ill may not receive MRI because monitoring equipment cannot be used in the scanner room. Other items that prevent MRI are an implanted insulin pump, bone-growth stimulator, internal hearing aid, cochlear implant, neurostimulator, metal eye prostheses, vena cava clot filter, an intrauterine device or diaphragm in place, some surgeries, claustrophobia, regular need for oxygen administration, and any metal device.

For persons with severe claustrophobia, open MRI is available. In open MRI, the patient is not completely enclosed in a chamber, which decreases the feeling of being enclosed in a small space.

Patient Care after MRI

There are no special patient instructions or teaching responsibilities after MRI unless the patient has received medication or a contrast agent. If the patient has received drugs or a contrast media, the instructions are the same as for other invasive imaging procedures.

Children are sometimes sedated for this examination. If this is the case, the patient is monitored throughout the examination and until fully recovered from the drug by a nurse proficient in this field. Sedating children requires special evaluation that will not be discussed in this text.

POSITRON EMISSION TOMOGRAPHY

Positron emission tomography (PET) combines the qualities of radionuclide imaging with CT to study blood flow and volume and protein metabolism. The body organ studies using this technique that have had great success to date are those of the brain, the heart, and the lungs. PET is able to assist in diagnosis of Alzheimer's disease, brain tumors, cardiac disease, and, most recently, the physiologic changes in psychiatric diseases (Fig. 16-8). It is one of the most innovative techniques currently used. Unfortunately, it is a very expensive procedure that requires sophisticated technology such as a cyclotron, a specialized chemical laboratory, computerized equipment, and a team of scientists and health care specialists to carry out the diagnostic procedures. More facilities are opting to install PET/CT scanners due to the high cost of the equipment and technology. The patient inhales or is injected with a radioisotope of an element that occurs naturally in the body such as oxygen, nitrogen, carbon, or fluorine.

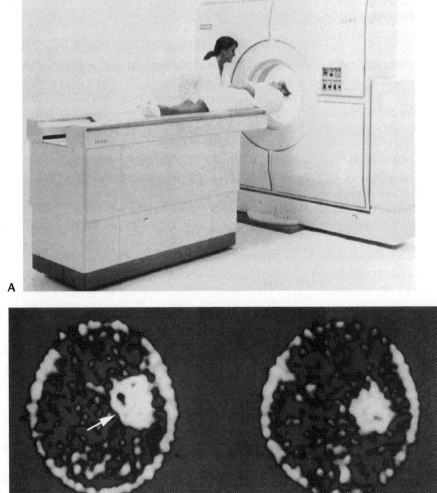

FIGURE 16-8 (A) PET scanner. **(B)** PET brain scan.

A

B

These isotopes emit subatomic particles called *positrons* (positively charged electrons).

Patient Care for PET

The patient or caregiver must have a clear explanation of the PET procedure. The patient must understand that there will be radiation exposure that is minimal and that he or she will receive the radioactive material either by injection or inhalation, depending on the organ to be studied. The examination will take from 30 to 90 minutes. An informed consent form is required by most institutions.

There is usually no food or fluid restriction before the examination; however, the patient should take no caffeine, nicotine, or alcohol for 24 hours. The patient should also receive no sedative or tranquilizing drugs. All these interfere with the examination. Diabetic patients may receive insulin 3 to 4 hours before the procedure. Patients who are pregnant or breastfeeding may be restricted from this examination. Immediately before the examination, the patient must be instructed to empty the bladder.

The patient receiving a brain scan must understand that he or she may be asked to perform an activity such as a recitation of a simple proverb or the pledge to the flag. This is so that brain activity during recall or cognitive processes can be assessed. The patient may also be blindfolded and wear earplugs to screen out external stimuli.

After the examination, instruct the patient to change positions slowly, and assist him or her to rise or leave the examining table because of possible dizziness due to orthostatic hypotension. Instruct the patient to increase fluid intake for 24 hours and to urinate frequently to eliminate the isotope from the body.

The patient receiving PET is often elderly and may have symptoms of dementia. If this is the case, the radiographer must recognize that the patient is unable to follow directions and may need to be closely guided through every aspect of the procedure. The strangeness of the environment may be frightening to a person with symptoms of dementia. Because excessive anxiety may affect the results of the examination, a family member or a familiar caretaker may need to remain with the patient to decrease his or her anxiety.

▮ NUCLEAR MEDICINE IMAGING

Nuclear medicine imaging is frequently the diagnostic imaging technique of choice to detect or rule out malignant lesions or to produce images that are not visible on standard radiographs. It may be used to visualize pathological conditions of the lungs, kidneys, heart, bones, thyroid, and other body organs.

Before the nuclear medicine examination, the patient may need to abstain from eating or drinking for several hours. The patient must sign a special consent form and must be informed that he or she will receive a small amount of a **radioisotope** and will be exposed to a minimal amount of radiation. He should be informed that the isotope will be excreted within 24 hours and there will be no residual radiation effects. Depending on the organ to be diagnosed, the patient may receive an intravenous injection of the isotope. He may also be given a radioactive tracer compound by inhalation or oral route. The patient should be told to expect to feel flushed for a short time after receiving the isotope.

Patients who are pregnant, have renal or hepatic disease, or are allergic to iodine should be carefully screened before being scheduled for this diagnostic procedure. Only one radionuclide procedure should be scheduled on one day because one may interfere with another.

> ### ◀))) CALL OUT!
>
> The patient must not receive more than one nuclear medicine procedure on one day. Other contrast media may interfere with the examination!

After initial preparation, the patient is taken to the nuclear medicine department for either dynamic or static scans, depending on the clinical symptoms. A tracer isotope and the contrast media are administered. The patient is placed on an examining table and expected to lie quietly while the test is in progress. This can be a problem for the elderly patient or for a person in pain.

The isotope accumulates in areas of pathology that are called "hot spots." If this is a bone scan, an area of decreased uptake of the radionuclide may indicate circulatory impairment and is called a "cold spot" (Fig. 16-9). If the total concentration of the radionuclide is less than normal, a diagnosis of a generalized renal disorder must be considered.

The standard imaging device in nuclear medicine is called the gamma camera. It does not move and produces a two-dimensional image. The newest nuclear imaging camera is three-dimensional. The third dimension has been achieved in gamma cameras through single photon emission computed tomography (SPECT). This has greatly increased the diagnostic ability of nuclear medicine imaging.

After nuclear medicine imaging, if an intravenous agent has been administered, assess the area for redness and swelling before discharging the patient. The patient must be cautioned to rise slowly to prevent postural hypotension. Do not allow the patient to leave the laboratory until the images are reviewed for clarity.

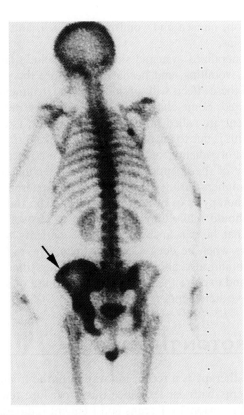

FIGURE 16-9   Bone scan: whole body.

Instruct the patient to resume his or her usual dietary and medication pattern unless contraindicated by the physician. Remind the patient that the radionuclide will be excreted within 24 hours and that the only precaution to be taken is to flush the commode immediately after each use.

Bone Scan

Bone scan images the skeleton by means of a scanning camera in order to diagnose malignant lesions of the skeletal system, degenerative bone infection, and unexplained bone pain. The scanner is able to detect "hot spots," as in radionuclide imaging. A radioactive tracer compound is administered intravenously approximately 3 hours before the scan. The patient is instructed to drink large amounts of water and to urinate immediately before the scan. The radiographer must explain this procedure in detail to the patient and alleviate any feeling of anxiety that the patient may have. This is particularly important if the scan is being performed to rule out cancer.

There should be no other radiographic examinations scheduled for 24 to 48 hours before or after this scan. A medical history, a history of allergic reactions, and a consent form must be signed.

After the bone scan, the patient must be instructed to increase fluid intake and notify the physician immediately if there is any sign of warmth, redness, or swelling

at the site of injection. The physician may prescribe pain medication if it is indicated.

Radiation Therapy

At least half of the patients with a diagnosis of cancer will receive external radiation therapy during the course of the disease. This form of treatment is used to cure the disease, to control malignant tumors that cannot be removed, to prevent spread of the tumor to the brain and spinal cord, and to decrease pain when the cancer metastasizes to the bones, brain, or soft tissues. Radiation therapists who work in the area of radiation therapy should receive specialized education; however, the radiography student may rotate to this area in the course of his or her education and must have some understanding of patient care in radiation therapy.

The intent of therapeutic radiation is not to kill all tumor cells immediately. All cells react differently, and some may repair the radiation-induced damage and begin to reproduce again. For this reason, radiation for treatment of cancer is administered in a series of divided doses for an established period of time. In this manner, tumor cells that survive initial radiation are eventually destroyed.

The size, location, and degree of sensitivity of the tumor to radiation are the deciding factors when the plan of therapy is devised. The sensitivity of the cells surrounding the tumor is also a factor in the plan.

When a patient's physician prescribes external radiation therapy, the patient is sent to the radiation treatment area for preparation known as treatment simulation. During this simulation, the patient is evaluated, and treatment is mimicked with machines that determine the exact treatment field, the volume of tissue to be radiated, and the radiation dosage necessary to accomplish the treatment purpose. When these decisions have been made, the patient's external skin is marked with indelible pen so that the same area of tissue receives the radiation therapy with each treatment. A plan of treatment is outlined for the patient, which usually extends daily for several weeks. The patient is instructed to refrain from removing or altering the markings. If they are accidentally removed, patients are asked not to redraw them, but to notify the radiation team so that they can reconstruct them according to plan.

At the time that the treatment plan is made, show the patient the treatment room. He or she should be allowed to ask any questions concerning the treatment. The treatment rooms are large and impersonal, and the patient must remain alone during the radiation treatment. Inform the patient that he or she can communicate by microphone with the radiation team and vice versa. Also inform the patient that the treatment table is somewhat uncomfortable and hard. If the patient is in pain, suggest that he or she receive pain medication 30 minutes before each treatment. Also explain to the patient that the radiation treatments themselves are painless and that there is no danger of the patient carrying radiation out of the treatment area.

Patient Care for Radiation Therapy

In caring for patients receiving radiation therapy, one must be aware that these patients are in various stages of the grieving process. They have received a diagnosis of a disease from which they may or may not recover. Some have hope of recovery and perhaps are in a phase of denial of the seriousness of their problem. Patients who are in this phase must never be confronted with their denial, since this may be their only means of coping with the problem. Others are in the later stages of the grieving process. Many have had radical surgical procedures that have altered their body image. This is particularly the case for a man or woman who has had reproductive organs or external genitalia altered by surgery during reproductive years.

Some patients receiving external radiation therapy are in the terminal stages of cancer and have metastasis of the disease to their bones. When this occurs, the structure of the bone weakens and becomes very fragile. There is a high incidence of pathological fractures with this condition. If one is caring for a person in the terminal stages of cancer, one must remember this and allow the patient to move at his or her own pace with as much assistance as necessary. The radiographer must be extremely cautious when lifting or moving cancer patients. Be certain to have adequate assistance to prevent abrupt, jarring, or pushing movements because this may cause fractures and a great deal of unnecessary pain for the patient. Allow the patient to direct all moves at his or her own pace.

Patients with cancer often have weakened immune systems. This must be taken into consideration because these patients are highly susceptible to infections. The health care team providing care must practice judicious medical asepsis and, when the occasion calls for it, meticulous surgical asepsis during patient care.

The radiographer must also remember that the patient undergoing a course of radiation therapy has localized toxic reactions to the treatment. This **toxicity** usually affects only the tissues surrounding the area being radiated, since the cells in the treatment area are destroyed by radiation. However, generalized systemic reactions may also occur. Some of the local reactions that may occur, depending on the irradiation site, are alopecia (loss of hair), erythema (redness and inflammation of the skin or mucous membranes), loss of appetite, alterations in oral mucous membranes (xerostomia and stomatitis), decreased salivation, difficulty swallowing, chest pain and cough, esophageal irritation, nausea and vomiting, diarrhea, and blood dyscrasias.

Generalized systemic side effects include fatigue, nausea, vomiting, and headache. Reassure the patient that all these effects will subside when the treatments are completed. Some changes in the area of the radiation treatment are called fibrous tissue formation (scar tissue). This is due to the destruction of the blood supply in the area of radiation, and that tissue will not regenerate.

Use of therapeutic communication techniques by radiographers caring for patients having external radiation therapy is of utmost importance. The radiographer should make himself available to answer questions that he can answer and assist patients to find answers when he does not know them. The radiographer should also allow patients to express their concerns and explore their feelings with the use of simple reflective statements.

■ PROTON THERAPY

Proton therapy is a recent innovation in the treatment of patients with cancer. Since this procedure requires three-dimensional CT scans and frequent radiographic images, the radiographer is directly involved in this therapy.

The benefit of proton therapy for treatment of malignant tumors is based on the fact that the proton works at the end of its desired pathway with very little effect on tissues that surround the area. In other words, the "scatter effect" that is such a problem in external radiation therapy is markedly decreased. This allows the dose to the tumor to be increased with no harmful effects to surrounding tissues. Proton therapy is currently being used in only a few medical centers, but it is expected to become the treatment of choice for several localized tumors of prostate, head and neck, and spinal cord tumors. Protocols for use of proton therapy are being added at this time for use in the treatment of tumors of the cervix, lungs, urinary bladder, and esophagus, and for melanomas. It is also used as a palliative measure in metastatic disease.

Patient Preparation for Proton Therapy

The patient preparation for proton therapy is preceded by a diagnostic workup that includes a three-dimensional CT scan to determine the area of treatment. An immobilization device is made to fit the contour of the patient's body with tumors below the neck, and if the head and neck are the areas of treatment, a form-fitted mask is made to fit the treatment area.

Meticulous patient positioning is ensured prior to each treatment with calculated calibrations, which are predetermined by the physicians, physicist, and dosimetrist. The patient must be instructed to lie still during treatment.

No metal can be worn by the patient in the treatment room. Inform the patient that he or she will be alone in the room but that the therapist will be in contact with him or her by microphone just outside. If claustrophobia or pain is a problem for the patient, a mild antianxiety or analgesic drug may be prescribed 20 to 30 minutes before treatment. Each treatment lasts approximately 15 minutes.

When caring for patients having proton therapy, one must understand that these patients, like patients receiving external radiation therapy, are in a stage of the grieving process because they have had a diagnosis of life-threatening illness. Their care requires extra sensitivity from the health care team, as described in the previous section.

■ MAMMOGRAPHY

Mammography is an imaging modality that is performed on a routine basis for prevention or early diagnosis of breast cancer and on an acute-care basis if a lesion, lump, or nodule found in the breast is suspected of being cancerous. The American Cancer Society (ACS) recommends that women age 40 and older have a screening mammogram every year and a yearly physical examination of the breasts.

Men do not usually receive routine mammograms for prevention of disease; however, if there is a family history of cancer of the breast or if any abnormality of the male breast is discovered, a mammogram is ordered.

A medical history is taken before an initial mammogram and updated each year that follows. If a patient has breast implants, the radiographer must be informed prior to the procedure.

No contrast media is used for routine mammography. The radiographer should instruct the patient to wear an item of clothing that can be easily removed to the waist. Deodorant or powders in the axillary region should not be used before the examination because they may prevent adequate visualization. The patient's breasts are exposed and positioned between an image receptor and a compression device. Radiographic images are taken from two projections (Fig. 16-10). During the procedure, the breasts are compressed tightly, to remove skin folds and air pockets. It is usually known by women presenting for mammogram that the procedure is most uncomfortable. They are therefore in a state of anxiety when they arrive for examination. If the patient is having the mammogram because of suspected pathology, the radiographer must ask the patient to identify the area that is suspect so that additional care is taken to obtain optimum images of that area. Make every effort to preserve patient privacy and minimize anxiety.

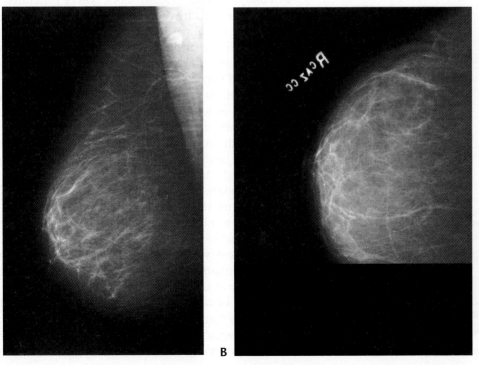

FIGURE 16-10
(**A**) Mammogram: medial lateral oblique projection.
(**B**) Mammogram: cranial caudad projection.

The patient may be asked to wait until the radiographic images are checked. The patient is notified of any need for follow-up care.

ARTHROGRAPHY

Arthrography is the diagnostic imaging examination of a joint. The indications for this procedure are continual complaints of incapacitating joint pain. The joints of the shoulder, knee, ankle, wrist, or hip can be visualized by this diagnostic imaging procedure (Fig. 16-11). Abnormalities that can be diagnosed are joint capsule abnormalities, synovial cysts, and joint and ligament pathological conditions. MRI is often the preferred method of diagnosing some joint conditions.

There is no restriction of food or fluids for arthrography. The patient's history of allergies to local anesthetics, iodine, and contrast agents must be taken. Pregnancy is a contraindication to having this procedure, since fluoroscopy is used. Explain the procedure to the patient and adequately answer any questions. A consent form is usually required to be signed.

The area where the joint will be punctured for instillation of contrast media must be cleansed as for surgical prep. The puncture area is anesthetized with a local anesthetic. The patient and staff wear protective clothing to shield them from radiation. A radiopaque contrast or air contrast or both are used to visualize the joint in question fluoroscopically while it is put through the range of motion and the contrast media fills the joint space. After administration of the contrast, the needle

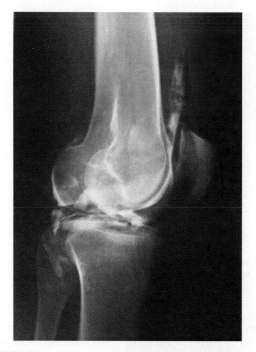

FIGURE 16-11   Knee arthrogram radiographic image.

is removed and the puncture may be sealed with collodium. Standard radiographs are taken during this time. If fluid is removed from the joint, it is collected in a sterile specimen tube and sent to the laboratory for analysis. The radiographer is responsible for its correct identification and safe arrival at the laboratory.

After arthrography, instruct the patient to rest the involved joint for several hours. If it is a knee or ankle joint, an Ace bandage may be applied to the site, and the patient should be instructed in the method of application and told to keep an Ace bandage on the site for several days. The patient should also be told that there may be some swelling or discomfort and possibly some crackling noise heard as the contrast is absorbed. The patient may be told to use ice applications for the swelling, and the physician may prescribe pain medication. Advise the patient to see the physician immediately if there is redness, warmth, or drainage at the site of needle insertion.

LITHOTRIPSY

Extracorporeal lithotripsy is a method of removing gallstones (biliary calculi, cholelithiasis), renal calculi (kidney stones, urolithiasis), and salivary stones (sialolithiasis). This is a noninvasive procedure that uses shock waves directed at calculi in the gallbladder, the common bile duct, the renal calyx, and the submandibular gland. The radiographer is a part of the team that conducts these procedures because fluoroscopic imaging is a component of the procedure.

For lithotripsy procedures performed for removal of biliary or renal calculi, shock waves generated by electric, piezoelectric, or electromagnetic discharge are directed at the stones that are meant to be fragmented. The calculi are broken into fragments and are then passed in the urine or dissolved in bile acid or saliva. Ultrasound may be used to visualize the calculi.

The patient who receives extracorporeal shockwave lithotripsy is usually treated on an outpatient basis, because there is no surgical incision or pretreatment care. If high total shock wave energy is used during the procedure to disintegrate the stones, the patient may receive a light anesthesia with a medication such as fentanyl or midazolam (Versed). The patient is usually discharged after the procedure, but he or she should be instructed to plan to be transported home by another person because he or she will be unable to drive.

A second type of lithotripsy procedure, called *intracorporeal lithotripsy*, is used to remove stones from the gallbladder or kidney after percutaneous insertion of an endoscope or nephroscope with visualization provided by use of a contrast agent and fluoroscopy. The stones are then fragmented with ultrasonic waves transmitted by an ultrasound probe placed near the stone. Another method of removing the pulverized stones is with a forceps or stone basket. The advent of laparoscopic cholecystectomy has reduced the use of this procedure.

Many of the patients who receive lithotripsy experience some discomfort depending on their pain tolerance. They may also be anxious and will require additional time for reassurance and instruction. Explain the treatment to patients in some detail. If there will be a contrast agent or other drugs administered, the usual drug history is required. Informed consent forms must also be signed. Pregnancy and the presence of a cardiac pacemaker are contraindications to having a lithotripsy procedure of any kind.

After the procedure, instruct patients to inform their physician of any excessive blood in the urine, decreasing urine output, fever, or increasing pain. They may eat and drink according to physician's orders. If the procedure was for renal calculi or if the patient received a contrast agent, fluid intake must be increased.

■ MYELOGRAPHY

Myelography (myelogram) is a radiographic examination of the spinal cord in which contrast media is injected into the subarachnoid or epidural spaces of the spinal cord. This examination is done to detect pathological conditions of the spinal cord such as a herniated intravertebral disc, tumors, malformation, and arthritic bone spurs. Other procedures that are less taxing often replace this diagnostic imaging procedure, and it is used less frequently than in the past (Fig. 16-12).

Patient Care and Education Preceding Myelography

A consent form must be signed by the patient or an appointed person before this procedure is begun. Assess the patient for potential allergic reaction to iodinated contrast media. Instruct the patient to increase clear fluid intake and omit solid food for 4 hours before the examination to be well hydrated and to not become nauseated because of food in the stomach. Food and fluid restrictions may vary depending on the contrast agent used. The patient should empty the bladder and bowels before this examination.

Also instruct the patient to stop taking all drugs 24 hours before the examination. Drugs that may enhance the possibility of seizure activity are particularly important to omit. This includes phenothiazines, tricyclic antidepressants, central nervous system stimulants, and amphetamines. Monoamine oxidase inhibitors must be discontinued 2 weeks before a myelogram. Patients with a diagnosis of diabetes mellitus must be instructed by their physician on how to prevent a hypoglycemic or hyperglycemic reaction during preparation for myelography.

Myelography should not be performed on patients with multiple sclerosis, inflammation of the meninges, Pott's disease, infections or bloody subarachnoid fluid, increased intracranial pressure, or a recent myelogram. Radiopaque contrast media are used for this procedure, so all precautions taken when these drugs are administered apply. Myelograms may also be contraindicated in patients who are prone to seizures. Seizure-prone

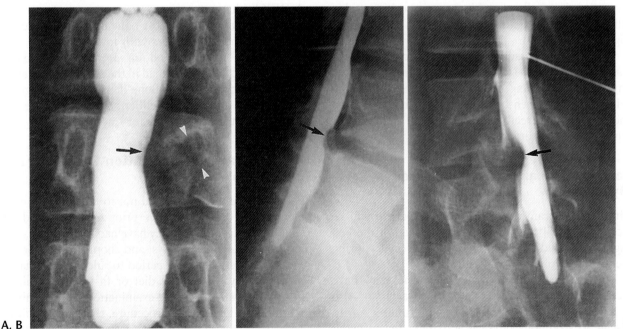

A, B   C

FIGURE 16-12 (**A**) Myelogram: neoplasm, L4. (**B** and **C**) Disc herniation, L4.

patients may receive medication to reduce the possibility of seizures before the examination. Physicians may order medication to reduce the patient's anxiety in preparation for this procedure.

The area into which the contrast media is to be injected intrathecally is shaved, if necessary, and prepped as for other sterile invasive procedures. The radiographer should inform the patient that the table will be tilted during the examination but that a footrest and shoulder harness will prevent a fall. The patient's privacy must be protected by having him or her wear pajamas or by taping a draw sheet in place to prevent it from sliding off during the table movement.

Baseline vital signs should be taken before the myelogram begins and then monitored during the examination. Inform the patient that the examination will take from 30 to 60 minutes to complete.

Intrathecal Drug Administration

Intrathecal (intraspinal) injections are given with a needle that is 3.5 inches long with a 16- to 25-gauge lumen. A stylet within the needle remains in place until the physician has completed the spinal puncture. When the needle is in the desired position in the spinal column, the stylet is removed, and the syringe containing the medication or contrast agent is attached to the needle.

The physician who is performing the special procedure or an anesthesiologist administers intrathecal drugs. An open sterile tray containing the necessary equipment and drugs will be available. The radiographer assists by obtaining any extra articles that the physician needs and placing them on the sterile field and positioning the patient. For lumbar myelography, the patient is usually placed in a prone position with a pillow under the abdomen to raise the lumbar area slightly (Fig. 16-13).

Report any unusual symptoms or complaints the patient has while the myelogram is in progress to the physician performing the procedure. Specimens of spinal fluid are often collected during this procedure and should be correctly labeled, bagged, and taken or sent to the laboratory immediately.

Patient Care and Education After Myelography

After a myelogram procedure, the out-patient will be monitored for 4 to 8 hours with the head of the bed slightly elevated at a 35- to 45-degree angle during recovery to avoid a spinal headache.

Inform the patient that he or she may have increased lumbar pain after a lumbar myelogram. Also encourage the patient to increase fluid intake, not to engage in strenuous physical activities, and to avoid bending for a couple of days. The radiographer should

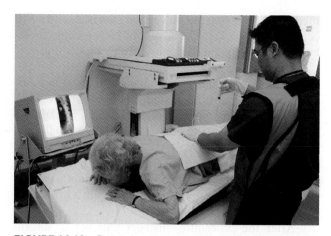

FIGURE 16-13 Patient receiving intrathecal drug administration as during myelography.

inform the patient to notify the physician immediately if he or she is unable to urinate or develops a fever, drowsiness, stiff neck, seizures, or paralysis. Other complications of myelography are arachnoiditis (inflammation of the delicate spinal cord covering) and meningitis. Any unusual reactions that the patient had to the contrast agent or in general are recorded on the patient's chart. Also record the time that the procedure began and ended, specimens sent to the laboratory, and the patient's tolerance of the procedure. Instructions given to the patient for postmyelogram care are included on the chart.

■ BONE DENSITY SCAN (DEXA)

A DEXA (dual-energy x-ray absorptiometry) scan is a quick, accurate, and painless bone density test used to measure bone mineral loss with low-dose x-rays. The examination is performed on an outpatient basis. Images are usually performed in the spine and hip areas to measure bone density. Bone density scans diagnose osteoporosis and other conditions that cause bone loss and a patient's susceptibility for fractures.

Patient Care and Education Preceding A Bone Density Scan

Patients should be instructed not to take calcium supplements at least 24 hours prior to the procedure; should be questioned if they have had any barium studies within the last few days; and should be questioned as to their last menstrual period to rule out any chance of pregnancy. No special diet or fasting is required. Inform the patient that the examination will take about 10 minutes. During the procedure, the patient will be asked to hold still and hold their breath for a few seconds to avoid blurring the images.

SUMMARY

Working in special procedures of diagnostic imaging, the radiographer is a member of a highly skilled technical team. As a member of this team, the radiographer must work with other team members to ensure positive patient outcomes from examinations and treatments. A successful outcome includes adequate patient preparation for the procedure and physical and emotional safety is it evolves.

Special procedures and radiographic imaging techniques in which the radiographer may participate involve specialized education. When working in these areas of patient care, the radiographer must be aware of the increased anxiety experienced by a patient who is about to undergo a complex procedure. The radiographer must not only be a highly skilled technologist but also have excellent therapeutic communication skills so that he is able to alleviate the patient's anxiety and fears.

Patients being examined by cardiac angiography, arteriography, CT, ultrasonography, MRI, PET, nuclear medicine imaging, mammography, arthrography, lithotripsy, myelography, and bone density scans require special preparation and teaching. The working technologist or the observing student radiographer in these areas of specialization must not neglect these aspects of patient care, since they are an important part of professional practice.

One half of the patients who are diagnosed as having cancer receive external radiation therapy for treatment or control of symptoms. When one chooses this area of specialization, he or she must understand that patients receiving this treatment are in varying stages of the grieving process and need extra time for communication. The radiographer must also realize that the cancer patient has an increased awareness of his or her body functions and focus on physical symptoms that he or she would ignore at other times. The radiographer should be available to discuss these problems with the patient whenever the patient desires. If time for communication when caring for the patient receiving external radiation therapy is omitted, a vital professional obligation is neglected.

Patients receiving proton therapy have also been informed that they have a life-threatening disease. They will need the same thoughtful care as someone receiving external radiation therapy.

When working in a special procedures area, the radiographer must recognize his or her responsibility in drug administration. He must learn the protocols for each procedure and understand potential problems so that he is prepared to take the correct action should problems occur.

CHAPTER 16 TEST

1. List ten potential areas of specialization for the radiography student.
2. Discuss patient care responsibilities before cardiac catheterization, angiography, or arteriography.
3. Explain the patient teaching that must follow cardiac catheterization, angiography, and arteriography.
4. What should the patient teaching before CT include?
5. A patient is to have a barium enema and an abdominal ultrasound examination. Explain how you as the radiographer will schedule these examinations.
6. Describe the common causes of anxiety before MRI. Explain how to alleviate these fears.
7. Explain the potential problems that may occur if an elderly demented patient is to have PET.
8. Describe the patient teaching needs of a patient who has had a nuclear medicine examination.
9. Explain the generalized systemic reactions that may occur when a patient is receiving radiation therapy for cancer treatment.
10. Describe the special care considerations necessary for a patient receiving radiation therapy or proton therapy.
11. State the American Cancer Society (ACS) guidelines for mammograms for women age 40 and older.
12. Define lithotripsy and explain the medical indications for this treatment.

References

Chapter 1

Agnes ME, Guralnik DB. *New World Webster's Dictionary* (4th ed.). Cleveland, OH: Books Worldwide, Inc., 2001.

American Heart Association. 2005 American Heart Association guidelines for cardiopulmonary resuscitation and emergency cardiovascular care. *Circulation*, 112 (24 Supplement) 1–211.

American Hospital Association. *The Patient Bill of Rights*. Chicago, IL: American Hospital Association, 1992.

American Hospital Association. *The Patient Care Partnership*. Chicago, IL: American Hospital Association, 2003.

American Registry of Radiologic Technologists. Standard of ethics. Available at: http://www.arrt.org/ethics/standardethic.pdf.

American Society of Radiologic Technologists. Practice standards, 2006. Available at: https://www.asrt.org/content/ProfResources/PracticeIssues/standards.aspx.

Chitty KK. *Professional Nursing: Concepts and Challenges* (4th ed.). St. Louis, MO: Elsevier Saunders Publishers, 2005.

Joint Commission for Accreditation of Healthcare Organizations. *Standards, Rights, Responsibilities, and Ethics*. Oakbrook Terrace, IL: Joint Commission for Accreditation of Healthcare Organizations, 1999.

Joint Review Committee on Education in Radiologic Technology (JRCERT), 2006. Available at: http://www.jrcert.org/acc_standards.html.

O'Neil J. Ethical decision making and the role of nursing. In: Deloughery G, ed.: *Issues and Trends in Nursing* (2nd ed.). St. Louis, MO: Mosby, 1995.

Smeltzer SC, Bare BG. *Brunner & Suddarth's Textbook of Medical-Surgical Nursing* (10th ed., Vol. 1). Philadelphia, PA: Lippincott Williams & Wilkins, 2004.

Timby BK, Smith NE. *Introductory to Medical-Surgical Nursing*. Philadelphia, PA: Lippincott Wilkins & Wilkins, 2007.

Chapter 2

Anderson ML, Collins PH. *Race, Class and Gender* (5th ed.). The Wadsworth Sociology Reader Series; Belmont, CA: Wadsworth, 2004.

Fejos P. Man, magic and medicine. In: Goldstone I, ed.: *Medicine and Anthropology*. New York, NY: International University Press, 1959.

Kubler-Ross E. *On Death and Dying*. New York, NY: Macmillan, 1969.

Northhouse PG, Northouse LL. *Health Communication, Strategies for Health Professionals* (2nd ed.). Norwalk, CT: Appelton & Lange, 1992.

Paul R. *Critical Thinking: How to Prepare Students for a Rapidly Changing World*. Dillon Beach, CA: Foundation for Critical Thinking, 1995.

Ramsden EL. *The Patient as a Person: Psychosocial Perspectives for the Health Care Professional*. Philadelphia, PA: WB Saunders, 1999.

Rankin SH, Stallings KD. *Patient Education, Principles and Practice* (4th ed.). Philadelphia, PA: Lippincott Williams & Wilkins, 2001.

Rubenfeld MG, Scheffer BK. *Critical Thinking in Nursing: An Interactive Approach*. Philadelphia, PA: J.B. Lippincott Co., 1995.

Thernstrom S, ed. *The Harvard Encyclopedia of American Ethnic Groups*. Cambridge, MA: Harvard University Press, 1980.

Chapter 3

Chitty KK. *Professional Nursing: Concepts and Challenges* (4th ed.). St. Louis, MO: Elsevier Saunders Publishers, 2005.

Craig M. *Essentials of Sonography and Patient Care* (2nd ed.). St. Louis, MO: Elsevier Saunders Publishers, 2006.

Dirckx JH, ed. *Stedman's Concise Medical Dictionary for the Health Professions* (4th ed.). Philadelphia, PA: Lippincott Williams & Wilkins, 2001.

Smeltzer S, et al. *Brunner & Suddarth's Textbook of Medical-Surgical Nursing* (11th ed.). Philadelphia, PA: Lippincott Williams & Wilkins, 2007.

Chapter 4

Curry K. Pertussis: a reemerging threat. *J Nurse Pract*. 2007; 3:97–100.

Diehl M. *Hepatitis C*. Ridgedale, MO: Nursing Education of America, 2002.

Gantz NM, et al. *Mannual of Clinical Problems in Infectious Disease* (5th ed.). Philadelphia, PA: Lippincott Williams & Wilkins, 2006.

Gladwin M, Trattler B. *Clinical Microbiology Made Ridiculously Simple* (2nd ed.). Miami, FL: MedMaster, Inc., 2000.

Herzberger S. *Killer Molds*. Ridgedale, MO: Nursing Education of America, 2003.

Mayhall CG. *Hospital Epidemiology and Infection Control* (3rd ed.). Philadelphia, PA: Lippincott Williams & Wilkins, 2004.

Nielsen RP, Van Slamlbrook ML, Diehl M. *Infection Control Update-2003*. Ridgedale, MO: Nursing Education of America, 2003.

Smeltzer SC, Bare BG. *Brunner & Suddarth's Textbook of Medical-Surgical Nursing* (10th ed., Vol. 1 and 2). Philadelphia, PA: Lippincott Williams & Wilkins, 2004.

Taylor C, et al. *Fundamentals of Nursing, The Art and Science of Nursing Care* (6th ed.). Philadelphia, PA: Lippincott Williams & Wilkins, 2005.

Wallace N. *Methicillin-Resistant Staphylococcus aureus (MRSA)*. Ridgedale, MO: Nursing Education of America, 2006

Washington W Jr. *Fundamentals of Nursing: The Art and Science of Nursing Care* (6th ed.). Philadelphia, PA: Lippincott Williams & Wilkins, 2006.

Chapter 5

Goodman J, Veeramachameni N, Winslow E. *The Washington Manual Surgery Survival Guide*. Philadelphia, PA: Lippincott Williams & Wilkins, 2003.

Phillips N. *Berry & Kohn's Operating Room Technique* (11th ed.). St. Louis, MO: Mosby, Elsevier, 2007.

Rothrock JC, McEwen DR. *Alexander's Care of the Patient in Surgery* (13th ed.). St. Louis, MO: Mosby, Elsevier, 2007.

Timby, BK, Smith NE. *Introductory Medical-Surgical Nursing* (9th ed.). Philadelphia, PA: Lippincott Williams & Wilkins, 2007.

Chapter 6

Chitty KK. *Professional Nursing: Concepts and Challenges* (4th ed.). St. Louis, MO: Elsevier Saunders Publishers, 2005.

Craig M. *Essentials of Sonography and Patient Care* (2nd ed.). St. Louis, MO: Elsevier Saunders Publishers, 2006.

Dirckx JH, ed. *Stedman's Concise Medical Dictionary for the Health Professions* (4th ed.). Philadelphia, PA: Lippincott Williams & Wilkins, 2001.

Chapter 7

Ellis KM. *EKG Plain and Simple: From Rhythm Strips to 12-Leads*. Upper Saddle River, NJ: Prentice Hall, 2002.

Karch A. *Lippincott's Nursing Drug Guide*. Philadelphia, PA: Lippincott Williams & Wilkins, 2007.

Roach SS. *Introductory Clinical Pharmacology* (7th ed.). Philadelphia, PA: Lippincott Williams & Wilkins, 2004.

Smeltzer SC, Bare BG. *Brunner & Suddarth's Textbook of Medical-Surgical Nursing* (10th ed., Vol. 1). Philadelphia, PA: Lippincott Williams & Wilkins, 2004.

Tait C. EZ *ECGs Booklet*. St. Louis, MO: Mosby-Year Book, Inc., 1994.

Chapter 8

American Heart Association. Guidelines 2005 for cardiopulmonary resuscitation. Available at: http://www.americanheart.org/presenter.jhtml?identifier=3035517.

Chitty KK. *Professional Nursing: Concepts and Challenges* (4th ed.). St. Louis, MO: Elsevier Saunders Publishers, 2005.

Dirckx JH, ed. *Stedman's Concise Medical Dictionary for the Health Professions* (4th ed.). Philadelphia, PA: Lippincott Williams & Wilkins, 2001.

Frank E, Long B, Smith B. *Merrill's Atlas of Radiographic Positioning & Procedures* (11th ed., Vol. 3). St. Louis, MO: Mosby Elsevier, 2007.

Smeltzer S, et al. *Brunner & Suddarth's Textbook of Medical-Surgical Nursing* (11th ed.). Philadelphia, PA: Lippincott Williams & Wilkins, 2007.

Chapter 9

Ballinger PW, Frank ED. *Merrill's Atlas of Radiographic Positions and Radiologic Procedures* (10th ed., Vol. 3). St. Louis, MO: Mosby, 2003.

Dirckx JH, ed. *Stedman's Concise Medical Dictionary for the Health Professions* (4th ed.). Philadelphia, PA: Lippincott Williams & Wilkins, 2001.

Drafke M, Nakayama H. *Trauma and Mobile Radiography* (2nd ed.). Philadelphia, PA: F.A. Davis, 2001.

Furlow B. Diagnostic imaging of traumatic brain injury. *Radiologic Technol*. 2006;78:145–155.

Kelley J. RTs in the ER, where every minute counts. *RT Image*. 2003;16:20–23.

Peart O. Mobile imaging: the equipment, techniques and complications. *RT Image*. 2002;15:12–15.

Weston H. The level 1 trauma center: an RT student's perspective. *RT Image*. 2005;18:17–18.

Chapter 10

Aberle L. Imaging kids (almost) without tears. *Advance for Imaging and Radiation Therapy Professionals*. 2006; 19:28–29.

Ballinger PW, Frank ED. *Merrill's Atlas of Radiographic Positions and Radiologic Procedures* (10th ed., Vol. 3). St. Louis, MO: Mosby, 2003.

Bontrager KL. *Textbook of Radiographic Positioning and Related Anatomy* (5th ed.). St. Louis, MO: Mosby, 2001.

Bryarly C. Embracing digital radiography. A health center changes the rules of pediatric imaging. *RT Image*. 2006; 19:12–13.

Dirckx JH, ed. *Stedman's Concise Medical Dictionary for the Health Professions* (4th ed.). Philadelphia, PA: Lippincott Williams & Wilkins, 2001.

Femia J. Techs offer advice on imaging chirldren with the Pigg-O-Stat. *Advance for Imaging and Radiation Therapy Professionals*. 2006;19:6, 25.

Knight S. Imaging little ones. *RT Image*. 2006;19:14–16.

Lorenzett JP. The role of the radiology professional in child abuse cases. *RT Image*. 2007;20:23–24.

Minigh J. Pediatric radiation protection. *Radiol Technol*. 2005;76:365–378.

Stinson J. Pediatric position and other "little" concerns. *RT Image*. 2007;20:20–21.

Storer A. Small patients, big ideas. *RT Image*. 2006;19:27–29.

Troiano LR. Imaging kids. *RT Image*. 2002;15:20–25.

Ward J. Kids in the new imaging world. *Advance for Imaging and Radiation Therapy Professionals*. 2006;19:14–18.

Chapter 11

Alzheimer's Association. *The Healthy Brian Initiative: A National Public Health Road Map to Maintaining Cognitive Health*. Available at: http://www.alz.org/national/documents/report_healthybraininitiative.pdf.

Davidhizar R, Shearer R, Giger JN. The challenges of cross-cultural communication. *RT Image*. 2002;15:18–23.

Dolan TG. Through the ages. *ASRT Scanner*. 2005;37:7–11.

Hosanksky A. Been there done that. *Caring Today*. 2006; September/October:20–21.

Immel MB. I'm old-I'm just fine with that. *Newsweek*. July 31, 2006, p. 18.

National Center on Elder Abuse. Newsletter, January 2007, Vol. 9, No. 3. Available at: http://www.ncea.aoa.gov/.

Moody EF. Alzheimer's is the death of the mind before the death of the body. Available at: http://www.efmoody.com/longterm/alzheimers.html.

Otto JM. 2005 White House Conference on Aging: background paper on elder abuse for delegates. Available at: http://www.apsnetwork.org/About/docs/WhiteHouseConf_ElderAbuse_2005.pdf.

Shams-Avari P. Linguistic and cultural competency. *Radiol Technol*. 2005;76:437–447.

Spieler G. Moving from pediatrics to geriatrics. *ASRT Scanner*. 2006;38:14–15.

Chapter 12

Chitty KK. *Professional Nursing: Concepts and Challenges* (4th ed.). St. Louis, MO: Elsevier Saunders Publishers, 2005.

Craig M. *Essentials of Sonography and Patient Care* (2nd ed.). St. Louis, MO: Elsevier Saunders Publishers, 2006.

Dirckx JH, ed. *Stedman's Concise Medical Dictionary for the Health Professions* (4th ed.). Philadelphia, PA: Lippincott Williams & Wilkins, 2001.

Robson WL, Leung A, Thomason M. Catheterization of the bladder in infants and children. In: *Clinical Pediatrics*. Thousand Oaks, CA: Sage Publications, 2006.

University of North Carolina Health Care System. Intermittent catheterization of the urinary bladder (adult and pediatric). In: *University of North Carolina Hospital Nursing Procedure Manual*, Chapel Hill, NC: University of North Carolina, 2005.

Chapter 13

Chitty KK. *Professional Nursing: Concepts and Challenges* (4th ed.). St. Louis, MO: Elsevier Saunders Publishers, 2005.

Dirckx JH, ed. *Stedman's Concise Medical Dictionary for the Health Professions* (4th ed.). Philadelphia, PA: Lippincott Williams & Wilkins, 2001.

Godderidge C. *Pediatric Imaging*. New York, NY: Harcourt Brace & Company, 1995.

Chapter 14

Chitty KK. *Professional Nursing: Concepts and Challenges* (4th ed.). St. Louis, MO: Elsevier Saunders Publishers, 2005.

Dirckx JH, ed. *Stedman's Concise Medical Dictionary for the Health Professions* (4th ed.). Philadelphia, PA: Lippincott Williams & Wilkins, 2001.

Chapter 16

Ballinger PW, Frank ED. *Merrill's Atlas of Radiographic Positions and Radiologic Procedures* (10th ed., Vol. 3). St. Louis, MO: Mosby, 2003.

Bushong SC. *Radiologic Science for Technologists* (8th ed.). St. Louis, MO: Mosby, 2001.

Chitty KK. *Professional Nursing: Concepts and Challenges* (4th ed.). St. Louis, MO: Elsevier Saunders Publishers, 2005.

Craig M. *Essentials of Sonography and Patient Care* (2nd ed.). St. Louis, MO: Elsevier Saunders Publishers, 2006.

Dirckx JH, ed. *Stedman's Concise Medical Dictionary for the Health Professions* (4th ed.). Philadelphia, PA: Lippincott Williams & Wilkins, 2001.

Yochum TR, Rowe LJ. *Essentials of Skeletal Radiology* (3rd ed.). Philadelphia, PA: Lippincott Williams & Wilkins, 2005.